AF366341

Actualización en infecciones relacionadas con el uso de catéteres vasculares

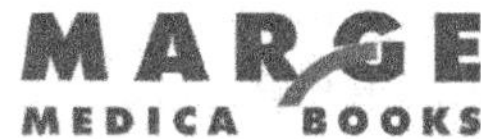

La edición de este libro se ha podido realizar por la colaboración de Novartis España, S.A. Los editores y la totalidad de los autores de los capítulos del sumario declaran que esta empresa no ha ejercido ninguna influencia sobre su contenido científico. Asimismo, el libro ha obtenido el aval científico de diferentes sociedades y redes de investigación cooperativa, sin implicaren ningún caso que la opinión de los autores sea considerada como oficial y representativa de cualquiera de dichas sociedades.

Actualización en infecciones relacionadas con el uso de catéteres vasculares

Coordinadores:
Dr. Benito Almirante
Dr. Albert Pahissa

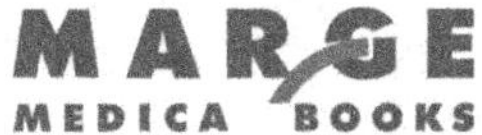

ACTUALIZACIÓN EN INFECCIONES RELACIONADAS CON EL USO DE CATÉTERES VASCULARES
Coordinadores: Dr. Benito Almirante, Dr. Albert Pahissa

1.ª edición 2013

© de esta edición, incluido el diseño de la cubierta, ICG Marge, SL

Edita: Marge Médica Books - València, 558, ático 2.ª - 08026 Barcelona (España)
www.marge.es - Tel. +34-932 449 130 - Fax +34-932 310 865

Director editorial: Hèctor Soler
Gestión editorial: Ana Soto
Edición: Neus Piñol, David Soler
Colaboración técnica: Carmen Company
Compaginación: Mercedes Lara
Impresión: Comgrafic

ISBN: 978-84-15340-71-3
Depósito Legal: B-5.404-2013

Índice

Autores

Benito Almirante
Servicio de Enfermedades Infecciosas
Hospital Universitari Vall d'Hebron
Universitat Autònoma de Barcelona
Barcelona

Francisco Álvarez Lerma
Servicio de Medicina Intensiva
Hospital Universitari del Mar
Parc de Salut
Barcelona

Francisco Anguita Santos
Servicio de Enfermedades Infecciosas
Hospital Universitario San Cecilio
Granada

Alejandra Bravo Molina
Servicio de Angiología y Cirugía
    Vascular
Hospital Universitario San Cecilio
Granada

Emilia Cercenado Mansilla
Servicio de Microbiología
    y Enfermedades Infecciosas
Hospital General Universitario Gregorio
    Marañón
Madrid
Facultad de Medicina
Universidad Complutense
Madrid

José Luís del Pozo León
Infectious Diseases Division
Clínica Universidad de Navarra
Pamplona (Spain)
Department of Clinical Microbiology
Clínica Universidad de Navarra
Pamplona (Spain)

Nuria Fernández -Hidalgo
Servei de Malalties Infeccioses
Hospital Universitari Vall d'Hebron
Universitat Autònoma de Barcelona
Barcelona

Jesús Fortún Abete
Servicio de Enfermedades Infecciosas
Hospital Universitario Ramón y Cajal
Madrid

Isabel García-Luque
Servicio de Microbiología
Hospital Universitario Virgen
    Macarena
Sevilla

Joan Gavaldà Santapau
Servei de Malalties Infeccioses
Hospital Universitari Vall d'Hebron
Universitat Autònoma de Barcelona
Barcelona

Jose Hernández Quero
Servicio de Enfermedades Infecciosas
Hospital Universitario San Cecilio
Granada

Ana Hornero López
Enfermería Clínica
Equipo de Control de Infección
    Hospitalaria
Hospital Universitario de Bellvitge
L'Hospitalet de Llobregat (Barcelona)

Francesc Marco Reverté
Servicio de Microbiología
Centro de Investigación en Salud
    Internacional
de Barcelona (CRESIB)
Hospital Clínic
Universitat de Barcelona
Barcelona

Yolanda Meije
Servei de Malalties Infeccioses
Hospital Universitari Vall d'Hebron
Universitat Autònoma de Barcelona
Barcelona

Josep Mensa Pueyo
Servicio de Enfermedades Infecciosas
Hospital Clínic
Universitat de Barcelona
Barcelona

Marta Montero Alonso
Unidad de Enfermedades Infecciosas
Hospital Universitario y Politécnico La Fe
Valencia

Albert Pahissa Berga
Servei de Malalties Infeccioses
Hospital Universitari Vall d'Hebron
Universitat Autònoma de Barcelona
Barcelona

Mercedes Palomar Martínez
Unidad de Críticos
Hospital Universitari Arnau de Vilanova
Lleida

Jorge Parra Ruiz
Servicio de Enfermedades Infecciosas
Hospital Universitario San Cecilio
Granada

Álvaro Pascual Hernández
Servicio de Microbiología
Hospital Universitario Virgen Macarena
Sevilla

Robin Patel
Division of Infectious Diseases
Department of Internal Medicine
Department of Laboratory Medicine
    and Pathology
Mayo Clinic, Rochester, Minnesota (USA)
Division of Clinical Microbiology
Department of Laboratory Medicine
    and Pathology
Mayo Clinic, Rochester, Minnesota (USA)

Cristina Pitart Ferré
Servicio de Microbiología
Centro de Investigación en Salud
    Internacional
de Barcelona (CRESIB)
Hospital Clínic
Universitat de Barcelona
Barcelona

Miquel Pujol Rojo
Servicio de Enfermedades Infecciosas
Equipo de Control de Infección
    Hospitalaria
Hospital Universitario de Bellvitge
L'Hospitalet de Llobregat (Barcelona)

José Manuel Rodríguez-Martínez
Servicio de Microbiología
Hospital Universitario Virgen Macarena
Sevilla

Dolors Rodríguez-Pardo
Servicio de Enfermedades Infecciosas
Hospital Universitari Vall d'Hebron
Universitat Autònoma de Barcelona
Barcelona

Miguel Salavert Lletí
Unidad de Enfermedades Infecciosas
Hospital Universitario y Politécnico La Fe
Valencia

Prólogo

El uso de dispositivos vasculares ha experimentado un enorme aumento en los últimos treinta años. La mayoría de los pacientes hospitalizados requieren algún catéter vascular durante parte o todo su ingreso, y además, cada día son más numerosos los enfermos portadores de catéteres venosos permanentes para diferentes tratamientos, como depuración renal, nutrición parenteral o quimioterapia.

Por desgracia, el uso de estos catéteres no se halla exento de efectos adversos y complicaciones, la mayoría infecciosas. De hecho, las bacteriemias relacionadas con catéteres vasculares se hallan entre las infecciones más frecuentes asociadas a los cuidados sanitarios, y conllevan una sustancial morbilidad, una mortalidad atribuible no despreciable y un aumento relevante de los costes sanitarios.

Un mejor conocimiento de la patogenia de estas infecciones, obtenido mediante la realización de gran número de estudios básicos, experimentales y clínicos, ha permitido el diseño y la aplicación de intervenciones dirigidas a reducir el riesgo de padecerlas. Diversas experiencias han mostrado disminuciones muy notables en la incidencia de la bacteriemia relacionada con catéteres vasculares tras la aplicación conjunta de diferentes medidas preventivas basadas en la evidencia científica, en especial en los pacientes ingresados en las unidades de cuidados intensivos (UCI). Más aún, hay datos que sugieren que podemos estar asistiendo a una tendencia global hacia una disminución de las bacteriemias relacionadas con catéteres vasculares, gracias a la generalización de la cultura de la prevención efectiva y de la seguridad de los pacientes. En este sentido, se considera de gran interés la extensión de las medidas preventivas a los pacientes ubicados fuera de las UCI, cuyo número absoluto es muy superior al de los pacientes graves, aunque obviamente tengan una menor incidencia de estas bacteriemias.

A pesar del éxito alcanzado por determinados programas, reforzando el concepto de que la bacteriemia relacionada con un catéter vascular constituye la infección nosocomial con mayor potencial de prevención, el problema sigue siendo relevante y merece la atención prioritaria de los profesionales del control de la infección. De aquí la importancia de los programas de vigilancia continuada como elemento fundamental para conocer las tendencias locales en las tasas de infección, establecer comparaciones entre centros *(benchmarking)*, indicar la oportunidad de instaurar determinadas estrategias preventivas y valorar los resultados de las intervenciones realizadas.

Recientemente se han publicado los resultados del indicador «bacteriemia de catéter» del Programa VINCat (Vigilancia de las Infecciones Nosocomiales en Cataluña), en el cual se realiza una monitorización continua de las bacteriemias relacionadas con catéteres vasculares en todas las unidades de hospitalización y para todos los tipos de catéteres vasculares, utilizando un sistema basado en los informes diarios de los hemocultivos positivos proporcionados por los laboratorios de microbiología de cada institución. En los 40 hospitales participantes, durante el período 2007-2010 se detectaron 2.977 bacteriemias. La incidencia acumulada de bacteriemias relacionadas con catéteres vasculares fue de 0,26 episodios por mil días de hospitalización, y claramente superior en los hospitales de mayor tamaño (0,36 por mil) que en los de menos de 200 camas (0,09 por mil). El 76 % de los episodios se asoció a catéteres venosos centrales, el 19 % a catéteres venosos periféricos y el 5 % restante a catéteres venosos centrales de inserción periférica. En las UCI se registraron el 34 % de los episodios (incidencia de 1,83 por mil), en las unidades convencionales médicas el 36 % (0,22 por mil) y en las quirúrgicas el 30 % restante (0,18 por mil). Durante los años analizados se observó una disminución importante (38,1 %; intervalo de confianza del 95 %: 29-46) de las tasas de bacteriemia relacionada con catéteres vasculares en los hospitales de mayor tamaño, lo que refuerza la importancia de la aplicación de medidas preventivas y de programas estandarizados de vigilancia.

El tratamiento más adecuado de la bacteriemia relacionada con un catéter vascular dependerá de la situación clínica del paciente, del tipo de catéter, de si éste puede o no ser retirado, del microorganismo causal y de su sensibilidad a los antimicrobianos. Diversos documentos de consenso y guías clínicas publicadas por sociedades científicas han establecido y actualizado las estrategias diagnósticas y terapéuticas de las bacteriemias relacionadas con catéteres vasculares. Sin embargo, algunos aspectos importantes en relación con la necesidad de retirar el catéter, las indicaciones de tratamiento local, la duración del tratamiento sistémico y la conducta en caso de bacteriemia persistente, entre otros, todavía no están resueltos. Asimismo, la relevancia de las biocapas bacterianas y sus mecanismos de resistencia, así como el papel de los nuevos antibióticos, son factores clave a considerar en el futuro inmediato.

Por los motivos señalados, creo que la publicación del libro *Actualización en infecciones relacionadas con el uso de catéteres vasculares,* editado por el Dr. Benito Almirante y el Dr. Albert Pahissa, es extraordinariamente oportuna y será, sin duda, de gran utilidad para los profesionales implicados en este notable problema de salud. El objetivo fundamental del libro es condensar en un solo volumen la información actual sobre los aspectos epidemiológicos, microbiológicos y clínicos más relevantes de estas infecciones, con la visión poliédrica de distintos especialistas e investigadores de amplia y reconocida experiencia. Es, pues, el momento de dar la bienvenida a esta obra, y la enhorabuena a los editores, por la feliz iniciativa, y a los autores por el trabajo realizado.

Dr. Francesc Gudiol
Director del Programa VINCat
Catedrático de Medicina
Universitat de Barcelona

Actualización en infecciones relacionadas con el uso de catéteres vasculares

Capítulo 1

A visual approach to biofilm related infections: from bench to bed

J.L. Del Pozo,[1,2] R. Patel[3,4]

[1] **Infectious Diseases Division**
Clínica Universidad de Navarra
Pamplona (Spain)

[2] **Department of Clinical Microbiology**
Clínica Universidad de Navarra
Pamplona (Spain)

[3] **Division of Infectious Diseases**
Department of Internal Medicine
Department of Laboratory Medicine and Pathology
Mayo Clinic, Rochester, Minnesota (USA)

[4] **Division of Clinical Microbiology**
Department of Laboratory Medicine and Pathology
Mayo Clinic, Rochester, Minnesota (USA)

Correspondencia:
José Luis Del Pozo, M.D., Ph.D.
jdelpozo@unav.es

Abstract

Bacteria that adhere to implanted medical devices or damaged tissue can become the cause of persistent infections. Biofilm microorganisms generally exhibit an altered growth and gene expression profile compared with that of planktonic or free-living microorganisms. Biofilm-associated infections have special clinical relevance, as they are generally resistant to antibiotic therapy and clearance by host defenses. Understanding the mechanisms involved in biofilm-associated antimicrobial resistance is key to the development of new therapeutic strategies.

Introduction

Bacterial cells have grown in the biofilm phenotype for billions of years, as a part of their successful strategy to colonize most of this planet and most of its life forms.[1] In natural aquatic ecosystems, surface-associated microorganisms vastly outnumber organisms in suspension.[2] Bacterial corrosion of metals is an economically important consequence of bacterial biofilm formation that illustrates several fascinating aspects of the structure and physiology of these adherent bacterial populations. From an evolutionary standpoint, the selective advantage of bacterial adhesion has been postulated to favor the localization of surface-bound bacterial populations in nutritionally favorable, non-hostile environments and, at the same time, provide some level of protection from external predation.[3] Bacterial populations living in this protected mode of growth produce planktonic cells, which have much reduced chances of survival.[4] A biofilm can be defined as a microbial-derived sessile community characterized by cells that are irreversibly attached to a substratum or interface or to each other, are embedded in a matrix of extracellular polymeric substances that they have produced, and exhibit an altered phenotype with respect to growth rate and gene transcription.

1   Biofilm-related infections

For many centuries humans have suffered from acute bacterial infections, in which planktonic cells of specialized pathogens mounted life-threatening attacks on our bodies. We have countered them with vaccines and antibiotics, and these acute diseases are now under some measure of control. However, organisms that have been successful for millions of years in the environment are now mounting successful attacks on human health. Obviously, they make full use of the biofilm strategy that has protected them so well in their native habitats.[4] According to the United States Centers for Disease Control and Prevention, more than 65 % of all infections in developed countries are caused by biofilm-associated microorganisms.[5] Infections ascribed to biofilms include endocarditis, osteomyelitis, sinusitis, urinary tract infections, chronic prostatitis, periodontitis, chronic lung infection in cystic fibrosis patients, middle-ear infections, and various nosocomial infections, especially those related to all known indwelling devices (figure 1).[6] These infections compromise quality of life, may be fatal, and are often traced to species of bacteria that are ubiquitous in water, air or soil, or on human skin. Biofilm-associated microorganisms behave differently from planktonic microorganisms with respect to growth rates and ability to resist host defenses and antimicrobial treatment.[7] Bacterial antigens at the biofilm surface stimulate the production of antibodies. These antibodies cannot penetrate the biofilm to resolve the infection, but they do form immune complexes at the biofilm surface and thus often damage the colonized tissue. When bacterial biofilms form on vascular surfaces, such as the endothelium of heart valves, they accrete blood components such as fibrin and platelets. Tissues adjacent to the biofilm may sustain collateral damage from immune complexes and invading neutrophils.[8]

Biofilm-related infections have the following unique characteristics:[9] *a)* they often have indolent pathogenic patterns with alternating quiescent and acute periods; *b)* there may be an initial response to antibiotic therapy, but relapses are frequent because bacteria

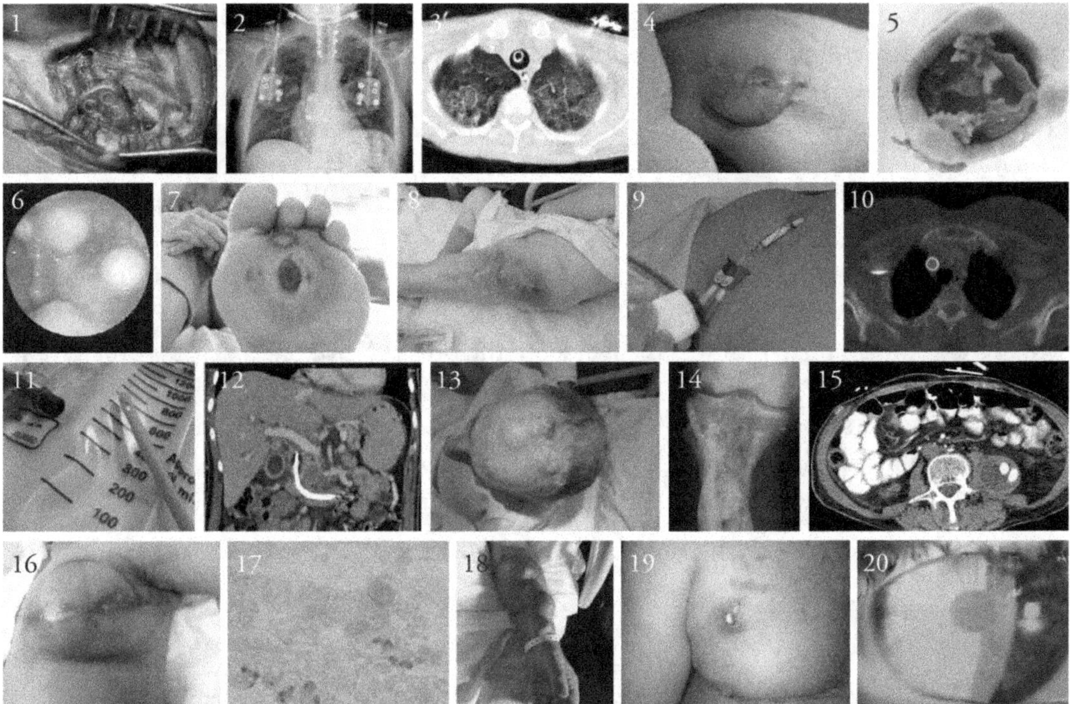

Figure 1. Diversity of biofilm-associated infections. 1) Cochlear implant infection. 2) Orthopedic hardware infection. 3) Ventilator associated pneumonia. 4) Pacemaker pocket infection. 5) Prosthetic valve endocarditis. 6) Chronic otitis media. 7) Diabetic foot infection. 8) Prosthetic hip infection. 9) Intravascular catheter infection. 10) Intravascular stent infection. 11) Urinary catheter infection. 12) Biliary stent infection. 13) Neurostimulation system infection. 14) Chronic osteomyelitis. 15) Aortoiliac bypass-associated abscess. 16) Breast implant infection. 17) Pulmonary infection in cystic fibrosis patient. Gram stain showing Gram-negative bacilli encased in an alginate matrix. 18) Arteriovenous fistula infection. 19) Port pocket related infection. 20) Contact lens-associated keratitis. Note: this figure does not show all types of biofilm-associated infections.

in biofilms are relatively protected from antibiotics; *c)* while these infections are often polymicrobial, the predominant bacteria are either common members of the autochthonous skin or bowel flora or very common environmental organisms; *d)* bacteria may be difficult to recover from adjacent fluids when the device is in place and from the device itself when it is removed.

2 Foreign body-related infections

The use of implanted medical devices has become an integral part of modern medicine. However, the implantation of a foreign body is a double-edged sword, as, besides the outstanding beneficial aspects, complications in the form of infections are regularly observed. Infections associated with indwelling medical devices affect millions of patients worldwide each year.[10] Microbial colonization of a foreign body has to be regarded as the crucial step in device-associated infection. Colonization of these devices can occur rapidly (i.e., within 24 hours) and may be enhanced by host-produced conditioning films (platelets, plasma, and tissue proteins).[11] Biofilms may be composed of a single species or multiple species, depending on the device and its anatomic location and duration of use in the patient. The most common causative organisms isolated in the context of device-related infections are staphylococci, which in turn have emerged as the most important nosocomial pathogens over the last decade.[12] Most infections associated with indwelling medical devices are caused by *Staphylococcus epidermidis*, an organism which produces few exotoxins and for which the ability to form biofilms is considered the primary virulence factor.[13] Small numbers of bacteria from the patient's skin or mucous membranes probably contaminate the device during the surgical implantation of the device. Other microorganisms commonly isolated from foreign body-related infections are *Staphylococcus aureus, Candida albicans, Pseudomonas aeruginosa, Klebsiella pneumoniae* and *Enterococcus faecalis* (figure 2).[9]

3   Biofilm architecture

Biofilms have been visualized using a variety of means, including light microscopy with computer enhancement, transmission electron microscopy, and scanning electron mi-

Gram positive cocci (70 %)	Gram negative bacilli (10-30 %)	Gram positive rods (10-20 %)	Fungi (1-5 %)	Mixed Biofilms (? %)
– Coagulase negative staphylococci – *Staphylococcus aureus* – *Streptococcus* species – Enterococci – Peptostreptococci	– *Pseudomonas aeruginosa* – *Serratia* species – *Klebsiella* species – *Escherichia coli*	– *Corynebacterium* species – *Propionibacterium acnes* – *Finegoldia magna*	– *Candida* species – *Aspergillus* species	– *Candida/* staphylococci – *Aspergillus/ Pseudomonas*

Figure 2. Microbiology of foreign body-related infections. Gram-positive cocci are involved in more than 70 % of foreign-body infections. Most infections associated with indwelling medical devices are caused by Staphylococcus epidermidis. *Note that culture-negative infections are not shown.*

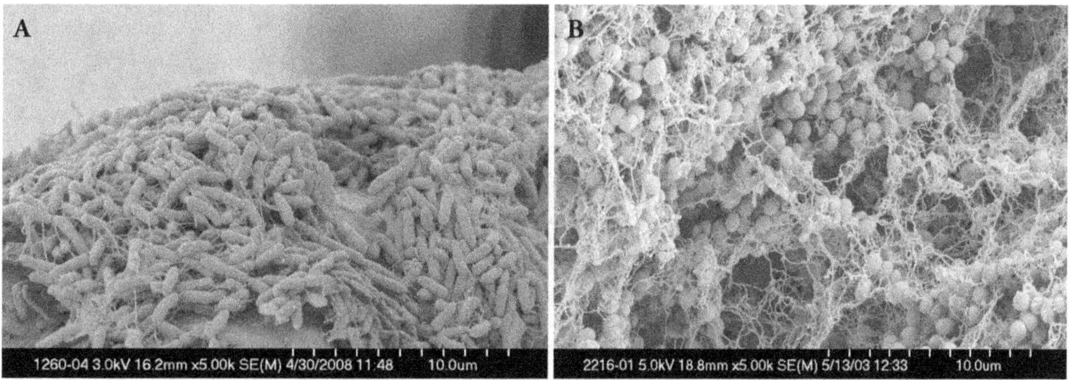

Figure 3. Scanning electron microscopy examples of biofilm. A) Chronic osteomyelitis: scanning electron micrograph showing a Pseudomonas aeruginosa *biofilm growing on the surface of a bone biopsy. B) Bloodstream catheter-related infection: scanning electron micrograph showing a* Staphylococcus aureus *biofilm growing on the surface of an intravascular catheter. Note: this technique utilizes graded solvents (alcohol, acetone, and xylene) to gradually dehydrate the specimen prior to examination. This dehydration process results in significant sample distortion and artifacts; the extracellular polymeric substances, which are approximately 95 % water, appear as fibers rather than as a thick gelatinous matrix surrounding the cells.*

croscopy (figure 3). Developed biofilms are not structurally homogeneous monolayers of microbial cells on a surface. Rather, they can be described as heterogeneous in both time and space. Bacterial biofilms are open structures composed of cells (15 % by volume) and of matrix material (85 % by volume), and the cells are located in matrix-enclosed "towers" and "mushrooms" (figure 4). Open water channels are interspersed between the microcolonies that contain the sessile cells. The extracellular polymeric substance is highly heterogeneous in its production between organisms and is influenced by growth conditions.[14] Biofilm matrix is the glue that holds the biofilm to the colonized surface and is a complex of exopolysaccharides, proteins and/or DNA of bacterial origin. Containing between 90 and 98 % water, the matrix expresses hydrodynamic properties. In most species, the matrix is predominantly anionic and creates an efficient scavenging system for trapping and concentrating essential minerals, nucleic acids, proteins, minerals, nutrients, etc. from the surrounding environment.[9] The porosity and channels throughout biofilms allow free diffusion of low-molecular-weight compounds such as fluorescein, which indicates that the spatial arrangement of cells, pores, and water channels within the biofilm permits access to nutrients as well as antibiotics. The cells within biofilms are more tightly packed at the surface and less densely packed near the periphery of the biofilm (i.e., pyramidal in shape). Once a biofilm has formed and the exopolysaccharide matrix has been secreted by the sessile cells, the resultant structure is highly viscoelastic and behaves in a rubbery manner.[7] When biofilms are formed in low shear environments, they have a low tensile strength and break easily, but biofilms formed under high shear conditions are strong and resistant to mechanical breakage. A structural characteristic

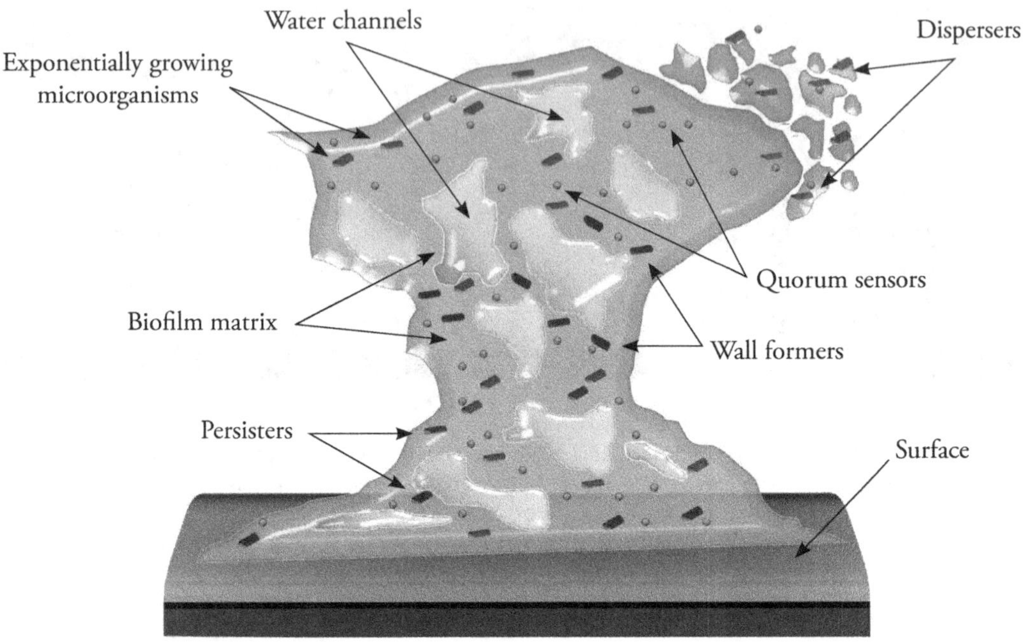

Figure 4. Biofilm composition and architecture. Biofilms are highly hydrated structures composed of 75 to 95 % noncellular material, including water channels and extracellular matrix.

of biofilms that has an impact on the outcome of certain chronic bacterial infections, such as native valve endocarditis, is the tendency of individual microcolonies to break off and/or detach when their tensile strength is exceeded.

4   Biofilm development

Biofilm formation is important because this mode of growth is associated with chronicity of associated infections, and with their inherent resistance to antimicrobial therapy. Virtually any surface, whether biotic or abiotic, is fair game for bacterial colonization and biofilm formation.[15] Microbial adherence to biomaterials depends on bacterial cell surface characteristics and on the nature of the polymer material.[13] Biofilm formation proceeds in distinct phases (figure 5):[16] first, the organism must be brought into close approximation of the surface, propelled either randomly (for example, by a stream of fluid flowing over a surface) or in a directed fashion via chemotaxis and motility. An opportune time for this to occur is when foreign bodies are implanted because this is often associated with some contact with skin microflora. Surface conditioning occurs, for example, when a foreign body is placed in the bloodstream and the native surface is modified by the adsorption of water, albumin, lipids, extracellular matrix molecules, complement, fibronectin, inorganic salts, etc.[17] Once a surface has been conditioned, its properties are permanently altered, so that the affinity of an organism for a native or a conditioned surface can be quite different.[18] The initial interaction between bacteria and the foreign body is determined by non-specific physicochemical properties of the implant and the bacterial cell. These forces include electrostatic and hydrophobic interactions, steric hindrance, van der Waals forces, temperature, and hydrodynamic forces.[19] The attachment of the bacterial cells to the device surface may occur very rapidly. Primary attachment of cells to a surface to be colonized is followed by bacterial accumulation in multiple layers. The second stage of adhesion is the anchoring (or locking) phase and employs molecularly mediated binding between specific adhesins and the surface. During this stage of adhesion, planktonic microorganisms can also stick to each other or different species of surface-bound organisms, forming aggregates on the substratum. This stage of biofilm formation is likely to be mediated in part by cell wall-associated adhesins, including microbial surface components recognizing adhesive matrix molecules. During the last phase of biofilm formation bacteria can detach from the cell community, a process that contributes to the pathogen's ability to colonize distant body sites.[20] *P. aeruginosa* and *Aggregatibacter actinomycetemcomitans* possess specific enzymes degrading the principal components of the biofilm matrix.[21] To improve their ability to cause a variety of human diseases and to occupy numerous niches within the host, staphylococci have developed quorum-sensing systems that enable cell-to-cell communication and regulation of numerous colonization and virulence factors. The staphylococcal accesso-

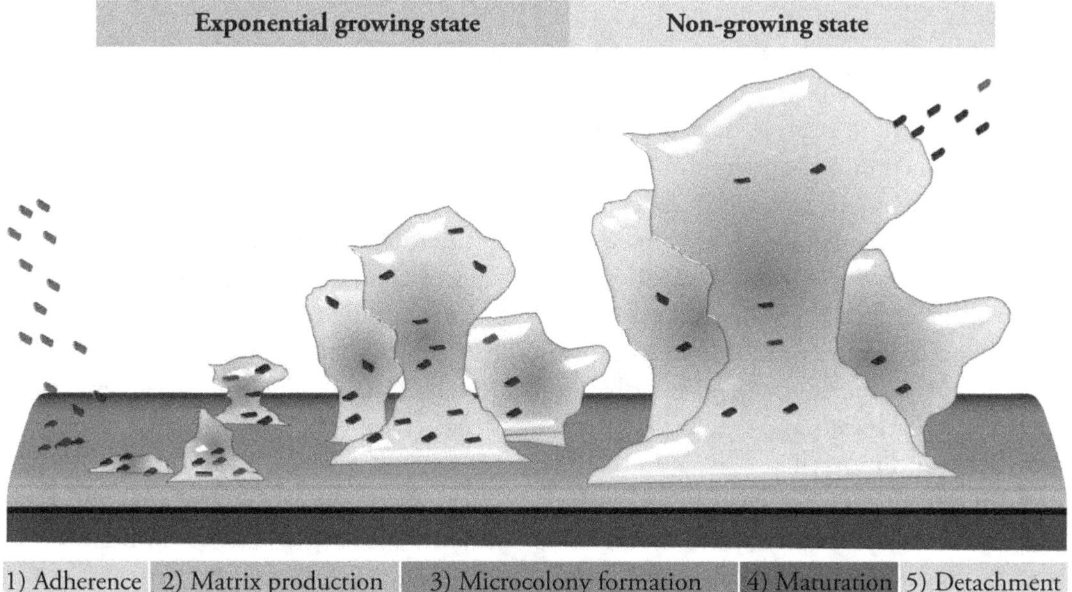

Figure 5. Phases of biofilm development. 1) Adherence: primary attachment of cells to a surface. 2) Extracellular matrix production: accumulation in multiple layers. 3) Microcolony formation. 4) Maturation. 5) Detachment (and colonization of new sites).

ry gene regulator (*agr*) quorum-sensing system decreases the expression of several cell surface proteins and increases the expression of many secreted virulence factors in the transition from late exponential growth to stationary phase in vitro.[22]

The genetic and molecular basis of biofilm formation is multifaceted.[23] Specific gene products are required for the initial association of bacteria with a surface. Dozens of new genes are turned on and others are turned off as bacteria move onto a surface, suggesting a pathway of differentiation. A hallmark of most staphylococcal biofilm formation is the production of the substance PIA (polysaccharide intercellular adhesin), a polysaccharide composed of b-1,6-linked N-acetylglucosamines with partly deacetylated residues, in which the cells are embedded and protected against the host's immune defense and antibiotic treatment. The genes encoding the synthesis apparatus for PIA are organized in the intercellular adhesion (*ica*) operon. This operon comprises four open reading frames: *icaA*, *icaD*, *icaB* and *icaC*. A regulator *icaR* controlling the transcription of *icaADBC* is located upstream of the *icaA* start codon.[22] *Ica* expression is modulated by various environmental conditions, appears to be controlled by SigB, and can be turned on and off by insertion sequence elements. Proteins have been identified that are also involved in biofilm formation, such as the accumulation-associated protein (AAP), the clumping factor A (ClfA), the staphylococcal surface protein (SSP1) and the biofilm-associated protein (Bap). Many virulence factors in *S. aureus* are controlled by *agr* and staphylococcal accessory regulator (sar). This regulation may be affected by the environment in which the organisms are grown.[24]

5   Antibiotic resistance of bacteria in biofilms

Biofilm formation represents a protected mode of growth that, by rendering bacterial cells less susceptible to antimicrobials and killing by host immune effector mechanisms, allows pathogens to survive in hostile environments and also to disperse to colonize new niches.[25] Treatment of biofilm-associated infections is increasingly problematic. Antimicrobial treatment can suppress symptoms of infection by killing free-floating bacteria shed from the attached population, but often fails to eradicate bacterial cells still embedded in the biofilm. When antimicrobial chemotherapy stops, the biofilm acts as a nidus for recurrence of infection (figure 6). The resulting failure of antimicrobial therapy regularly demands the removal of the infected biomaterial, leading to substantial morbidity and mortality.

While the molecular basis of the resistance of biofilm bacteria to clearance by antibodies and phagocytes remains obscure, it is unequivocally a general phenomenon that biofilms persist in spite of the vigorous immunological and inflammatory reactions of the infected host. Antimicrobial concentrations sufficient to destroy planktonic-organisms are generally inadequate to destroy biofilm organisms, especially those deep within the biofilm, potentially selecting for resistant subpopulations.[26] The familiar mechanisms

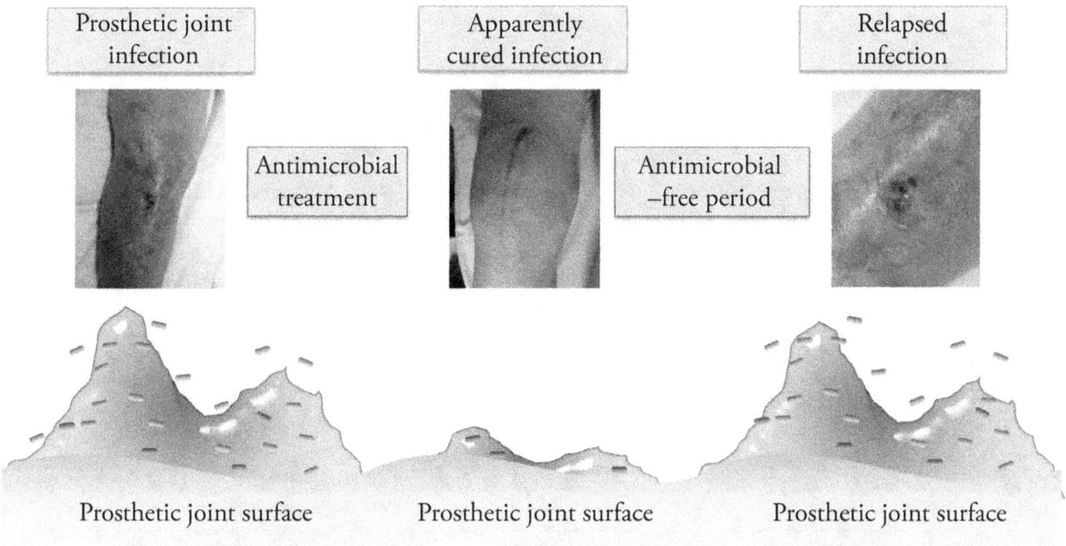

Figure 6. The challenge of treating biofilm-associated infections. Antibiotic treatment will kill most biofilm and planktonic cells, leaving only so-called persisters alive. Persisters that are contained in the biofilm can survive both the onslaught of antibiotic treatment and the immune system. After the antibiotic concentration is reduced, persisters can repopulate the biofilm, which will shed new planktonic cells, resulting in relapsed biofilm infection.

of antibiotic resistance, such as efflux pumps, antibiotic-modifying enzymes, and target mutations, do not seem to be responsible for the protection of bacteria in a biofilm. When bacteria are dispersed from a biofilm they usually rapidly become susceptible to antibiotics (figure 7), which suggests that resistance of bacteria in biofilms is not acquired via mutations or mobile genetic elements.[27]

The mechanisms of resistance to antibiotics in bacterial biofilms are described in figure 8. The most well-established mechanism of antibiotic resistance is that a subpopulation of microorganisms in a biofilm forms a unique, and highly protected, phenotypic state called persisters. Since persisters are dormant and have little or no cell-wall synthesis, translation or topoisomerase activity, antibiotics are unable to corrupt the function of their target molecules.[28] In this way tolerance enables resistance to killing by antibiotics, but at the price of non-proliferation.[26] Examination of *Escherichia coli* persister-cell formation over time shows that few of these cells are formed in early exponential phase, followed by a sharp increase in persister-cell formation in mid-exponential phase, reaching a maximum of ~1 % of cells forming persisters in the non-growing stationary phase.[26] Expression profiling of RNA from isolated persister cells reveals down-regulation of transcription of genes involved in energy production and non-essential functions such as flagellar synthesis, indicating that persisters are dormant, consistent with their

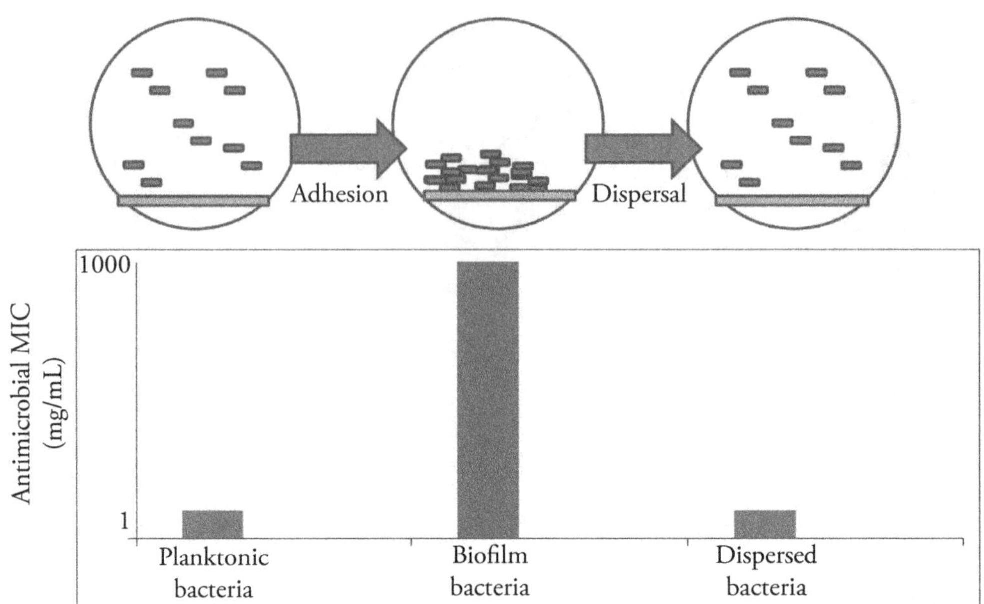

Figure 7. Biofilm-related antimicrobial resistance. When microorganisms band together in a biofilm, they are protected from killing by antimicrobial agents. However, planktonic cells that are dispersed from these biofilms are, in most cases, fully susceptible to antimicrobial agents.

phenotype of slow or non-growth.[29] The second mode of antimicrobial resistance relates to the altered chemical microenvironment within the biofilm.[30] The microenvironment of the biofilm or the metabolic state of the bacteria within the biofilm negates the antimicrobial efficacy of agents with in vitro activity. The growth potential of any bacterial biofilm is limited by the availability of nutrients in the immediate environment, the perfusion of those nutrients to cells within the biofilm, and the removal of waste. In terms of microenvironment, it is likely that the same factors that adversely influence antimicrobial activity in vitro, including pH, pCO_2, pO_2, divalent cation concentration, hydration level, and pyrimidine concentration, will also produce undesirable effects at the deepest layers of a bacterial biofilm. Besides, bacteria can transfer extrachromosomal genetic elements within biofilms. Resistance plasmids may therefore be transferred within biofilms on indwelling medical devices. Finally, there is the possibility of slow or incomplete penetration of antibiotics into the biofilm. Although this seems intuitive, it has been shown, with a few exceptions, that antibiotics do penetrates into biofilms.[31]

6 Laboratory testing of biofilm antimicrobial susceptibility

In the laboratory, microbiologists select planktonic bacteria for almost every application from the bulk solution of a broth growth medium or the water surface of an agar plate,

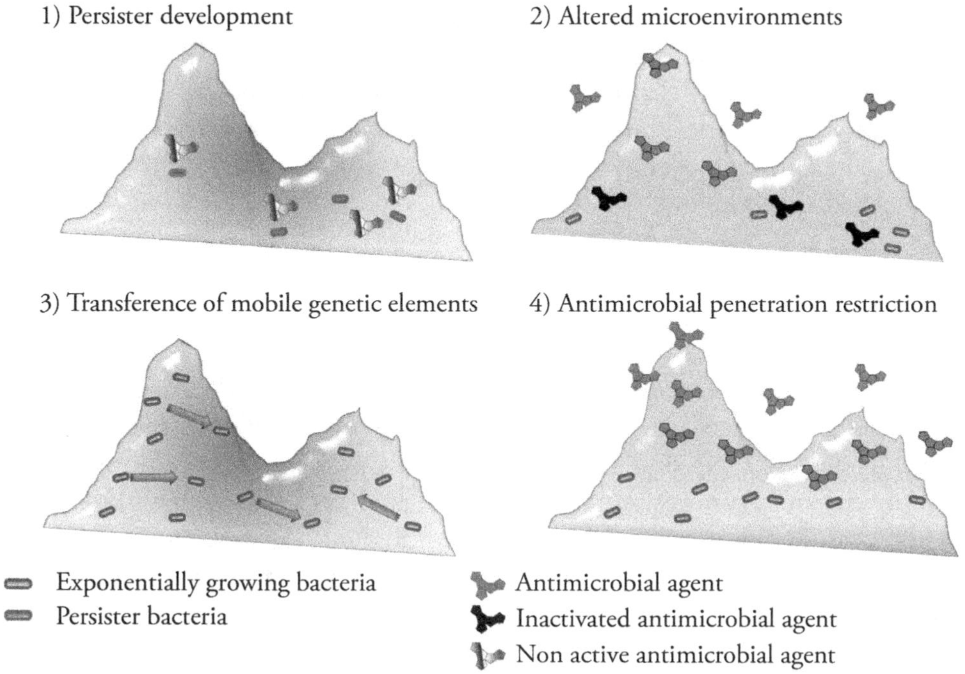

1) Persister development

2) Altered microenvironments

3) Transference of mobile genetic elements

4) Antimicrobial penetration restriction

- Exponentially growing bacteria
- Persister bacteria
- Antimicrobial agent
- Inactivated antimicrobial agent
- Non active antimicrobial agent

Figure 8. Antimicrobial biofilm resistance mechanisms. 1) Slow or incomplete penetration of the antibiotic into the biofilm. 2) Altered chemical microenvironment within the biofilm. 3) A subpopulation of microorganisms in the biofilm form a unique and highly protected, phenotypic state called a persister state. 4) Transfer of extrachromosomal genetic elements.

whereas the more naturally occurring biofilm bacteria grow at interfaces under varying nutrient conditions, and at times under high shear forces. The laboratory environment does not typically reflect the natural life cycle of pathogenic bacteria. Standard Clinical and Laboratory Standards Institute (CLSI) broth microdilution and agar dilution methods, as well as *E-test®* and disk diffusion approaches for susceptibility testing cannot accurately estimate antimicrobial efficacy against biofilms, because these techniques are based on the exposure of planktonic organisms to the antimicrobial agent. A variety of in vitro models and devices have been developed for research and/or commercial applications but would require substantial evaluation, standardization, and education prior to routine use in the clinical microbiology laboratory.

7 New therapeutic strategies

Intervention strategies currently used for biofilm control are either *a)* prevent initial device contamination, *b)* minimize initial microbial cell attachment to the device, *c)* penetrate the biofilm matrix and kill the biofilm-associated cells, or *d)* remove the device (and any associated device). It became clear early on that novel, innovative therapeutic as well as prophylactic strategies are required to cope with biomaterial-associated infections. More work is needed to fully elucidate antimicrobial resistance mechanisms in biofilms and develop new therapeutic strategies. Numerous biofilm control strategies have been proposed.[32] To be clinically effective, anti-biofilm therapies would have to thwart more than one mechanism simultaneously (figure 9).[6]

7.1 New biomaterials

The attractive properties of antimicrobial polymers are likely to lead to the development of products with sterile surfaces that will prevent the growth of biofilms on catheters and indwelling devices.[33] No single material absolutely prevents colonization, including silicone, polyurethane, composite biomaterials, or hydrogel-coated materials. Staphylococcal adhesins involved in attachment to conditioned surfaces related to implanted biomaterials have attracted considerable attention, as these may provide a means of blocking staphylococcal attachment entirely, thus preventing devastating device-related

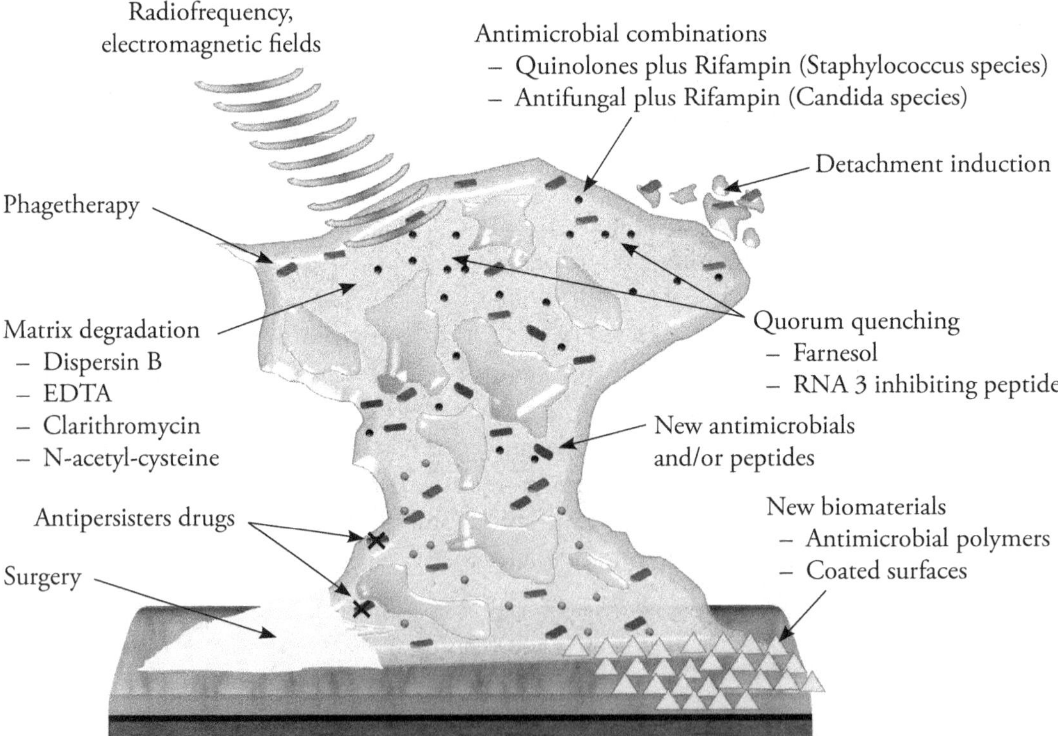

Figure 9. Treatment approach to biofilm disease. Anti-biofilm therapies might have to target more than one site simultaneously to be clinically effective.

biofilm infection from its outset. In a study by Kamal *et al.*,[34] catheters coated with a cationic surfactant (tridodecylmethylammonium chloride), which was in turn used to bond cephalosporin to the surface, were less likely to become colonized than were untreated catheters. Darouiche[35] found that catheters impregnated with minocycline and rifampin were less likely to be colonized than those impregnated with chlorhexidine and silver sulfadiazine.

7.2   Quorum quenching

Davies *et al.*[36] demonstrated the role of acyl-homoserine lactones (HSL) in *P. aeruginosa* biofilms and showed that HSL-knockouts were deficient in biofilm architecture and much more readily detached than wild-type organisms. A greater understanding of cell-to-cell communication within biofilms may lead to better predictability of biofilm processes such as detachment, as well as more effective control strategies.[37,38]

7.3   Targeting the extracellular matrix

Anticipating that matrix is especially important for mediating intercellular adhesion and stabilization of the complex cell architecture, much effort has been made to unravel the chemical composition and structural resolution of exopolysaccharides produced by *S. epidermidis* and *S. aureus*.[39] Combinations of antibiotics and dextranase have been reported to be effective for eradicating biofilm bacteria.[36] Yasuda *et al.*[40] investigated the interaction between clarithromycin and biofilms formed by *P. aeruginosa* and presented the new finding that treatment of the biofilms with clarithromycin resulted in the eradication of the slime-like structure by means of inhibition of production of some polysaccharides of *P. aeruginosa* or destruction of exopolysaccharides. Interactions between clarithromycin and biofilms formed by *S. epidermidis* were investigated using a clarithromycin-resistant strain. Treatment of the colonization with a relatively low concentration of clarithromycin resulted in the eradication of the slime-like structure and a decrease in the quantity of hexose. Another result was increased penetration of antibiotics through the *S. epidermidis* biofilm.[41] Therefore, antibiotic activity against bacteria in a biofilm may be enhanced by clarithromycin. Future work will focus on specific enzymes dedicated to breaking down the extracellular biofilm matrix, allowing bacteria to actively remodel the biofilm structure in order to adapt to changing environmental conditions. A major component of the extracellular matrix of several bacteria (e.g., *S. aureus, S. epidermidis, E. coli*) is a linear polymer of *N*-acetylglucosamine residues in β (1,6)-linkage called PIA. Kaplan *et al.*[21] reported that *A. actinomycetemcomitans* produces a soluble glycoside hydrolase called dispersin B, which degrades PIA. It is possible that dispersin B could be used to detach PIA-containing biofilms from the surface of colonized biomaterials.

7.4   Anti-persister strategies

The need for compounds that could eradicate persisters is obvious. Identifying the genes responsible for persister formation and maintenance should lead to drugs that disable persisters and might allow conventional antibiotics to eradicate an infection.

7.5   Strategies to enhance the activity of conventional antimicrobial agents.

Several physical approaches to biofilm eradication are being evaluated, including the use of an electrical current,[42,43] radiofrequency electrical current,[44] electromagnetic fields, and ultrasound, alone or in combination with antimicrobial therapy. These strategies are in preclinical stages of development.

References

1. Davey ME, O'Toole GA. Microbial biofilms: from ecology to molecular genetics. Microbiol Mol Biol Rev2000; 64: 847-67.
2. Zobell CE. The effect of solid surfaces upon bacterial activity. J Bacteriol. 1943; 46: 39-56.
3. Costerton JW. Overview of microbial biofilms. J Ind Microbiol. 1995; 15: 137-40.
4. Fux CA, Costerton JW, Stewart PS, Stoodley P. Survival strategies of infectious biofilms. Trends Microbiol. 2005; 13: 34-40.
5. Hall-Stoodley L, Costerton JW, Stoodley P. Bacterial biofilms: from the natural environment to infectious diseases. Nat Rev Microbiol. 2004; 2: 95-108.
6. del Pozo JL, Patel R. The challenge of treating biofilm-associated bacterial infections. Clin Pharmacol Ther. 2007; 82: 204-9.
7. Donlan RM. Biofilms and device-associated infections. Emerg Infect Dis. 2001; 7: 277-81.
8. Hoiby N, Ciofu O, Johansen HK, Song ZJ, Moser C, Jensen PO, *et al*. The clinical impact of bacterial biofilms. Int J Oral Sci. 2011; 3: 55-65.
9. Costerton JW, Stewart PS, Greenberg EP. Bacterial biofilms: a common cause of persistent infections. Science. 1999; 284: 1318-22.
10. Fux CA, Stoodley P, Hall-Stoodley L, Costerton JW. Bacterial biofilms: a diagnostic and therapeutic challenge. Expert Rev Anti Infect Ther. 2003; 1: 667-83.
11. Raad, II, Bodey GP. Infectious complications of indwelling vascular catheters. Clin Infect Dis. 1992; 15: 197-208.
12. Rohde H, Burandt EC, Siemssen N, Frommelt L, Burdelski C, Wurster S, *et al*. Polysaccharide intercellular adhesin or protein factors in biofilm accumulation of Staphylococcus epidermidis and Staphylococcus aureus isolated from prosthetic hip and knee joint infections. Biomaterials. 2007; 28: 1711-20.
13. Patel JD, Ebert M, Ward R, Anderson JM. S. epidermidis biofilm formation: effects of biomaterial surface chemistry and serum proteins. J Biomed Mater Res A. 2007; 80: 742-51.
14. Uhlinger DJ, White DC. Relationship between physiological status and formation of extracellular polysaccharide glycocalyx in Pseudomonas atlantica. Appl Environ Microbiol. 1983; 45: 64-70.
15. Gristina AG, Shibata Y, Giridhar G, Kreger A, Myrvik QN. The glycocalyx, biofilm, microbes, and resistant infection. Semin Arthroplasty. 1994; 5: 160-70.
16. Rohde H, Frankenberger S, Zahringer U, Mack D. Structure, function and contribution of polysaccharide intercellular adhesin (PIA) to Staphylococcus epidermidis biofilm formation and pathogenesis of biomaterial-associated infections. Eur J Cell Biol. 2010; 89: 103-11.

17. Dunne WM, Jr. Bacterial adhesion: seen any good biofilms lately? Clin Microbiol Rev. 2002; 15: 155-66.

18. Wang IW, Anderson JM, Marchant RE. Staphylococcus epidermidis adhesion to hydrophobic biomedical polymer is mediated by platelets. J Infect Dis. 1993; 167: 329-36.

19. Gotz F. Staphylococcus and biofilms. Mol Microbiol. 2002; 43: 1367-78.

20. Chambless JD, Stewart PS. A three-dimensional computer model analysis of three hypothetical biofilm detachment mechanisms. Biotechnol Bioeng. 2007; 97: 1573-84.

21. Kaplan JB, Ragunath C, Ramasubbu N, Fine DH. Detachment of Actinobacillus actinomycetemcomitans biofilm cells by an endogenous beta-hexosaminidase activity. J Bacteriol. 2003; 185: 4693-8.

22. Vuong C, Otto M. Staphylococcus epidermidis infections. Microbes Infect. 2002; 4: 481-9.

23. Jager S, Jonas B, Pfanzelt D, Horstkotte MA, Rohde H, Mack D, *et al*. Regulation of biofilm formation by sigma B is a common mechanism in Staphylococcus epidermidis and is not mediated by transcriptional regulation of sarA. Int J Artif Organs. 2009; 32: 584-91.

24. Pratten J, Foster SJ, Chan PF, Wilson M, Nair SP. Staphylococcus aureus accessory regulators: expression within biofilms and effect on adhesion. Microbes Infect. 2001; 3: 633-7.

25. Mack D, Rohde H, Harris LG, Davies AP, Horstkotte MA, Knobloch JK. Biofilm formation in medical device-related infection. Int J Artif Organs. 2006; 29: 343-59.

26. Lewis K. Riddle of biofilm resistance. Antimicrob Agents Chemother. 2001; 45: 999-1007.

27. Anwar H, van Biesen T, Dasgupta M, Lam K, Costerton JW. Interaction of biofilm bacteria with antibiotics in a novel in vitro chemostat system. Antimicrob Agents Chemother. 1989; 33: 1824-6.

28. Knobloch JK, Von Osten H, Horstkotte MA, Rohde H, Mack D. Biofilm formation is not necessary for development of quinolone-resistant "persister" cells in an attached Staphylococcus epidermidis population. Int J Artif Organs. 2008; 31: 752-60.

29. Balaban N, Giacometti A, Cirioni O, Gov Y, Ghiselli R, Mocchegiani F, *et al*. Use of the quorum-sensing inhibitor RNAIII-inhibiting peptide to prevent biofilm formation in vivo by drug-resistant Staphylococcus epidermidis. J Infect Dis. 2003; 187: 625-30.

30. Walters MC, 3rd, Roe F, Bugnicourt A, Franklin MJ, Stewart PS. Contributions of antibiotic penetration, oxygen limitation, and low metabolic activity to tolerance of Pseudomonas aeruginosa biofilms to ciprofloxacin and tobramycin. Antimicrob Agents Chemother. 2003; 47: 317-23.

31. Stewart PS, Davison WM, Steenbergen JN. Daptomycin rapidly penetrates a Staphylococcus epidermidis biofilm. Antimicrob Agents Chemother. 2009; 53: 3505-7.

32. Stewart PS. New ways to stop biofilm infections. Lancet. 2003; 361: 97.

33. Carlson RP, Taffs R, Davison WM, Stewart PS. Anti-biofilm properties of chitosan-coated surfaces. J Biomater Sci Polym Ed. 2008; 19: 1035-46.

34. Kamal GD, Pfaller MA, Rempe LE, Jebson PJ. Reduced intravascular catheter infection by antibiotic bonding. A prospective, randomized, controlled trial. JAMA. 1991; 265: 2364-8.

35. Darouiche RO. Treatment of infections associated with surgical implants. N Engl J Med. 2004; 350: 1422-9.

36. Davies DG, Parsek MR, Pearson JP, Iglewski BH, Costerton JW, Greenberg EP. The involvement of cell-to-cell signals in the development of a bacterial biofilm. Science. 1998; 280: 295-8.

37. Dong YH, Zhang LH. Quorum sensing and quorum-quenching enzymes. J Microbiol. 2005; 43 Spec No: 101-9.

38. Cirioni O, Giacometti A, Ghiselli R, Dell'Acqua G, Orlando F, Mocchegiani F, *et al*. RNAIII-inhibiting peptide significantly reduces bacterial load and enhances the effect of antibiotics in the treatment of central venous catheter-associated Staphylococcus aureus infections. J Infect Dis. 2006; 193: 180-6.

39. Xavier JB, Picioreanu C, Rani SA, van Loosdrecht MC, Stewart PS. Biofilm-control strategies based on enzymic disruption of the extracellular polymeric substance matrix – a modelling study. Microbiology. 2005; 151: 3817-32.

40. Yasuda H, Ajiki Y, Koga T, Kawada H, Yokota T. Interaction between biofilms formed by Pseudomonas aeruginosa and clarithromycin. Antimicrob Agents Chemother. 1993; 37: 1749-55.

41. Yasuda H, Ajiki Y, Koga T, Yokota T. Interaction between clarithromycin and biofilms formed by Staphylococcus epidermidis. Antimicrob Agents Chemother. 1994; 38: 138-41.

42. del Pozo JL, Rouse MS, Mandrekar JN, Sampedro MF, Steckelberg JM, Patel R. Effect of electrical current on the activities of antimicrobial agents against Pseudomonas aeruginosa, Staphylococcus aureus and Staphylococcus epidermidis biofilms. Antimicrob Agents Chemother. 2009; 53: 35-40.

43. del Pozo JL, Rouse MS, Mandrekar JN, Steckelberg JM, Patel R. The electricidal effect: reduction of Staphylococcus and Pseudomonas biofilms by prolonged exposure to low-intensity electrical current. Antimicrob Agents Chemother. 2009; 53: 41-5.

44. Caubet R, Pedarros-Caubet F, Chu M, Freye E, de Belem Rodrigues M, Moreau JM, *et al.* A radio frequency electric current enhances antibiotic efficacy against bacterial biofilms. Antimicrob Agents Chemother. 2004; 48: 4662-4.

Capítulo 2

Actividad de los antimicrobianos sobre los materiales protésicos

J.M. Rodríguez-Martínez, I. García-Luque, A. Pascual

Servicio de Microbiología
Hospital Universitario Virgen Macarena
Sevilla

Correspondencia:
Dr. Álvaro Pascual
apascual@us.es

Sinopsis

La formación de las biocapas bacterianas es un fenómeno de gran complejidad, sujeto a numerosos factores ambientales. La actividad de los antimicrobianos frente a las biocapas bacterianas se ve dificultada por numerosos factores que dependen del microorganismo, del biomaterial y del propio antimicrobiano. El desarrollo de modelos experimentales que mimeticen en la medida de lo posible la situación *in vivo* es esencial. Sólo de esta manera podremos evitar la retirada de dispositivos protésicos en situaciones en las que un tratamiento antimicrobiano podría destruir las biocapas bacterianas.

Introducción

El uso de dispositivos protésicos en humanos ha aumentado considerablemente en los últimos años. Entre ellos destacan los sistemas de drenaje de líquido cefalorraquídeo, los dispositivos intravasculares, las válvulas protésicas cardíacas, las prótesis ortopédicas, los dispositivos de ventilación asistida, los sistemas de drenaje de las vías urinarias, los catéteres para hemodiálisis, y los implantes oculares y dentarios. Su uso generalizado ha contribuido a la aparición de infecciones relacionadas con la formación de biocapas bacterianas en sus superficies. El tratamiento de estas infecciones es muy complejo, y su éxito depende, entre otros factores, del uso de antimicrobianos y de la retirada del cuerpo extraño implantado.

Las biocapas bacterianas son resistentes a una amplia variedad de agentes antimicrobianos, antisépticos y desinfectantes. El concepto convencional de resistencia antimicrobiana se refiere a la adquirida por las bacterias planctónicas mediante inactivación de los antimicrobianos, modificación de la diana sobre la que éstos actúan o disminución del fármaco en el interior de la bacteria. Todos estos mecanismos están mediados por mutaciones o por la adquisición de uno o más genes en intercambios genéticos. Como se describirá en este capítulo, los mecanismos por los cuales las bacterias presentes en las biocapas bacterianas se hacen resistentes y modifican la eficacia de los antimicrobianos son diversos, y atienden, en principio, a las características estructurales y fisiológicas de la propia biocapa.

La resistencia de las biocapas bacterianas a los agentes antimicrobianos tiene importantes consecuencias clínicas, ya que en la actualidad más del 60 % de las infecciones bacterianas están asociadas a la formación de biocapas.[1] En la tabla 1 se muestran los principales ejemplos de infecciones relacionadas con material protésico en las que están involucradas las biocapas bacterianas.[2-6]

El mecanismo por el cual las bacterias presentes en las biocapas presentan resistencia múltiple parece ser multifactorial y puede variar de unas especies a otras. Se ha propuesto una amplia variedad de estrategias para combatir este tipo de infecciones. El propósito de este capítulo es dar una visión general sobre la actividad de los principales grupos de antimicrobianos frente a las biocapas bacterianas (principalmente producidas por el género *Staphylococcus)*, describir los mecanismos de resistencia presentes en los microorganismos que en ellas se encuentran (que conducen al fracaso terapéutico) y las diversas estrategias alternativas para combatir este tipo de infecciones.

1   Eficacia de los antimicrobianos sobre los materiales protésicos

El tratamiento de las infecciones asociadas a materiales protésicos es complicado, y a menudo resulta necesario combinar antibioticoterapia prolongada y procedimientos quirúrgicos que, con frecuencia, comportan la retirada del dispositivo. En determinadas circunstancias, por la naturaleza del implante o el estado grave del paciente, esto no es posible y la única alternativa terapéutica es el uso de antimicrobianos durante largos periodos de tiempo.[7] La principal razón de la resistencia de estos microorganismos a los tratamientos antimicrobianos convencionales es que las superficies de los biomateriales, con independencia de su composición y naturaleza, son colonizadas por bacterias que se recubren con unos exopolímeros de naturaleza principalmente polisacárida, que las protegen de la acción de los antimicrobianos y de los mecanismos de defensa del huésped;[8,9] es lo que se denomina biocapa bacteriana.

Para que un antimicrobiano sea eficaz frente a una biocapa bacteriana ha de penetrar a través de su densa matriz, mantener una actividad bactericida en las distintas condi-

Mecanismo de resistencia	Especies bacterianas	Principales antimicrobianos afectados	Infecciones asociadas a materiales protésicos
Impermeabilidad de las biocapas a los agentes antimicrobianos	*P. aeruginosa*	Aminoglucósidos, betalactámicos	Neumonía asociada a aparatos de ventilación mecánica o a tubos endotraqueales, cistitis por catéter urinario, endoftalmitis por lentes de contacto, infecciones asociadas a catéteres endovasculares
	S. epidermidis, S. aureus	Vancomicina, teicoplanina	Infecciones asociadas a sistemas de drenaje de líquido cefalorraquídeo, catéteres endovasculares, válvulas cardíacas mecánicas, implantes ortopédicos y suturas
Tasa alterada de crecimiento	*P. aeruginosa, E. coli*	Betalactámicos	Neumonía asociada a aparatos de ventilación mecánica o tubos endotraqueales, cistitis por catéter urinario, endoftalmitis por lentes de contacto, infecciones asociadas a catéteres endovasculares
	S. epidermidis, S. aureus	Fluoroquinolonas	Infecciones asociadas a sistemas de drenaje de líquido cefalorraquídeo, catéteres endovasculares, válvulas cardíacas mecánicas, implantes ortopédicos y suturas
El microambiente de las biocapas afecta a la actividad antibacteriana	Característica general de las biocapas	Aminoglucósidos, macrolidos, tetraciclinas	
Mecanismos de resistencia expresados en bacterias planctónicas	*P. aeruginosa*	Azitromicina, betalactámicos, tobramicina	Neumonía asociada a aparatos de ventilación mecánica o a tubos endotraqueales, cistitis por catéter urinario, endoftalmitis por lentes de contacto, infecciones asociadas a catéteres endovasculares
Elementos genéticos de transferencia horizontal	*Enterobacteriaceae*	Betalactámicos, aminoglucósidos	Neumonía asociada a aparatos de ventilación mecánica o a tubos endotraqueales, cistitis por catéter urinario, endoftalmitis por lentes de contacto, infecciones asociadas a catéteres endovasculares

Tabla 1. Mecanismos de resistencia a los antimicrobianos en las biocapas bacterianas y principales infecciones asociadas a materiales protésicos.

ciones microambientales existentes en su interior y frente a unas bacterias en una fase de crecimiento muy lento, y presentar una baja tasa de desarrollo de resistencias. Antimicrobianos con bajo peso molecular que difundan fácilmente a través de la biocapa y que tengan como diana procesos básicos de la célula, como la síntesis de proteínas o de ácidos nucleicos, pueden ser candidatos para el tratamiento de estas infecciones.[10] En la actualidad no hay fármaco ni tratamiento que cumplan totalmente estos requisitos. Los estudios realizados *in vitro* ponen de manifiesto una gran variabilidad en los resultados, que dependen, entre otros factores, de la cepa, del biomaterial utilizado y de la localización de la infección. Por otra parte, no hay estudios clínicos aleatorizados y es reducido el número de ensayos clínicos que se han realizado. De los antimicrobianos disponibles en la actualidad, la rifampicina parece ser uno de los más efectivos cuando se utiliza en tratamiento combinado. Tanto *in vitro* como en modelos experimentales y en ensayos clínicos, muestra una aceptable actividad bactericida frente a bacterias en fase lenta de crecimiento, y tiene capacidad de difundirse a través de las biocapas. Sin embargo, el rápido desarrollo de resistencias obliga a no utilizarla en monoterapia.[11]

La mayoría de las infecciones asociadas a dispositivos médicos se deben a microorganismos grampositivos, y entre ellos *Staphylococcus aureus* y *Staphylococcus epidermidis* son los más prevalentes. Datos clínicos y de laboratorio han puesto recientemente de manifiesto la aparición de un nuevo fenotipo, tanto en *S. aureus* como en *S. epidermidis,* llamado «variantes de colonias pequeñas», que podría ser la causa de las infecciones persistentes y explicar, al menos en parte, los numerosos fracasos terapéuticos observados en las infecciones relacionadas con materiales protésicos.[12] El aumento de estas infecciones producidas por cepas de estafilococos resistentes a la meticilina ha requerido el uso de glucopéptidos, en especial de la vancomicina, con distintos resultados. Son varios los estudios que han evaluado la eficacia de la vancomicina frente a biocapas de *S. aureus* y *S. epidermidis,* y en la mayoría no se ha conseguido demostrar una eliminación total del microorganismo.[1,13,14] La limitada actividad de la vancomicina frente a las biocapas bacterianas justifica su asociación con otros antimicrobianos, como la rifampicina, la gentamicina o la clindamicina, lo que permite una mayor penetración del fármaco y un aumento de la muerte celular.[9,15] En los últimos años se han descrito cepas de *S. aureus* con sensibilidad disminuida a la vancomicina (VISA, *vancomycin-intermediate S. aureus),* y un aumento paulatino de la concentración mínima inhibitoria (CMI) de la vancomicina (CMI de hasta 1,5-2 mg/l) frente a ellas, que podrían explicar algunos fracasos terapéuticos.[16] Diversos estudios *in vitro* han demostrado que ciertas alteraciones en la funcionalidad del gen *agr* en el locus δ inducen, en *S. aureus,* heterorresistencia o sensibilidad disminuida a la vancomicina.[17] La posible relación entre disfuncionalidad del gen *agr* y fenotipo hVISA se ha analizado en varios estudios, con gran número de cepas de *S. aureus* resistente a la meticilina (SARM) asociadas a bacteriemias, y los resultados han sido contradictorios.[18] El linezolid, la daptomicina y la tigeciclina son antimicrobianos con diferentes mecanismos de acción que presentan actividad frente a un amplio espectro de bacterias grampositivas, incluidas las multirresistentes, como los estafilocos resistentes a la meticilina y con sensibilidad disminuida a la vancomicina. Su excelente actividad *in vitro,* así como sus propiedades farmacodinámicas, hacen que estos antimicrobianos, solos o asociados a rifampicina, deban valorarse como posibles alternativas en el tratamiento de las infecciones relacionadas con dispositivos médicos.[19]

El linezolid pertenece al grupo de las oxazolidinonas, y es la única de ellas aprobada para uso clínico. Las oxazolidinonas son fármacos semisintéticos que han mostrado actividad *in vitro* frente a bacterias grampositivas, incluyendo SARM y *S. epidermidis.* Actúan sobre la síntesis proteica, impidiendo el ensamblado de las dos subunidades de los ribosomas bacterianos. Este mecanismo no es compartido con otros fármacos que actúan del mismo modo, lo cual es importante desde el punto de vista del desarrollo de resistencias. Tanto *in vitro* como en modelos animales, el linezolid se ha mostrado activo frente a biocapas estafilocócicas.[20] En estudios *in vitro* llevados a cabo en nuestro laboratorio, el linezolid mostró mayor actividad que la vancomicina frente a biocapas de *S. epidermidis* formadas sobre catéteres de silicona.[21] En modelos que simulan tratamientos antimicrobianos con sellado del catéter los resultados son contradictorios, y parecen depender de las cepas y de los biomateriales.[22,23] El linezolid fue más activo que la vancomicina frente a biocapas de *S. epidermidis* formadas sobre catéteres de poliuretano, pero esta diferencia de actividad no se observó con algunas cepas de SARM.[22,24] En función de los resultados obtenidos puede asegurarse que, en general, el linezolid es activo frente a las biocapas estafilocócicas tras un tiempo de exposición prolongado (de cuatro a siete días). En cortos períodos de exposición, la actividad ha resultado ser dependiente de la cepa y del biomaterial ensayado. En un modelo experimental de infección por cuerpo extraño con una cepa de SARM, el linezolid asociado a rifampicina mostró una mayor actividad que solo, con unos porcentajes de erradicación del 60 % y el 50 %, respectivamente.[25]

La daptomicina es un lipopéptido cíclico con rápida actividad bactericida frente a microorganismos grampositivos, incluyendo los estafilococos resistentes a la meticilina. Se inserta en la membrana celular, induce su despolarización y provoca la muerte celular. Cuando se habla de biocapas bacterianas, el hecho de presentar actividad frente a bacterias tanto en fase estacionaria de crecimiento como metabólicamente inertes es una extraordinaria ventaja frente a otros antimicrobianos que, para ejercer su acción, necesitan bacterias metabólicamente activas. Su exclusivo mecanismo de acción y su gran actividad bactericida hacen de la daptomicina un buen candidato para el tratamiento de las infecciones asociadas a materiales protésicos.[26,27] Además, estudios de permeabilidad bacteriana han demostrado que penetra rápidamente a través de biocapas de *S. epidermidis.*[28] Diversos estudios *in vitro* han puesto de manifiesto que la daptomicina es más eficaz que otros antimicrobianos activos frente a las biocapas estafilocócicas. En un estudio con aislados clínicos de SARM, mostró una mayor actividad que la clindamicina, el linezolid, la tigeciclina y la vancomicina sobre las biocapas estafilocócicas.[19] En un modelo dinámico desarrollado por nuestro grupo, utilizando catéteres de poliuretano como sustrato para la formación de biocapas de *S. epidermidis*, la daptomicina también presentó una gran actividad, muy superior a la de la vancomicina.[29] En la figura 1 se muestran, con microscopía electrónica de barrido, las biocapas de *S. epidermidis* formadas sobre catéteres de poliuretano utilizando este dispositivo, y el efecto de la exposición a daptomicina durante 72 horas. Diversos modelos animales de infección relacionada con materiales protésicos han demostrado la eficacia de la daptomicina, tanto para prevenir la colonización como para el tratamiento de las infecciones por *S. aureus* y *S. epidermidis* resistentes a la meticilina.[30,31] Son pocos los estudios *in vitro* que han evaluado la eficacia de la asociación de daptomicina y rifampicina frente a las biocapas estafilocócicas. En biocapas de *S. aureus,* la rifampicina retrasó la actividad bactericida de la daptomicina, con un efecto dependiente de la cepa.[32] En un modelo animal de infección relacionada con material protésico, la actividad de la daptomicina asociada a rifampicina frente a biocapas de *S. epidermidis* fue significativamente más alta que cuando se administraba sola. En este estudio, la rifampicina sola mostró la misma actividad que asociada a daptomicina, lo que sugiere que la función de la daptomicina podría limitarse a impedir el desarrollo de resistencias a la rifampicina.[33] Por otra parte, son prometedores los resultados de varios estudios que han utilizado daptomicina en monoterapia para el tratamiento de infecciones como endocarditis y osteomielitis, en las cuales pueden estar involucradas biocapas.[34]

La tigeciclina es una glicilciclina, derivada de la minociclina, con actividad frente a grampositivos. Presenta un sustituyente glicilamido que previene la acción de las bombas de flujo, causa fundamental de la resistencia a las tetraciclinas.[35] Este antimicrobiano, al igual que las restantes tetraciclinas, actúa inhibiendo la síntesis proteica, y por tanto es otro posible candidato para el tratamiento de las infecciones relacionas con biocapas. Aunque son pocos los estudios *in vitro* realizados, ponen de manifiesto que la tigeciclina presenta una moderada actividad bactericida frente a biocapas de *S. aureus* y *S. epider-*

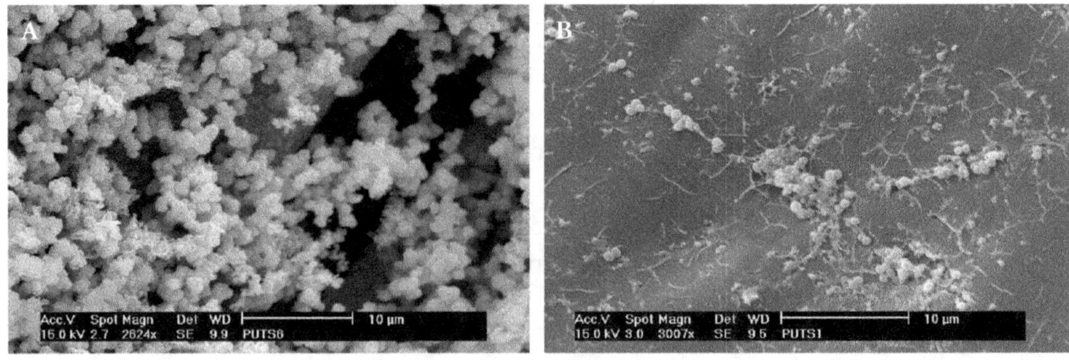

Figura 1. Microscopía electrónica de barrido de las biocapas de 72 horas de S. epidermidis *sobre catéteres de poliuretano, usando el dispositivo diseñado por nuestro grupo. Sin antimicrobiano (A) y expuesto a 7,5 mg/l de daptomicina (B).*

midis.[36,37] En un modelo *in vitro* que simulaba tratamientos antimicrobianos con sellado del catéter, la tigeciclina erradicó la biocapa de *S. aureus* tras dos días de exposición durante cuatro horas al día. Al asociar rifampicina a la tigeciclina, la erradicación se produjo en el primer día de tratamiento.[23]

2   Mecanismos de resistencia a los antimicrobianos en materiales protésicos

Las características estructurales y fisiológicas de las biocapas confieren una resistencia innata tanto a los antimicrobianos como a los desinfectantes y a los germicidas. Las bacterias de las biocapas son resistentes a los agentes antimicrobianos por mecanismos adicionales y diferentes a los de las células planctónicas. Generalmente, la concentración de antimicrobiano requerida para lograr una actividad bactericida frente a las biocapas suele ser muy superior a la de las bacterias planctónicas.[5] Otra característica importante es que las bacterias que forman parte de las biocapas recuperan la sensibilidad original de la cepa bacteriana una vez que se liberan de ella y vuelven a su estado de célula planctónica.[4] Teniendo en cuenta todos estos aspectos, parece probable que la resistencia de las biocapas a los antimicrobianos no se deba a mecanismos codificados genéticamente ni tampoco a la selección de mutantes resistentes presentes en subpoblaciones. Como ejemplo, en los pacientes con dispositivos médicos sobre los que crecen biocapas bacterianas, los altos grados de resistencia desaparecen cuando éstos son retirados. Se ha demostrado que la resistencia en este tipo de estructuras es multifactorial, varía de unas especies a otras y se debe, en primer lugar, a las características fisiológicas de las bacterias individuales de la biocapa, así como a la ultraestructura de ésta.[1]

A continuación se detallan los mecanismos de resistencia en las biocapas bacterianas mejor conocidos que afectan a la actividad de los principales grupos de antimicrobianos (véase la figura 2).

2.1   *Impermeabilidad de las biocapas a los antimicrobianos*

El primer paso para que los antimicrobianos ejerzan su actividad es que alcancen su diana. Las biocapas disponen de una estructura, denominada glicocálix, que protege a las bacterias infectantes de los sistemas de defensa del paciente, así como de la difusión de los antimicrobianos hacia las dianas celulares, con lo cual actúa como una barrera que impide o reduce el transporte de los fármacos al interior de la biocapa (véase la tabla 1).

A modo de ejemplo, se ha demostrado que el alginato embebido en las biocapas de *Pseudomonas aeruginosa* impide el transporte del imipenem y de la tobramicina, y estas biocapas son hasta mil veces más resistentes en comparación con la forma de vida planctónica.[38] En otros estudios se ha investigado la penetración de las fluoroquinolonas, los betalactámicos, los macrólidos y los aminoglucósidos en biocapas producidas por

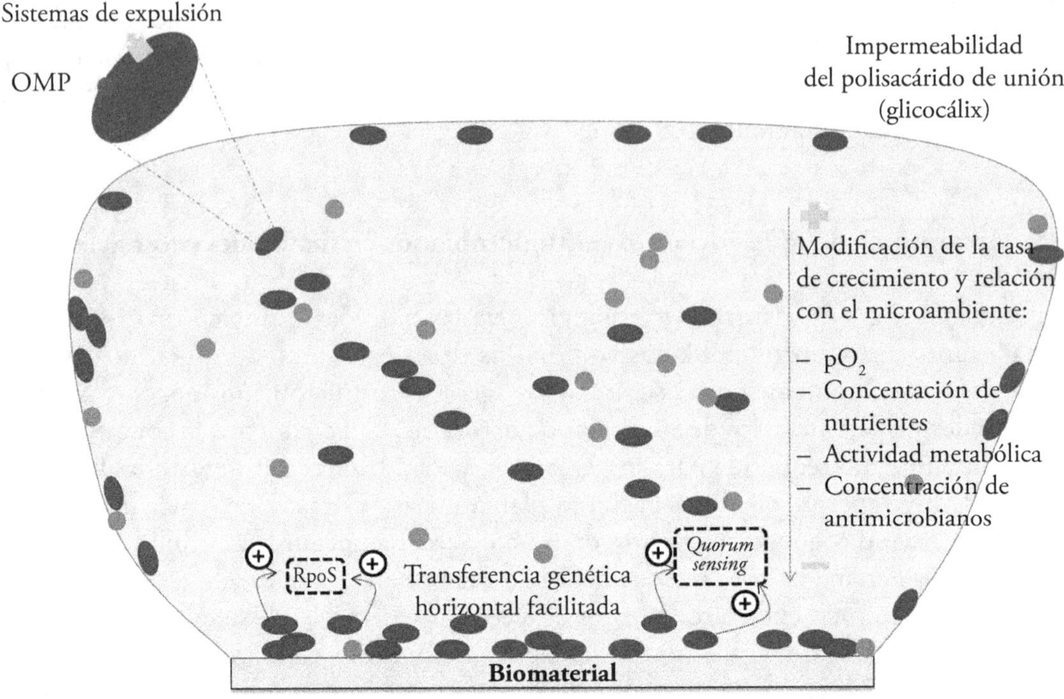

*Figura 2. Representación de los principales mecanismos de resistencia a los antimicrobianos
en las biocapas bacterianas. OMP: proteinas de la membrana externa.*

P. aeruginosa. Parece que los macrólidos son los que mejor atraviesan estas biocapas, seguidos de las fluoroquinolonas y los betalactámicos.[39] En *P. aeruginosa* y *Escherichia coli,* el ciprofloxacino y la amoxicilina-ácido clavulánico presentan una mayor actividad *in vitro* que la fosfomicina y el cotrimoxazol;[40] además, el ciprofloxacino y la amoxicilina-ácido clavulánico presentan las mayores tasas de penetración en las biocapas bacterianas maduras.

En *S. epidermidis,* patógeno asociado frecuentemente con las biocapas formadas en los catéteres endovasculares, la producción de *slime* tiene un efecto similar, aunque no del mismo modo para todos los antimicrobianos.[41] Por ejemplo, la vancomicina y la teicoplanina se afectan más que la rifampicina y la clindamicina. Del mismo modo, y de acuerdo con estudios realizados por nuestro grupo, el linezolid presenta una mayor actividad que la vancomicina frente a biocapas de *S. epidermidis* sobre catéteres de silicona, y este efecto se debe, al menos en parte, a la capacidad del linezolid para concentrarse en las biocapas en comparación con la vancomicina.[42]

La actividad antimicrobiana es dependiente de la estructura de la biocapa bacteriana, de las características bioquímicas de los componentes del glicocálix, de la especie bacteriana y del tamaño y las características químicas del antimicrobiano en cuestión. Todos estos datos realzan la importancia de la impermeabilidad de las biocapas en la reducción de la actividad de los antimicrobianos.[43]

2.2 Alteraciones del crecimiento bacteriano en las biocapas

El segundo mecanismo propuesto para la resistencia antimicrobiana de las biocapas bacterianas está relacionado con la tasa de crecimiento de las bacterias. En las biocapas, las bacterias presentan una tasa de crecimiento más lenta y, por tanto, un metabolismo muy limitado en comparación con las células planctónicas, con lo que se retrasa la acción de los antimicrobianos y se alargan los tiempos de tratamiento (véase la tabla 1). En el interior de las biocapas bacterianas los nutrientes son limitados, lo cual lleva a un retraso en el crecimiento. Del mismo modo, la transición de la fase exponencial a la fase estacionaria se acompaña de un aumento de la resistencia.[44] Diversos autores han desarrollado modelos para caracterizar experimentalmente la relación entre la disponibilidad de nutrientes y el estado de crecimiento de las biocapas. La penetración de glucosa y oxígeno se reduce en las biocapas y, por ejemplo, la actividad catalasa aumenta a niveles similares a los encontrados en fase estacionaria en las células planctónicas.[45] Mediante microscopía electrónica se ha podido apreciar que la acción de la ampicilina afectó a la biocapa superficialmente, pero no a su interior. Estos resultados indican que la limitación de nutrientes genera diferentes regiones en las biocapas con mayor y menor tasa de crecimiento, y las regiones con menor tasa de crecimiento presentan menos sensibilidad a la actividad bactericida de los antimicrobianos.

Diversos autores han evaluado el efecto de la tasa de crecimiento sobre la sensibilidad a determinados antimicrobianos (betalactámicos y fluoroquinolonas). En *P. aeruginosa*, la acción bactericida de los betalactámicos se ve afectada por la tasa de crecimiento, mientras que la actividad de las fluoroquinolonas es mayor e independiente de ésta.[46,47] Tal situación parece similar en las bacterias grampositivas. En las biocapas de *S. epidermidis,* la tasa de crecimiento afecta notablemente a la sensibilidad antimicrobiana, y se ha correlacionado con la actividad del ciprofloxacino.[48]

2.3 Efecto del microambiente de las biocapas en la actividad antimicrobiana

El microambiente en el interior de las biocapas es un factor que afecta a la actividad antimicrobiana *in vitro* debido a diferentes variables, como la pO_2, la pCO_2, la concentración de cationes divalentes, el grado de hidratación, el pH y las concentraciones de pirimidinas, que producen efectos adversos en la acción de los antimicrobianos en el interior de la biocapa, donde las condiciones ácido-básicas y aeróbicas-anaeróbicas pueden variar (véase la tabla 1).[49,50] Las limitaciones de oxígeno pueden reducir la sensibilidad a la tobramicina en las biocapas de *P. aeruginosa*. Presiones relativamente altas de CO_2 pueden afectar a la actividad de los aminoglucósidos, los macrólidos y las tetraciclinas. Por otro lado, la naturaleza polianiónica del exopolisacárido de alginato producido por *P. aeruginosa*, debido a su capacidad para concentrar cationes divalentes, puede alterar la actividad de antimicrobianos como los aminoglucósidos y las tetraciclinas.[49-52]

2.4 Mecanismos de resistencia a los antimicrobianos presentes en las bacterias planctónicas

En principio, la resistencia a los antimicrobianos de las bacterias en las biocapas parecía independiente de los mecanismos de resistencia expresados por las bacterias planctónicas, como los sistemas de expulsión activa, las mutaciones en las dianas celulares o las enzimas modificantes. Las primeras observaciones indicaban que estos mecanismos no eran suficientes para explicar los grados de resistencia alcanzados por los microorganismos presentes en las biocapas bacterianas. Sin embargo, estas evidencias no excluyen la posibilidad de que los mecanismos convencionales de resistencia se expresen en las biocapas y contribuyan a la resistencia antimicrobiana en ellas detectada. Se ha demostrado que la desrepresión de la betalactamasa cromosómica y la expresión de los sistemas de expulsión activa MexAB-OprM y MexCD-OprJ en biocapas de *P. aeruginosa* contribuyen de manera específica a la persistencia de la infección en tratamientos con betalactámicos y azitromicina, respectivamente.[53,54] También en relación con *P. aeruginosa* se ha descrito un mecanismo de tolerancia en las biocapas, por el cual los glucanos periplásmicos interaccionan y secuestran a la tobramicina e impiden que alcance su diana.[55] Este mecanismo abre la posibilidad de que las biocapas no sean simplemente barreras de difusión para los antimicrobianos, sino que más bien estas comunidades bacterianas emplean diferentes mecanismos para resistir la acción de los antimicrobianos (véase la tabla 1).

2.5 Papel de los elementos genéticos de transferencia horizontal

Las biocapas son estructuras idóneas para que se produzcan fenómenos de transferencia de genes horizontalmente, debido a la acumulación de microorganismos y a la estabilización física de éstos. Los plásmidos, por un mecanismo de conjugación, pueden transferir genes entre microorganismos de la misma especie o de especies diferentes. Al mismo tiempo, los productos de los genes necesarios para la maquinaria de conjugación promueven el contacto célula-célula, con lo cual pueden facilitar el proceso de formación de las biocapas bacterianas, lo que denota su importancia clínica. Teniendo en cuenta este razonamiento, parece plausible confirmar que las biocapas, en las cuales pueden convivir bacterias de diferentes especies, son ambientes ideales para la transferencia horizontal de genes, dependiente del contacto célula-célula, y favorecen la diseminación de genes de resistencia a los antimicrobianos y de factores de virulencia en diferentes microorganismos relacionados con la formación de biocapas.[56-59]

2.6 Papel del biomaterial en la inducción de resistencias

Muchos de los biomateriales usados en clínica presentan superficies hidrófobas que facilitan la unión inespecífica de las bacterias. Posteriormente, la unión de modo específico se produce mediante adhesinas que fijan al microorganismo a la superficie de un modo estable. Por tanto, la composición del biomaterial tiene importancia en la adherencia bacteriana. Además, se ha demostrado que los biomateriales pueden inducir resistencia, si bien este fenómeno sólo se ha descrito con sondas de látex siliconizado y *P. aeruginosa*. En relación con este fenómeno, se observó que la actividad del imipenem frente a *P. aeruginosa* disminuye hasta 16 veces cuando crece en un medio previamente incubado con sondas de látex siliconizado, con lo cual el microorganismo se hace resistente a los carbapenémicos. Este proceso está causado por la disminución de la expresión de una porina *(oprD2)* que es la vía de entrada de los carbapenémicos para alcanzar su diana. A pesar de que el látex siliconizado se utiliza para la fabricación de numerosos dispositivos de uso sanitario, se desconoce la relevancia de este fenómeno en la epidemiología de la resistencia al imipenem en el ambiente hospitalario.[60,61]

3 Nuevas estrategias frente a las biocapas bacterianas

Considerando la resistencia de las biocapas a los tratamientos antimicrobianos convencionales, es necesario encontrar nuevas estrategias para la prevención y el tratamiento de las infecciones asociadas a materiales protésicos. Se están evaluando diversas alternativas al tratamiento clásico, pero debido a la complejidad de las biocapas y a los muchos factores que intervienen en su formación, aún no son aplicables a la práctica clínica. Algunas van dirigidas a prevenir la formación de la biocapa, impidiendo la adherencia del microorganismo al biomaterial, y otras a destruirla, bien por acción directa o de manera indirecta debilitando su estructura y haciéndolas más sensibles a la acción de los antimicrobianos.

Entre las medidas dirigidas a prevenir las infecciones asociadas a las biocapas, cabe destacar los ensayos clínicos que han demostrado que el uso de catéteres impregnados con biocidas o antimicrobianos, como clorhexidina/sulfadiazina argéntica o minociclina/rifampicina, bloquean la adherencia bacteriana e impiden la formación de la biocapa.[62] También se están evaluando nuevas medidas preventivas, como el uso de moléculas antisentido, que silencien los genes que codifican la adherencia y la formación de las biocapas estafilocócicas, o de inhibidores del *quorum sensing,* que bloqueen la comunicación entre bacterias dentro de la biocapa, pero los resultados obtenidos hasta la fecha son controvertidos.[63,64] Para poder avanzar en muchos aspectos relacionados con este tema es necesario profundizar en el conocimiento de la estructura de las biocapas y de los múltiples factores involucrados en su formación.

Hay varias estrategias en estudio dirigidas al tratamiento de estas infecciones, con resultados prometedores. Se ha comprobado que el uso de corriente eléctrica de baja intensidad y de ultrasonidos disgrega la estructura de la biocapa y aumenta la eficacia de los antibióticos *in vitro*.[65,66] El uso de bacteriófagos es otra posible medida para controlar la estructura de la biocapa. Éstos infectarían a la bacteria e inducirían la producción de una polimerasa que hidrolizaría sustancias presentes en la matriz.[67] También se han realizado estudios con enzimas como la DNasaI y la dispersina B, y se ha observado que los tratamientos con ellas hacen que las biocapas sean más sensibles a los biocidas.[68]

Otra posible opción terapéutica para eliminar la biocapa es el uso de terapia fotodinámica en combinación con antimicrobianos. Ésta se basa en la acción combinada de la luz visible y de un compuesto fotosensibilizador que genera radicales de oxígeno, que son tóxicos para las bacterias. Los ensayos realizados con biocapas de *S. aureus* sobre implantes accesibles a la luz visible muestran resultados prometedores.[69,70] En la práctica clínica, la terapia fotodinámica puede ser un tratamiento complementario. Su eficacia depende de las propiedades farmacocinéticas y de la capacidad de penetrar del fotosensibilizador, de la idoneidad de la longitud de onda y del tiempo de irradiación, junto con la inherente limitación de la técnica en cuanto a la accesibilidad del implante mediante fibra óptica.

4   Técnicas y limitaciones para el estudio de la actividad de los antimicrobianos sobre materiales protésicos

Los parámetros normalmente utilizados para establecer la actividad de los antimicrobianos en el tratamiento clínico de las infecciones son la CMI y la concentración mínima bactericida (CMB). Estos valores se determinan mediante métodos estandarizados y utilizando bacterias en suspensión. Muchos estudios han demostrado que las CMB frente a las bacterias sésiles son muy superiores a las que requieren las planctónicas, por lo que en las infecciones relacionadas con materiales protésicos es necesario disponer de otros parámetros que reflejen mejor la actividad antimicrobiana.[9] Nuevos conceptos, como las concentraciones mínimas inhibitorias y erradicadoras de las biocapas, son más representativos de la actividad de los antibióticos que los clásicos de CMI y CMB.[71] La metodología para determinar estos parámetros no se encuentra estandarizada, por lo que es difícil su extrapolación a la práctica clínica.

La formación y el desarrollo de la biocapa es un proceso muy complejo, en el cual influyen muchas variables relacionadas con la localización de la infección, la composición del biomaterial, las características del fluido en que se encuentra inmerso y las condiciones inherentes a la propia bacteria adherida (fase de crecimiento y actividad metabólica).[72] Debido al elevado número de variables, los estudios que evalúan *in vitro* la actividad antimicrobiana frente a ellas son reducidos y difíciles de comparar. Muchos utilizan biocapas muy jóvenes y tiempos de incubación muy cortos, o biomateriales que no se utilizan en la práctica clínica, condiciones todas que se encuentran muy lejos de la situación *in vivo*.[10,19,21,36] Hay algunos estudios *in vitro* que utilizan modelos que permiten una mayor aproximación a las condiciones *in vivo* y estudian las biocapas de forma dinámica, para determinar la actividad de los antimicrobianos sobre ellas. También permiten establecer un modelo de «sellado antibiótico» que simula el tratamiento conservador de las colonizaciones endoluminales de los catéteres vasculares de larga duración.[22,23,73]

A la mayoría de los biomateriales que se usan en biomedicina, en especial a los de naturaleza polimérica, se les añaden diferentes aditivos dirigidos a mejorar su flexibilidad o biocompatibilidad. Se ha comprobado que algunos de estos aditivos pueden afectar de manera significativa a la actividad de los antimicrobianos.[60] Los biomateriales metálicos y las aleaciones metálicas utilizados para la fabricación de las prótesis ortopédicas sufren una serie de procesos superficiales dirigidos a evitar su corrosión y mejorar su biocompatibilidad, que pueden afectar a la formación de las biocapas. Todo ello justifica la necesidad de utilizar, en la medida de lo posible, los mismos biomateriales utilizados en la práctica médica. Con frecuencia la composición de estos biomateriales es secreto industrial, y suele ser difícil disponer de muestras que se adapten al dispositivo, por lo que la disponibilidad de biomateriales reales es muy limitada. Nuestro grupo ha desarrollado un dispositivo que permite evaluar *in vitro,* de manera dinámica, la actividad de un antimicrobiano durante largos períodos de tiempo frente a biocapas maduras formadas sobre segmentos de catéteres de uso clínico, modelo que reproduce muchos de los parámetros que influyen en la interacción *in vivo* de la bacteria, el antimicrobiano y el biomaterial.[29]

Bibliografía

1. Costerton JW, Stewart PS, Greenberg EP. Bacterial biofilms: a common cause of persistent infections. Science. 1999; 284: 1318-22.
2. De Carvalho CC. Biofilms: new ideas for an old problem. Recent Pat Biotechnol. 2012; 6: 13-22.
3. Leroy O, Meybeck A, Sarraz-Bournet B, d'Elia P, Legout L. Vascular graft infections. Curr Opin Infect Dis. 2012; 25: 154-8.
4. Fux CA, Costerton JW, Stewart PS, Stoodley P. Survival strategies of infectious biofilms. Trends Microbiol. 2005; 13: 34-40.
5. Peters BM, Jabra-Rizk MA, O'May GA, Costerton JW, Shirtliff ME. Polymicrobial interactions: impact on pathogenesis and human disease. Clin Microbiol Rev. 2012; 25: 193-213.
6. Singh PK, Schaefer AL, Parsek MR, Moninger TO, Welsh MJ, Greenberg EP. Quorum-sensing signals indicate that cystic fibrosis lungs are infected with bacterial biofilms. Nature. 2000; 407: 762-4.
7. Raad I, Hanna H, Maki D. Intravascular catheter-related infections: advances in diagnosis, prevention, and management. Lancet Infect Dis. 2007; 7: 645-57.
8. Rodríguez-Martínez JM, Pascual A. Actividad de los antimicrobianos en biocapas bacterianas. Enferm Infecc Microbiol Clin. 2008; 26: 107-14.
9. Kiedrowski MR, Horswill AR. New approaches for treating staphylococcal biofilm infections. Ann N Y Acad Sci. 2011; 1241: 104-21.
10. Saginur R, Stdenis M, Ferris W, Aaron SD, Chan F, Lee C, et al. Multiple combination bactericidal testing of staphylococcal biofilms from implant-associated infections. Antimicrob Agents Chemother. 2006; 50: 55-61.
11. Neut D, Van der Mei HC, Bulstra SK, Busscher HJ. The role of small-colony variants in failure to diagnose and treat biofilm infections in orthopedics. Acta Orthop. 2007; 78: 299-308.
12. Mermel LA, Allon M, Bouza E, Craven DE, Flynn P, O'Grady NP, et al. Clinical practice guidelines for the diagnosis and management of intravascular catheter-related infection: 2009 update by the Infectious Diseases Society of America. Clin Infect Dis. 2009; 49: 1-45.
13. Monzón M, Oteiza C, Leiva J, Lamata M, Amorena B. Biofilm testing of Staphylococcus epidermidis clinical isolates: low performance of vancomycin in relation to other antibiotics. Diagn Microbiol Infect Dis. 2002; 44: 319-24.
14. Rose WE, Poppens PT. Impact of biofilm on the in vitro activity of vancomycin alone and in combination with tigecycline and rifampicin against Staphylococcus aureus. J Antimicrob Chemother. 2009; 63: 485-8.

15. Deresinski S. Vancomycin in combination with other antibiotics for the treatment of serious methicillin-resistant Staphylococcus aureus infections. Clin Infect Dis. 2009; 49: 1072-9.

16. Howden BP, Davies JK, Johnson PD, Stinear TP, Grayson ML. Reduced vancomycin susceptibility in Staphylococcus aureus, including vancomycin-intermediate and heterogeneous vancomycin-intermediate strains: resistance mechanisms, laboratory detection, and clinical implications. Clin Microbiol Rev. 2010; 23: 99-139.

17. Harigaya Y, Ngo D, Lesse AJ, Huang V, Tsuji BT. Characterization of heterogeneous vancomycin-intermediate resistance, MIC and accessory gene regulator (agr) dysfunction among clinical bloodstream isolates of Staphyloccocus aureus. BMC Infect Dis. 2011; 11: 287.

18. Butterfield JM, Tsuji BT, Brown J, Ashley ED, Hardy D, Brown K, *et al.* Predictors of agr dysfunction in methicillin-resistant Staphylococcus aureus (MRSA) isolates among patients with MRSA bloodstream infections. Antimicrob Agents Chemother. 2011; 55: 5433-7.

19. Smith K, Pérez A, Ramage G, Gemmell CG, Lang S. Comparison of biofilm-associated cell survival following in vitro exposure of meticillin-resistant Staphylococcus aureus biofilms to the antibiotics clindamycin, daptomycin, linezolid, tigecycline and vancomycin. Int J Antimicrob Agents. 2009; 33: 374-8.

20. Leach KL, Brickner SJ, Noe MC, Miller PF. Linezolid, the first oxazolidinone antibacterial agent. Ann NY Acad Sci. 2011; 1222: 49-54.

21. Rodríguez-Martínez JM, Ballesta S, García I, Conejo MC, Pascual A. Actividad y permeabilidad de linezolid y vancomicina en biocapas de Staphylococcus epidermidis. Enferm Infecc Microbiol Clin. 2007; 25: 425-8.

22. Curtin J, Cormican M, Fleming G, Keelehan J, Colleran E. Linezolid compared with eperezolid, vancomycin, and gentamicin in an in vitro model of antimicrobial lock therapy for Staphylococcus epidermidis central venous catheter-related biofilm infections. Antimicrob Agents Chemother. 2003; 47: 3145-8.

23. Raad I, Hanna H, Jiang Y, Dvorak T, Reitzel R, Chaiban G, *et al.* Comparative activities of daptomycin, linezolid, and tigecycline against catheter-related methicillin-resistant Staphylococcus bacteremic isolates embedded in biofilm. Antimicrob Agents Chemother. 2007; 51: 1656-60.

24. Fernández-Hidalgo N, Gavaldà J, Almirante B, Martín MT, Onrubia PL, Gomis X, *et al.* Evaluation of linezolid, vancomycin, gentamicin and ciprofloxacin in a rabbit model of antibiotic-lock technique for Staphylococcus aureus catheter-related infection. J Antimicrob Chemother. 2010; 65: 525-30.

25. Baldoni D, Haschke M, Rajacic Z, Zimmerli W, Trampuz A. Linezolid alone or combined with rifampin against methicillin-resistant Staphylococcus aureus in experimental foreign-body infection. Antimicrob Agents Chemother. 2009; 53: 1142-8.

26. Rybak MJ. The efficacy and safety of daptomycin: first in a new class of antibiotics for Gram-positive bacteria. Clin Microbiol Infect. 2006; 12 (Suppl 1): 24-32.

27. Eisenstein BI. Treatment of staphylococcal infections with cyclic lipopeptides. Clin Microbiol Infect. 2008; 14 (Suppl 2): 10-6.

28. Stewart PS, Davison WM, Steenbergen JN. Daptomycin rapidly penetrates a Staphylococcus epidermidis biofilm. Antimicrob Agents Chemother. 2009; 5: 3505-7.

29. García I, Conejo MC, Ojeda A, Rodríguez-Baño J, Pascual A. A dynamic in vitro model for evaluating antimicrobial activity against bacterial biofilms using a new device and clinical-used catheters. J Microbiol Methods. 2010; 83: 307-11.

30. Domínguez-Herrera J, Docobo-Pérez F, López-Rojas R, Pichardo C, Ruiz-Valderas R, Lepe JA, *et al.* Efficacy of daptomycin versus vancomycin in an experimental model of foreign-body and systemic infection caused by biofilm producers and methicillin-resistant Staphylococcus epidermidis. Antimicrob Agents Chemother. 2012; 56: 613-7.

31. Garrigós C, Murillo O, Euba G, Verdaguer R, Tubau F, Cabellos C, *et al.* Efficacy of usual and high doses of daptomycin in combination with rifampin versus alternative therapies in experimental foreign-body infection by methicillin-resistant Staphylococcus aureus. Antimicrob Agents Chemother. 2010; 54: 5251-6.

32. LaPlante KL, Woodmansee S. Activities of daptomycin and vancomycin alone and in combination with rifampin and gentamicin against biofilm-forming methicillin-resistant

Staphylococcus aureus isolates in an experimental model of endocarditis. Antimicrob Agents Chemother. 2009; 53: 3880-6.

33. Olson ME, Slater SR, Rupp ME, Fey PD. Rifampicin enhances activity of daptomycin and vancomycin against both a polysaccharide intercellular adhesion (PIA)-dependent and -independent Staphylococcus epidermidis biofilm. J Antimicrob Chemother. 2010; 65: 2164-71.

34. Falagas ME, Kapaskelis AM, Kouranos VD, Kakisi OK, Athanassa Z, Karageorgopoulos DE. Outcome of antimicrobial therapy in documented biofilm-associated infections: a review of the available clinical evidence. Drugs. 2009; 69: 1351-61.

35. Projan SJ. Preclinical pharmacology of GAR-936, a novel glycylcycline antibacterial agent. Pharmacotherapy. 2000; 20: 219S-223S.

36. Aslam S, Trautner BW, Ramanathan V, Darouiche RO. Combination of tigecycline and N-acetylcysteine reduces biofilm-embedded bacteria on vascular catheters. Antimicrob Agents Chemother. 2007; 51: 1556-8.

37. Cafiso V, Bertuccio T, Spina D, Purrello S, Stefani S. Tigecycline inhibition of a mature biofilm in clinical isolates of Staphylococcus aureus: comparison with other drugs. FEMS Immunol Med Microbiol. 2010; 59: 466-9.

38. Coquet L, Junter GA, Jouenne T. Resistance of artificial biofilms of Pseudomonas aeruginosa to imipenem and tobramycin. J Antimicrob Chemother. 1998; 42: 755-60.

39. Bdi-Ali A, Mohammadi-Mehr M, Agha AY. Bactericidal activity of various antibiotics against biofilm-producing Pseudomonas aeruginosa. Int J Antimicrob Agents. 2006; 27: 196-200.

40. Rodríguez-Martínez JM, Ballesta S, Pascual A. Activity and penetration of fosfomycin, ciprofloxacin, amoxicillin/clavulanic acid and co-trimoxazole in Escherichia coli and Pseudomonas aeruginosa biofilms. Int J Antimicrob Agents. 2007; 30: 366-8.

41. Hatch RA, Schiller NL. Alginate lyase promotes diffusion of aminoglycosides through the extracellular polysaccharide of mucoid Pseudomonas aeruginosa. Antimicrob Agents Chemother. 1998; 42: 974-7.

42. Rodríguez-Martínez JM, Ballesta S, García I, Conejo MC, Pascual A. Activity and penetration of linezolid and vancomycin against Staphylococcus epidermidis biofilms. Enferm Infecc Microbiol Clin. 2007; 25: 425-8.

43. Rodríguez-Martínez JM, Pascual A. Antimicrobial resistance in bacterial biofilms. Rev Med Microbiol. 2006; 17: 65-76.

44. Lewis K. Persister cells. Annu Rev Microbiol. 2010; 64: 357-72.

45. Anderl JN, Zahller J, Roe F, Stewart PS. Role of nutrient limitation and stationary-phase existence in Klebsiella pneumoniae biofilm resistance to ampicillin and ciprofloxacin. Antimicrob Agents Chemother. 2003; 47: 1251-6.

46. Tanaka G, Shigeta M, Komatsuzawa H, Sugai M, Suginaka H, Usui T. Effect of the growth rate of Pseudomonas aeruginosa biofilms on the susceptibility to antimicrobial agents: beta-lactams and fluoroquinolones. Chemotherapy. 1999; 45: 28-36.

47. Karatan E, Watnick P. Signals, regulatory networks, and materials that build and break bacterial biofilms. Microbiol Mol Biol Rev. 2009; 73: 310-47.

48. Dubar V, López I, Gosset P, Aerts C, Voisin C, Wallaert B. The penetration of co-trimoxazole into alveolar macrophages and its effect on inflammatory and immunoregulatory functions. J Antimicrob Chemother. 1990; 26: 791-802.

49. Frei E, Hodgkiss-Harlow K, Rossi PJ, Edmiston CE Jr, Bandyk DF. Microbial pathogenesis of bacterial biofilms: a causative factor of vascular surgical site infection. Vasc Endovascular Surg. 2011; 45: 688-96.

50. Costerton JW, Montanaro L, Arciola CR. Bacterial communications in implant infections: a target for an intelligence war. Int J Artif Organs. 2007; 30: 757-63.

51. Field TR, White A, Elborn JS, Tunney MM. Effect of oxygen limitation on the in vitro antimicrobial susceptibility of clinical isolates of Pseudomonas aeruginosa grown planktonically and as biofilms. Eur J Clin Microbiol Infect Dis. 2005; 24: 677-87.

52. Borriello G, Werner E, Roe F, Kim AM, Ehrlich GD, Stewart PS. Oxygen limitation contributes to antibiotic tolerance of Pseudomonas aeruginosa in biofilms. Antimicrob Agents Chemother. 2004; 48: 2659-64.

53. Bagge N, Ciofu O, Skovgaard LT, Hoiby N. Rapid development in vitro and in vivo of resistance to ceftazidime in biofilm-growing Pseudomonas aeruginosa due to chromosomal beta-lactamase. APMIS. 2000; 108: 589-600.

54. Gillis RJ, White KG, Choi KH, Wagner VE, Schweizer HP, Iglewski BH. Molecular basis of azithromycin-resistant Pseudomonas aeruginosa biofilms. Antimicrob Agents Chemother. 2005; 49: 3858-67.

55. Mah TF, Pitts B, Pellock B, Walker GC, Stewart PS, O'Toole GA. A genetic basis for Pseudomonas aeruginosa biofilm antibiotic resistance. Nature. 2003; 426: 306-10.

56. Ghigo JM. Natural conjugative plasmids induce bacterial biofilm development. Nature. 2001; 412: 442-5.

57. Molin S, Tolker-Nielsen T. Gene transfer occurs with enhanced efficiency in biofilms and induces enhanced stabilisation of the biofilm structure. Curr Opin Biotechnol. 2003; 14: 255-61.

58. Reisner A, Holler BM, Molin S, Zechner EL. Synergistic effects in mixed Escherichia coli biofilms: conjugative plasmid transfer drives biofilm expansion. J Bacteriol. 2006; 188: 3582-8.

59. Cook L, Chatterjee A, Barnes A, Yarwood J, Hu WS, Dunny G. Biofilm growth alters regulation of conjugation by a bacterial pheromone. Mol Microbiol. 2011; 81: 1499-510.

60. Conejo MC, García I, Martínez-Martínez L, Picabea L, Pascual A. Zinc eluted from siliconized latex urinary catheters decreases OprD expression, causing carbapenem resistance in Pseudomonas aeruginosa. Antimicrob Agents Chemother. 2003; 47: 2313-5.

61. Perron K, Caille O, Rossier C, Van DC, Dumas JL, Kohler T. CzcR-CzcS, a two-component system involved in heavy metal and carbapenem resistance in Pseudomonas aeruginosa. J Biol Chem. 2004; 279: 8761-8.

62. Casey AL, Mermel LA, Nightingale P, Elliott TS. Antimicrobial central venous catheters in adults: a systematic review and meta-analysis. Lancet Infect Dis. 2008; 8: 763-76.

63. Costerton WJ, Montanaro L, Balaban N, Arciola CR. Prospecting gene therapy of implant infections. Int J Artif Organs. 2009; 32: 689-95.

64. Balaban N, Cirioni O, Giacometti A, Ghiselli R, Braunstein JB, Silvestri C, et al. Treatment of Staphylococcus aureus biofilm infection by the quorum-sensing inhibitor RIP. Antimicrob Agents Chemother. 2007; 51: 2226-9.

65. Del Pozo JL, Rouse MS, Mandrekar JN, Sampedro MF, Steckelberg JM, Patel R. Effect of electrical current on the activities of antimicrobial agents against Pseudomonas aeruginosa, Staphylococcus aureus, and Staphylococcus epidermidis biofilms. Antimicrob Agents Chemother. 2009; 53: 35-40.

66. Bigelow TA, Northagen T, Hill TM, Sailer FC. The destruction of Escherichia coli biofilms using high-intensity focused ultrasound. Ultrasound Med Biol. 2009; 35: 1026-31.

67. Curtin JJ, Donlan RM. Using bacteriophages to reduce formation of catheter-associated biofilms by Staphylococcus epidermidis. Antimicrob Agents Chemother. 2006; 50: 1268-75.

68. Kaplan JB. Therapeutic potential of biofilm-dispersing enzymes. Int J Artif Organs. 2009; 32: 545-5.

69. Sbarra MS, Arciola CR, Di Poto A, Saino E, Rohde H, Speziale P, et al. The photodynamic effect of tetra-substituted N-methyl-pyridyl-porphine combined with the action of vancomycin or host defense mechanisms disrupts Staphylococcus epidermidis biofilms. Int J Artif Organs. 2009; 32: 574-83.

70. Di Poto A, Sbarra MS, Provenza G, Visai L, Speziale P. The effect of photodynamic treatment combined with antibiotic action or host defense mechanisms on Staphylococcus aureus biofilms. Biomaterials. 2009; 30: 3158-66.

71. Furustrand Tafin U, Majic I, Zalila Belkhodja C, Betrisey B, Corvec S, Zimmerli W, et al. Gentamicin improves the activities of daptomycin and vancomycin against Enterococcus faecalis in vitro and in an experimental foreign-body infection model. Antimicrob Agents Chemother. 2011; 55: 4821-7.

72. Donlan RM. Biofilms: microbial life on surfaces. Emerg Infect Dis. 2002; 8: 881-90.

73. Raad I, Hanna H, Dvorak T, Chaiban G, Hachem R. Optimal antimicrobial catheter lock solution, using different combinations of minocycline, EDTA, and 25-percent ethanol, rapidly eradicates organisms embedded in biofilm. Antimicrob Agents Chemother. 2007; 51: 78-83.

Capítulo 3

Actividad antimicrobiana de los nuevos fármacos activos frente a bacterias grampositivas

E. Cercenado

Servicio de Microbiología y Enfermedades Infecciosas
Hospital General Universitario Gregorio Marañón
Madrid
Facultad de Medicina
Universidad Complutense
Madrid

Correspondencia:
Dra. Emilia Cercenado
ecercenado@terra.es

Introducción

La resistencia a los antimicrobianos continúa siendo un problema de salud pública, con graves consecuencias clínicas y económicas. El aumento de la resistencia bacteriana a los antimicrobianos no sólo conlleva un mayor fracaso clínico y una mayor morbilidad y mortalidad para los pacientes infectados por estos microorganismos, sino que supone además un aumento de los costes hospitalarios debido a los mayores cuidados sanitarios que requieren estos pacientes y al mayor tiempo de hospitalización.

Entre los factores que contribuyen a la resistencia a los antimicrobianos se incluyen el amplio uso que se hace de ellos, el envejecimiento de la población, el aumento del número de pacientes inmunodeprimidos y la mayor utilización de dispositivos médicos, principalmente en las unidades de cuidados intensivos (UCI).[1,2]

En el caso de las bacterias grampositivas, en las dos últimas décadas se ha observado un progresivo aumento en su incidencia, debido tanto al ascenso de los patógenos clásicos *(Staphylococcus aureus, Enterococcus* spp., *Streptococcus pneumoniae, Streptococcus pyogenes)*[3-5] como al mayor número de infecciones producidas por otras especies previamente consideradas menos patógenas (estafilococos coagulasa negativos, estreptococos del grupo *viridans* y corinebacterias) en pacientes inmunodeprimidos y en ancianos que con frecuencia son portadores de dispositivos intravasculares y de materiales protésicos.[6,7] Paralelamente, también se ha producido un incremento de la resistencia de estos microorganismos a los antibióticos de primera elección utilizados para su tratamiento. En la actualidad, la resistencia de *S. aureus* y de otros estafilococos coagulasa negativos a la meticilina, las fluoroquinolonas y los macrólidos, la pérdida de eficacia de la vancomicina frente a los estafilococos, la multirresistencia de los enterococos, y la emergente resistencia al linezolid de los estafilococos y los enterococos, son los principales problemas terapéuticos.[8-10] Por desgracia, el desarrollo de nuevos antimicrobianos siempre ha ido por detrás del desarrollo de resistencias por parte de las bacterias. No obstante, en el caso de las infecciones por bacterias grampositivas multirresistentes, se dispone de varias alternativas terapéuticas ya comercializadas y algunas más que están en fase de desarrollo e investigación.[11]

Hasta muy recientemente la vancomicina se consideraba el fármaco de elección para el tratamiento de las infecciones graves o invasivas por *S. aureus* resistente a la meticilina (SARM), por estafilococos coagulasa negativos resistentes a la meticilina, por enterococos multirresistentes o por corinebacterias, debido a su relativamente buen perfil de seguridad, su estabilidad frente al desarrollo de resistencia y, durante muchos años, por la falta de otros antimicrobianos alternativos. Sin embargo, la emergencia de cepas de enterococos resistentes a la vancomicina, principalmente en Estados Unidos y con menos frecuencia en Europa, y la emergencia de cepas de *S. aureus* con sensibilidad intermedia (VISA, *vancomycin-intermediate S. aureus)* o resistentes a la vancomicina (VRSA, *vancomycin-resistant S. aureus*), creó la necesidad de nuevos agentes antimicrobianos con actividad frente a estas bacterias. En años recientes, el desarrollo y la aprobación de nuevos antimicrobianos con mayor actividad que la vancomicina frente a SARM y a otros grampositivos multirresistentes, junto con las numerosas descripciones de fracasos clínicos con vancomicina debido a su baja penetración en ciertos tejidos (como el pulmonar), a su lenta actividad bactericida y al posible aumento de sus concentraciones mínimas inhibitorias (CMI) frente a cepas de SARM causantes de infecciones graves, han cuestionado la eficacia de la vancomicina a la vez que se ha producido un aumento del uso de nuevos antimicrobianos, como el linezolid y la daptomicina.[12]

En los últimos años hemos asistido a un gran impulso en el desarrollo de agentes antimicrobianos con actividad frente a bacterias grampositivas multirresistentes, y varios de ellos han sido aprobados para el tratamiento de las infecciones producidas por estos microorganismos, como el linezolid, la daptomicina, la tigeciclina y la quinupristina-dalfopristina, si bien el uso de esta última ha sido desautorizado recientemente en España. Además, hay otros en desarrollo e investigación, o pendientes de autorización por las agencias reguladoras, como la telavancina, la oritavancina, la dalbavancina, el ceftobiprol, la ceftarolina y el iclaprim, que han demostrado buena actividad *in vitro* frente a SARM y otras bacterias grampositivas. Las estructuras moleculares de todos estos antimicrobianos se muestran en la figura 1, y en la tabla 1 se presenta un resumen de su actividad frente a los microorganismos grampositivos de mayor interés clínico.

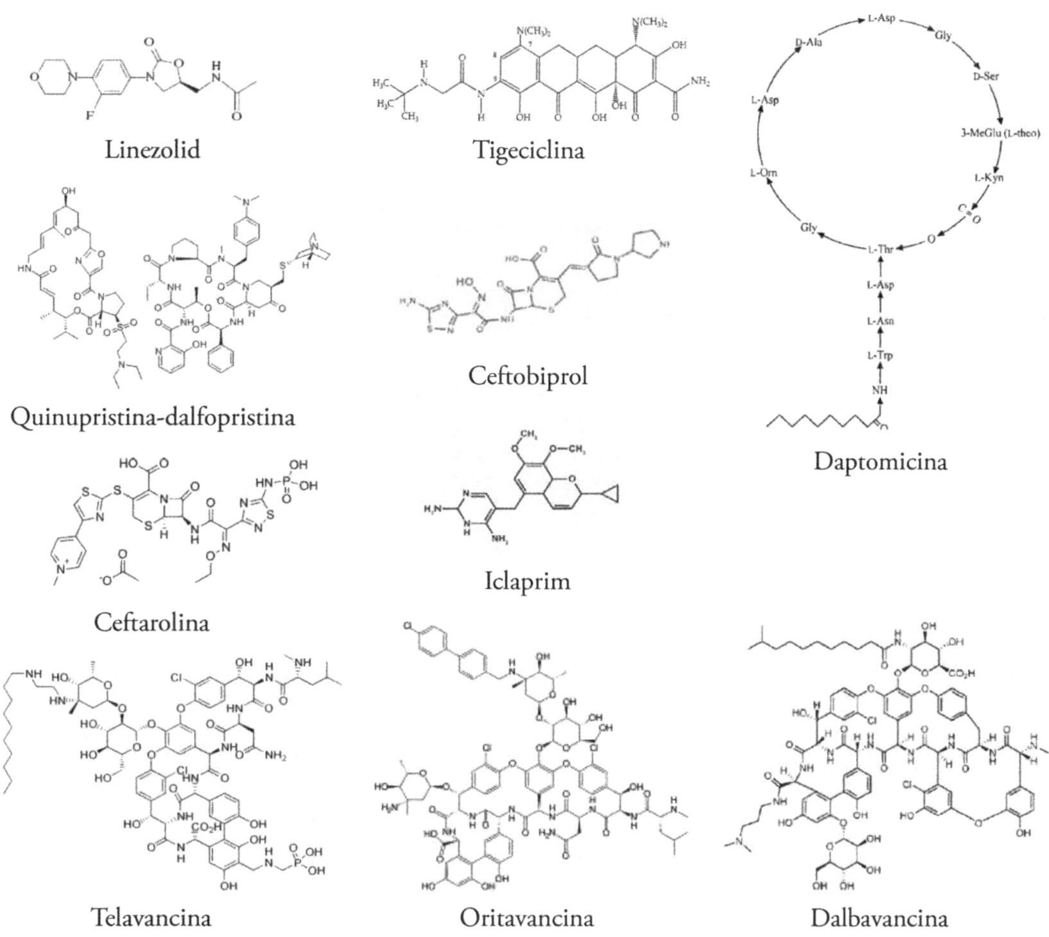

Figura 1. Estructuras químicas de los nuevos antimicrobianos activos frente a microorganismos grampositivos multirresistentes.

1 Linezolid

El linezolid es una oxazolidinona sintética que inhibe el inicio de la síntesis proteica en la subunidad 50S del ribosoma, en concreto en la subunidad 23S del RNA ribosómico. Aunque es un antibiótico bacteriostático, frente a algunos microorganismos puede comportarse como bactericida. Su uso está aprobado para el tratamiento de infecciones complicadas de la piel y los tejidos blandos, y para la neumonía nosocomial y comunitaria causada por patógenos sensibles a este antimicrobiano. El linezolid es activo frente a cepas de SARM, enterococos resistentes a la vancomicina y *S. pneumoniae* multirresistente. Se administra por vía intravenosa u oral a dosis de 600 mg cada 12 horas. Es el primer antimicrobiano aprobado para el tratamiento por vía oral de las infecciones por SARM y por enterococos resistentes a la vancomicina.[13]

Microorganismos[a]	Linezolid	Daptomicina	Tigeciclina	Q/D	Telavancina	Oritavancina	Dalbavancina	Ceftobiprol	Ceftarolina	Iclaprim
S. aureus										
Meticilina S	2	0,5	0,5	0,5	0,5	0,12	0,06	0,5-1	0,25	0,12
Meticilina R	2	0,5	0,5	1	0,25	0,12	0,06	1-4	1	0,12
Estafilococos coagulasa negativos										
Meticilina S	1	0,5	0,5	≤0,25	0,5	0,25	0,06	0,25	0,12	ND
Meticilina R	1	0,5	0,5	0,5	0,5	0,25	0,06	1-2	0,5	ND
Enterococcus spp.	2	2	0,12	1[b]	1[c]	0,25	0,12[c]	2-4[d]	4[d]	4[d]
S. pneumoniae	1	0,25	≤0,12	0,5	0,03	0,004	≤0,03	≤0,03-2[e]	≤0,03-0,12[e]	0,06[f]
Streptococcus grupo *viridans*	1	1	≤0,12	1	0,06	0,03	≤0,03	0,25-1[e]	0,25-2[e]	ND
Estreptococos beta hemolíticos	1	0,25	≤0,12	0,5	0,06	0,25	≤0,03	≤0,03	≤0,03	0,03-0,25

Q/D: quinupristina-dalfopristina; S: sensible; R: resistente; ND: no determinado.
[a] Datos obtenidos de las referencias 15, 25, 40, 41, 45, 49, 57, 61, 68, 71, 75, 79 y 80.
[b] Solamente incluye *E. faecium.*
[c] No incluye cepas resistentes a la vancomicina.
[d] Solamente incluye *E. faecalis.*
[e] Incluye cepas resistentes a la penicilina.
[f] Solamente incluye cepas sensibles al cotrimoxazol.

Tabla 1. Actividad in vitro (CMI$_{90}$ en mg/l) de los nuevos antimicrobianos activos frente a microorganismos grampositivos.

1.1　*Actividad antimicrobiana*

El linezolid tiene un amplio espectro de actividad frente a la mayoría de los patógenos grampositivos, incluyendo *S. aureus* y estafilococos coagulasa negativos sensibles y resistentes a la meticilina, *Enterococcus faecalis*, *Enterococcus faecium*, *S. pneumoniae*, estreptococos del grupo *viridans* y otros estreptococos, incluyendo los beta hemolíticos, y otros patógenos grampositivos aerobios y anaerobios aislados con menor frecuencia como causa de infecciones, entre los que se incluyen *Corynebacterium* spp., *Bacillus* spp., *Listeria monocytogenes, Rhodococcus* spp., *Erysipelothrix rhusopathiae, Clostridium difficile, Clostridium perfringens, Peptostreptococcus* spp. y diferentes especies de *Nocardia* y de micobacterias. El linezolid es bacteriostático frente a estafilococos y enterococos, pero ha demostrado actividad bactericida *in vitro* frente a algunos estreptococos.[14]

Como el linezolid es un antibiótico completamente sintético, es probable que ésta sea la razón de que su actividad se haya mantenido uniforme en numerosos estudios realizados frente a microorganismos diana desde su aprobación y comercialización, hace ya más de una década. No obstante, se han comunicado cepas de estafilococos, enterococos y estreptococos resistentes al linezolid, así como brotes nosocomiales producidos por enterococos, enterococos resistentes a la vancomicina, SARM y estafilococos coagulasa negativos resistentes a este antimicrobiano.[15-18] La resistencia al linezolid en estafilococos y en enterococos se debe principalmente a mutaciones en la diana de la subunidad 23S del RNA ribosómico, entre las cuales las mutaciones G2576T, G2447T y T2504A son las más frecuentes. Además, también se ha descrito otro tipo de resistencia menos frecuente y transferible que está mediada por el gen *cfr*, que codifica la producción de una metiltransferasa que altera la diana al producir una metilación en la posición A2503 de la subunidad 23S del RNA ribosómico. Un tercer mecanismo de resistencia descrito son las mutaciones en las proteínas ribosómicas L3 y L4.[19,20] En un reciente caso de *S. pneumoniae* resistente al linezolid, la resistencia se debió a mutaciones en la proteína L4.[15]

Desde la aprobación del linezolid para su uso en clínica se han realizado continuos estudios para vigilar la emergencia de resistencias, tanto en Estados Unidos como en Europa. En Estados Unidos, el programa de vigilancia LEADER *(Linezolid Experience and Accurate Determination of Resistance)*, que comenzó en 2004, monitoriza anualmente la actividad del linezolid, su espectro y las tasas de resistencia de los microorganismos grampositivos más relevantes en patología humana. En el último estudio realizado en 2010, la CMI_{90} del linezolid frente a 6.801 cepas analizadas fue de 1 mg/l, y globalmente la resistencia al linezolid fue del 0,38 % ($CMI \geq 4$ mg/l). En comparación con estudios realizados en años anteriores, esta cifra de resistencia se mantuvo estable en los últimos cinco años y osciló entre el 0,34 % de 2009 y el 0,45 % de 2006. En el caso de *S. aureus*, sólo el 0,06 % de las cepas fueron resistentes al linezolid ($CMI \geq 8$ mg/l), y se detectaron dos cepas de SARM portadoras del gen *cfr* con una CMI de linezolid de 4 mg/l (sensibilidad disminuida). Asimismo, se detectó resistencia al linezolid en el

0,75 % de los enterococos y el 1,48 % de los estafilococos coagulasa negativos, lo que demuestra que este antimicrobiano mantiene una excelente actividad *in vitro* frente a los patógenos grampositivos en ese país. Todos los estreptococos del grupo *viridans* y beta hemolíticos fueron sensibles al linezolid, y por vez primera se detectó una cepa de *S. pneumoniae* resistente a él.[15] En un estudio que analizó 5.754 cepas recogidas en los cinco continentes en 2009, la resistencia al linezolid fue del 0,14 % y sólo se detectó en estafilococos coagulasa negativos y en enterococos.[21] En España se han descrito ocasionalmente cepas de SARM resistentes al linezolid en varios hospitales, como casos aislados o como parte de brotes hospitalarios.[17,18] En estudios multicéntricos que han analizado su actividad frente a más de 800 cepas de SARM se han detectado casos concretos de cepas resistentes.[8,22] La resistencia de SARM al linezolid se ha descrito en general en pacientes tratados con este antimicrobiano durante largos periodos de tiempo, pero también como consecuencia de la diseminación plasmídica del gen *cfr* o por diseminación clonal entre pacientes hospitalizados, sobre todo en la UCI, que se ha visto favorecida por la presión selectiva ejercida por este antibiótico.[19] Asimismo, en los estudios multicéntricos antes citados, realizados en 2006 y 2008, la resistencia de los estafilococos coagulasa negativos al linezolid fue muy baja y osciló entre el 0,25 % y el 0,5 %, y en otro estudio realizado en 2010 se observó un aumento de la resistencia desde el 0,2 % en 2006 al 4,3 % en 2010 (p < 0,001),[23] lo que indica que aunque la resistencia todavía no es muy frecuente parece haber aumentado en los últimos años. Finalmente, también se han descrito en España cepas de *E. faecium* y *E. faecalis* resistentes al linezolid, y brotes producidos por estos microorganismos, pero hasta el momento no se han detectado cepas de estreptococos resistentes a este antimicrobiano.[18,24]

En conclusión, aunque el uso clínico de linezolid se aprobó en el año 2000 y desde entonces se ha utilizado ampliamente, la resistencia sigue siendo poco frecuente, salvo las notables excepciones de resistencia en SARM, enterococos resistentes a la vancomicina y estafilococos coagulasa negativos causantes de brotes nosocomiales. Por ello, es necesario que los laboratorios de microbiología realicen una determinación sistemática de la sensibilidad a este antimicrobiano, así como estudios de vigilancia, para ver las tendencias de resistencia en las diferentes especies bacterianas y detectar precozmente brotes producidos por microorganismos resistentes. Es más probable que la resistencia al linezolid entre los grampositivos aparezca en determinados pacientes expuestos al fármaco durante largo tiempo o por transmisión de clones resistentes entre pacientes, o entre éstos y el personal sanitario, incluso en ausencia de presión selectiva ejercida por el uso del fármaco. Además, el linezolid debería usarse con precaución en aquellas infecciones en que se produzca una baja penetración del fármaco y en las asociadas a cuerpos extraños, y en los pacientes profundamente inmunodeprimidos o en hemodiálisis, en quienes pueden reducirse las concentraciones séricas de linezolid, ya que todas estas situaciones aumentan el riesgo de selección de resistencia.[19]

Actualmente están en desarrollo dos nuevos antimicrobianos (tedizolid y radezolid) que son activos frente a cepas resistentes al linezolid. El tedizolid es una prometedora alternativa, principalmente frente a las cepas que presentan el mecanismo de resistencia transferible al linezolid mediado por el gen *cfr*.[20]

2   Daptomicina

La daptomicina es un lipopéptido cíclico que actúa sobre la membrana celular bacteriana y produce su despolarización, lo que resulta en una rápida actividad bactericida. Presenta actividad bactericida dependiente de la concentración frente a *S. aureus* y estafilococos coagulasa negativos sensibles y resistentes a la meticilina, VRSA, *S. pneumoniae* resistente a la penicilina y enterococos resistentes a la ampicilina y la vancomicina. Su uso está aprobado a dosis de 4 mg/kg al día por vía parenteral para el tratamiento de las infecciones de la piel y los tejidos blandos, y a dosis de 6 mg/kg al día para el tratamiento de la bacteriemia y la endocarditis derecha por *S. aureus*, aunque recientemente se ha demostrado[25] una mayor eficacia clínica con dosis de hasta 10 mg/kg al día sin un aumento de los efectos adversos. La daptomicina no puede utilizarse para el tratamiento de la neumonía, ya que se inactiva por el surfactante pulmonar. Es el único antimicrobiano con actividad bactericida *in vitro* frente a los enterococos resistentes a la vancomicina aprobado para su uso en clínica.[26,27]

2.1   Actividad antimicrobiana

La daptomicina es activa frente a un amplia variedad de microorganismos grampositivos, incluyendo cepas multirresistentes de estafilococos, enterococos, estreptococos y bacilos grampositivos aerobios. No se ha establecido una definición microbiológica de resistencia a la daptomicina en *S. aureus*, pero se consideran sensibles todas las cepas frente a las cuales la CMI de daptomicina es ≤ 1 mg/l. Por el contrario, se consideran no sensibles aquellas para las que la CMI de daptomicina es > 1 mg/l. En el caso de los enterococos, se consideran sensibles las cepas cuya CMI de daptomicina es ≤ 4 mg/l.[28]

En diferentes estudios multicéntricos se ha demostrado que la daptomicina presenta una buena actividad *in vitro* frente a los microorganismos grampositivos. En un estudio realizado en Estados Unidos[29] con 12.443 cepas de grampositivos causantes de infecciones graves, incluyendo un 55,9 % de cepas de SARM, un 74 % de cepas de estafilococos coagulasa negativos resistentes a la meticilina, un 5,4 % de cepas de *E. faecalis* y un 75,4 % de cepas de *E. faecium* resistentes a la vancomicina, los valores de CMI_{90} para *S. aureus* y estafilococos coagulasa negativos (sensibles y resistentes a la meticilina), estreptococos beta hemolíticos, estreptococos del grupo *viridans* y enterococos fueron, respectivamente, 0,5, 0,25, 0,5 y 2 mg/l. En general, el 99,9 % de las cepas de *S. aureus*, el 100 % de las de *E. faecalis* y el 99,5 % de las de *E. faecium* fueron sensibles a la daptomicina. En este estudio, solamente ocho cepas de *S. aureus* (0,1 %) se consideraron no sensibles a la daptomicina, con una CMI de 2 mg/l (siete cepas) o de 4 mg/l (una cepa). En el caso de los estafilococos coagulasa negativos, se detectaron seis cepas (0,5 %) no sensibles a la daptomicina (CMI ≥ 2 mg/l). En cuanto a los enterococos, la más alta CMI de daptomicina detectada fue de 8 mg/l (cuatro cepas), y la resistencia a la vancomicina no influyó negativamente en la actividad de la daptomicina. Todos los estreptococos beta hemolíticos fueron sensibles a la daptomicina, así como los estreptococos del grupo *viridans*, pero frente a estos últimos los valores de CMI fueron ligeramente superiores a los obtenidos para los beta hemolíticos.[29]

En Europa, en diversos estudios multicéntricos[30] realizados entre 2003 y 2009, en los que participaron hasta 15 países, que analizaron la actividad de la daptomicina frente a 36.769 cepas de microorganismos grampositivos causantes de infecciones graves, el porcentaje de cepas no sensibles fue inferior al 0,1 %. La CMI_{90} frente a *S. aureus* y a los estafilococos coagulasa negativos, incluyendo cepas sensibles y resistentes a la meticilina, fue de 0,5 mg/l. El 100 % de las cepas de *E. faecalis* (sensibles y resistentes a la vancomicina) fueron sensibles a la daptomicina (CMI_{90} = 1 mg/l), y en el caso de *E. faecium* sensibles a la vancomicina el 99,7 % fueron sensibles a la daptomicina, mientras que entre las cepas resistentes a la vancomicina el 99,1 % fueron sensibles a la daptomicina. Del mismo modo, el 100 % de los estreptococos beta hemolíticos y el 99,8 % de las cepas de estreptococos del grupo *viridans* fueron sensibles a la daptomicina.[30] En España, según los datos publicados en dos estudios multicéntricos realizados en 2006 y 2008,[8,22] la actividad de la daptomicina fue excelente frente a *S. aureus* y frente a los estafilococos coagulasa negativos. Solamente se detectó un aislado de SARM con sensibilidad disminuida a la daptomicina (CMI = 2 mg/l), y no se halló ninguna cepa de estafilococos coagulasa negativos con resistencia o sensibilidad disminuida a la daptomicina en ninguno de los estudios, que en total analizaban más de mil cepas.

Aunque los diferentes estudios multicéntricos han demostrado que la daptomicina es muy activa frente a *S. aureus*, se han detectado cepas para las cuales la CMI de daptomicina está por encima de los valores considerados de sensibilidad. Son muy poco frecuentes las cepas de *S. aureus* no sensibles a la daptomicina (CMI ≥ 2 mg/l), pero se han detectado algunas durante tratamientos prolongados con vancomicina, con daptomicina o con ambas, especialmente en pacientes portadores de catéteres intravenosos o con otros dispositivos protésicos, y en pacientes con endocarditis, tromboflebitis, osteomielitis o artritis séptica y con focos sin drenar. También se han descrito cepas de *S. aureus* no sensibles a la daptomicina en pacientes que nunca habían recibido daptomicina y en otros que no habían recibido ningún antibiótico.[28] Asimismo, se ha documentado una asociación entre la sensibilidad disminuida a la vancomicina y la sensibilidad disminuida a la daptomicina. La exposición de *S. aureus* a la vancomicina tiene una influencia sobre la fisiología global del microorganismo, lo que resulta en importantes alteraciones metabólicas y fisiológicas que afectan, en consecuencia, a la actividad de la daptomicina. Así, se ha comunicado que la asociación entre los aumentos de las CMI de la vancomicina y de la daptomicina parece deberse al engrosamiento de la pared celular, lo que impide la difusión de la daptomicina a través de la pared hasta su diana en la membrana celular.[31,32] En las cepas con CMI altas se han detectado mutaciones en los genes *mprF* (que codifica una lisil-fosfatidil-glicerol sintetasa), *yycG* (que codifica una histidina cinasa), *rpoB* y *rpoC* (que codifican las subunidades β y β', respectivamente, de la RNA polimerasa), y *cls2* (que codifica una cardiolipina sintetasa). Estas enzimas están involucradas en la síntesis de los fosfolípidos de la membrana celular bacteriana, y mutaciones en ellas dan lugar a un aumento de la carga positiva de la membrana, alterando el contenido de fosfolípidos de ésta, lo que contribuye a su desestructuración y a la resistencia (no sensibilidad) a la daptomicina.[28] De manera concreta también se han descrito cepas de *E. faecalis* y de *E. faecium* resistentes a la daptomicina, en general en el transcurso de tratamientos prolongados con estos antimicrobianos por bacteremia y endocarditis. En estos casos se han detectado mutaciones en genes relacionados con el metabolismo de los fosfolípidos *(cls, gdpD)* y de las proteínas de la membrana celular *(liaF)*, que llevan a alteraciones en el potencial y en la permeabilidad de la membrana.[33] También se ha comunicado el desarrollo de resistencia a la daptomicina (CMI > 256 mg/l) durante el tratamiento de una bacteriemia por *Corynebacterium jeikeium* en un paciente inmunodeprimido.[34]

En definitiva, la daptomicina sigue siendo un antimicrobiano con una buena actividad bactericida frente a microorganismos grampositivos multirresistentes y, a pesar de llevar varios años de utilización clínica, las cepas no sensibles a este antibiótico siguen siendo muy poco frecuentes. No obstante, es prudente realizar una monitorización continuada de la resistencia, en especial en aquellos pacientes tratados durante largo tiempo con este antimicrobiano y en los que presentan focos sin drenar que pueden contribuir al desarrollo de resistencia.

3 Tigeciclina

La tigeciclina es una glicilciclina cuyo mecanismo de acción consiste en la unión a la subunidad 30S ribosómica, con el consiguiente bloqueo de la entrada de moléculas de aminoacil-RNA de transferencia en el sitio A del ribosoma, inhibiendo así la síntesis de proteínas y dando como resultado un efecto bacteriostático. La tigeciclina es activa frente a numerosos microorganismos grampositivos aerobios y anaerobios, incluyendo SARM y enterococos resistentes a la vancomicina, y también frente a muchos microorganismos aerobios y anaerobios gramnegativos, microorganismos atípicos (micoplasmas, clamidias, *Legionella* spp.), *Nocardia* spp. y micobacterias de crecimiento rápido. También es activa frente a los microorganismos resistentes a las tetraciclinas clásicas (tetraciclina, minociclina, doxiciclina), ya que no se afecta por los mecanismos conocidos de resistencia a éstas. La tigeciclina está indicada para el tratamiento de las infecciones complicadas de la piel y los tejidos blandos, y de la infección intraabdominal complicada.

Se administra por vía parenteral a una dosis inicial de 100 mg, seguida de 50 mg cada 12 horas, y se le han asociado como efectos adversos relativamente frecuentes náuseas y vómitos tras su administración. Las concentraciones que alcanza en sangre no son altas (C_{max} = 0,9 mg/l), pero presenta una buena penetración en los tejidos, donde alcanza mayores concentraciones.[35,36]

3.1 Actividad antimicrobiana

La tigeciclina presenta una buena actividad *in vitro* frente a una amplia variedad de microorganismos grampositivos multirresistentes de importancia clínica, incluyendo *S. aureus* y estafilococos coagulasa negativos sensibles y resistentes a la meticilina, enterococos sensibles y resistentes a la vancomicina, *S. pneumoniae* y estreptococos del grupo *viridans* sensibles y resistentes a la penicilina y a los macrólidos, estreptococos beta hemolíticos y corinebacterias. Su actividad frente a microorganismos grampositivos anaerobios incluye, entre otros, *Peptostreptococcus* spp., *Gemella* spp., *Propionibacterium* spp.y *Clostridium* spp. Aunque su acción es bacteriostática, puede comportarse como bactericida frente a *S. pneumoniae*.[37-39]

Las CMI de tigeciclina frente a la mayoría de los estafilococos, enterococos y estreptococos oscilan entre 0,06 y 0,5 mg/l. En un estudio realizado con una colección de 10.127 estafilococos, estreptococos y enterococos procedentes de muestras clínicas de todo el mundo, la tigeciclina inhibió todos los aislados estudiados con una concentración ≤ 2 mg/l. Mostró igual actividad frente a *S. aureus* y a los estafilococos coagulasa negativos sensibles y resistentes a la meticilina, con una CMI_{90} de 0,5 mg/l. La CMI_{90} de tigeciclina frente a *S. pneumoniae*, estreptococos del grupo *viridans* y estreptococos beta hemolíticos fue ≤ 0,12 mg/l.[40] Otros estudios[37,38] han comunicado valores similares de CMI de tigeciclina, que oscilan entre 0,06 y 1 mg/l frente a *S. aureus* sensibles y resistentes a la meticilina, y valores de CMI_{90} de 0,25 mg/l y 0,5 mg/l frente a cepas sensibles y resistentes a la meticilina, respectivamente. Asimismo, estos estudios han demostrado una excelente actividad frente a *S. pneumoniae* (intervalo de CMI: ≤ 0,016-0,5 mg/l), y frente a *S. pyogenes* y *Streptococcus agalactiae*, incluyendo cepas resistentes a la tetraciclina y a los macrólidos (CMI_{90} = 0,06 mg/l). En estudios multicéntricos realizados en España, todas las cepas de *S. aureus* y de estafilococos coagulasa negativos estudiadas fueron uniformemente sensibles a la tigeciclina.[8] La tigeciclina también es activa *in vitro* frente a los enterococos resistentes a la vancomicina (fenotipos VanA, VanB y VanC) y los estafilococos con sensibilidad disminuida a los glucopéptidos (*S. aureus* y estafilococos coagulasa negativos). En un estudio que evaluó 157 cepas con estas características, todas se inhibieron con concentraciones entre ≤ 0,03 y 1 mg/l, incluyendo las que eran resistentes a la tetraciclina, y el 90 % se inhibieron con 0,5 mg/l de tigeciclina. La CMI_{90} de tigeciclina frente a los estafilococos coagulasa negativos fue de 0,5 mg/l, para los enterococos fue de 0,12 mg/l y todas las cepas de *S. aureus* resultaron inhibidas con 1 mg/l de tigeciclina.[41] En cuanto a su actividad frente a los bacilos grampositivos, la CMI_{90} es más alta que para los estafilococos (2 mg/l), y puede alcanzar hasta 4 mg/l frente a cepas de *C. jeikeium*.[42] Finalmente, aunque la resistencia a la tigeciclina entre los microorganismos grampositivos es anecdótica, se ha descrito en cepas de SARM debido a la expresión de bombas de expulsión activa.[43]

Cabe concluir que la tigeciclina es un antimicrobiano con una buena actividad frente a microorganismos grampositivos multirresistentes, aunque por la baja concentración que alcanza en sangre y por su intervalo de CMI_{90} frente a SARM (0,25-1 mg/l), no se recomienda su uso en pacientes con bacteriemia o con sospecha de ella. Por otra parte, como la tigeciclina es activa frente a bacterias grampositivas y gramnegativas multirresistentes, puede utilizarse en infecciones mixtas.

4   Quinupristina-dalfopristina

La quinupristina-dalfopristina es un antimicrobiano que se desarrolló en la década de 1990 para el tratamiento de las infecciones complicadas de la piel y los tejidos blandos. Este antimicrobiano está constituido por una mezcla 30:70 de una estreptogramina B (quinupristina) y una estreptogramina A (dalfopristina), y su mecanismo de acción es la inhibición de la síntesis de proteínas. La actividad sinérgica de la combinación se debe a un cambio conformacional en el ribosoma bacteriano producido tras la unión de la dalfopristina a éste. Aunque los componentes individuales son bacteriostáticos, la asociación actúa de modo sinérgico y en general se comporta como bactericida frente a los aislados sensibles a los dos componentes. Al ser más potente la asociación, es incluso activa cuando hay resistencia bacteriana a uno de los dos componentes. Esta asociación de antimicrobianos es activa frente a estafilococos, neumococos, estreptococos beta hemolíticos y *E. faecium* (incluyendo cepas resistentes a la vancomicina), pero no tiene actividad frente a *E. faecalis* ni otras especies de enterococos. En Estados Unidos, la quinupristina-dalfopristina se aprobó para el tratamiento de las infecciones complicadas de la piel y los tejidos blandos causadas por *S. pyogenes* y por *S. aureus* sensibles a la meticilina (no para SARM), y para las infecciones graves por *E. faecium* resistentes a la vancomicina y asociadas con bacteriemia. En España se aprobó para el tratamiento de infecciones de la piel y los tejidos blandos, aunque actualmente está revocada la autorización para su uso. La dosis recomendada es de 7,5 mg/kg cada 8 horas por vía parenteral. El uso clínico de este agente es complicado porque presenta interacciones con los fármacos que se metabolizan por la vía del citocromo P450; además, es muy frecuente la intolerancia venosa cuando se administra por una vena periférica y es frecuente la aparición de mialgias y artralgias que pueden ser graves. Este antibiótico es incompatible con solución salina, por lo que ha de administrarse en dextrosa al 5 %.[44]

4.1 Actividad antimicrobiana

La quinupristina-dalfopristina es un antimicrobiano activo frente a estafilococos (*S. aureus* y estafilococos coagulasa negativos) sensibles y resistentes a la meticilina, *S. pneumoniae* (sensibles y resistentes a la penicilina), estreptococos beta hemolíticos y *E. faecium*. Es inactiva frente a *E. faecalis* y otras especies de enterococos. Su inactividad frente a *E. faecalis* se debe a la expresión de una bomba de expulsión activa, intrínseca en esta especie, que le confiere resistencia a la dalfopristina. Asimismo, es bactericida *in vitro* frente a neumococos y algunas cepas de estafilococos, pero no frente a las resistentes a la eritromicina y la clindamicina ni tampoco frente a *E. faecium* resistente a la vancomicina, ni frente a aquellas cepas con alto grado de resistencia a la eritromicina. Aunque esta asociación de estreptograminas es activa *in vitro* frente a la mayoría de las cepas de SARM y también es bactericida frente a muchas de ellas, no está aprobado su uso para el tratamiento de las infecciones por SARM. A pesar de ello, durante su desarrollo clínico se utilizó con éxito para el tratamiento de algunas infecciones graves por SARM.[44]

Varios estudios multicéntricos han analizado la actividad de la quinupritina-dalfopristina frente a cepas procedentes de América y de Europa. En un estudio realizado en 200 centros de Estados Unidos y Canadá[45] se analizó la actividad de este antimicrobiano frente a 28.029 cocos grampositivos, incluyendo cepas de SARM, de *E. faecium* resistente a la vancomicina y de neumococos resistentes a la penicilina. En general, más del 90 % de los grampositivos fueron sensibles. Las CMI_{90} frente a cepas de *S. aureus* sensibles y resistentes a la meticilina fueron de 0,5 y 1 mg/l, respectivamente, y frente a *E. faecium* resistente a la vancomicina la CMI_{90} fue de 1 mg/l. El 0,2 % de las cepas de *E. faecium* resistentes a la vancomicina lo fueron también a la quinupristina-dalfopristina. En el caso de *S. pneumoniae,* la CMI_{90} fue de 0,75 mg/l, con independencia de la resistencia a la penicilina o a los macrólidos.[45] Diversos estudios[46,47] *in vitro* realizados en Europa con cepas recogidas durante la pasada década demostraron que la mayoría de *S. aureus,* incluyendo SARM, así como los estafilococos coagulasa negativos, los neumococos y *E. faecium,* eran sensibles. En un estudio de vigilancia realizado en 20 hospitales de Europa,[46] en el cual se analizaron 3.653 cepas clínicas de neumococos, estafilococos y enterococos (incluyendo cepas resistentes a la vancomicina), la CMI_{90} frente a *S. pneumoniae* fue de 1 mg/l (incluyendo cepas resistentes a la penicilina); frente a *S. aureus* sensibles y resistentes a la meticilina fue de 0,5 mg/l y 1 mg/l, respectivamente; frente a estafilococos coagulasa negativos sensibles y resistentes a la meticilina fue de 0,5 mg/l; y frente a *E. faecium* fue de 4 mg/l. Sólo 35 de las 3.052 cepas de *S. aureus* recogidas durante este estudio fueron resistentes. En cuanto a *S. aureus* con sensibilidad intermedia a la vancomicina, en diferentes estudios[47,48] algunas cepas eran sensibles y otras resistentes.

En general, casi todos los estreptococos que se han analizado en estudios multicéntricos han sido sensibles a este antimicrobiano, aunque ocasionalmente se han detectado algunas cepas de estreptococos del grupo *viridans* resistentes procedentes de Asia (96 % sensibles). Por el contrario, la mayoría de las cepas de *E. faecium* resistentes a la vancomicina han sido sensibles.[49]Aunque en algunos estudios iniciales el 94,3 % de las cepas de *E. faecium* resistentes a la vancomicina eran sensibles a la quinupristina-dalfopristina,[45] en otros estudios de vigilancia más recientes se han encontrado unas tasas de sensibilidad más bajas.[50]

Según los datos publicados en varios estudios multicéntricos realizados en 2006 y 2008 en España,[8,22] la gran mayoría de las cepas de *S. aureus* y de estafilococos coagulasa negativos analizados fueron sensibles a la quinupristina-dalfopristina. Solamente en un estudio el 0,5 % de las cepas de *S. aureus* fueron resistentes. Sin embargo, en el caso de *E. faecium*, España es uno de los países con los índices más altos de resistencia (23 % a 45 %).[51]

Es relativamente frecuente la emergencia de resistencia durante el tratamiento con este antimicrobiano, en especial en los pacientes con infecciones graves por *E. faecium* resistente a la vancomicina. La resistencia se debe a enzimas inactivantes de los dos componentes individuales (mediada por los genes *vat),* a bombas de expulsión activa (mediada por el gen *lsa)* o a modificaciones en la diana (genes *erm),* y todos estos mecanismos pueden ser transferibles en elementos genéticos móviles. En cepas de *E. faecium* se han detectado diferentes enzimas que inactivan a la dalfopristina y dan lugar a resistencia.[44]

Si bien los datos de actividad *in vitro* de la quinupristina-dalfopristina indican que es eficaz frente a microorganismos grampositivos multirresistentes, los problemas de irritación venosa asociados a su administración parenteral, sus numerosas interacciones medicamentosas, la baja prevalencia de enterococos resistentes a la vancomicina en Europa y en España, y la disponibilidad actual de otros agentes alternativos, han hecho que su uso sea muy limitado, aunque no deja de ser una alternativa terapéutica válida frente a estos microorganismos.

5　Telavancina

La telavancina es un antibiótico lipoglucopéptido derivado de la vancomicina con actividad frente a microorganismos grampositivos multirresistentes, incluyendo SARM, pero no es activa frente a todos los fenotipos de enterococos resistentes a la vancomicina. Presenta un mecanismo de acción dual, ya que inhibe la síntesis del peptidoglucano, y en consecuencia de la pared celular, y además produce una despolarización de la membrana celular. Como consecuencia de este mecanismo de acción, es rápidamente bactericida. Es un potente inhibidor de la síntesis del peptidoglucano, ya que se une a sus precursores pentapeptídicos en el terminal D-Ala-D-Ala, de igual modo que la vancomicina, pero con una afinidad diez veces superior a la de ésta. Por otro lado, interacciona con la membrana celular y ello proporciona una unión más fuerte con los precursores del peptidoglucano al localizar la molécula en la superficie celular de la bacteria. Además, desencadena una rápida alteración del potencial de la membrana celular, dependiente de la concentración, mediante la formación de poros en ésta y la liberación de iones potasio y adenosina trifosfato del citoplasma. Actualmente está aprobada en Estados Unidos para el tratamiento de las infecciones complicadas de la piel y los tejidos blandos causadas por microorganismos grampositivos, y en Europa está en proceso de autorización para el tratamiento de la neumonía nosocomial producida por SARM. Se administra por vía intravenosa a dosis de 10 mg/kg cada 24 horas. Se excreta por vía renal, por lo que requiere ajuste de dosis en los pacientes con insuficiencia renal, aunque no requiere la determinación de sus concentraciones séricas. La telavancina es más nefrotóxica que la vancomicina, pero presenta menos reacciones adversas relacionadas con la administración parenteral que esta última.[52,53]

5.1 Actividad antimicrobiana

La telavancina es activa frente a *S. aureus* y estafilococos coagulasa negativos sensibles y resistentes a la meticilina (intervalo de CMI_{90}: 0,25-0,5 mg/l), frente a cepas de estafilococos con sensibilidad intermedia o heterorresistentes a la vancomicina ($CMI_{90} = 1$ mg/l), frente a cepas resistentes al linezolid y con sensibilidad disminuida a la daptomicina (intervalo de CMI_{90}: 0,25-0,5 mg/l). También ha demostrado actividad ($CMI = 2$-4 mg/l) sobre dos de las escasas cepas de *S. aureus* resistentes a la vancomicina que se han descrito en el mundo, aunque debido al limitado número de aislados estudiados no puede concluirse que sea universalmente activa frente a dichas cepas. Es activa frente a enterococos sensibles a la vancomicina (intervalo de CMI_{90}: 0,25-1 mg/l), pero no tiene actividad frente a los enterococos resistentes a la vancomicina con los fenotipos VanA (CMI_{90} 8 mg/l) y VanB, aunque puede presentar cierta actividad frente a los fenotipos VanB y VanC, dependiendo de las concentraciones de fármaco libre que se alcancen. También es muy activa frente a los neumococos y los estreptococos beta hemolíticos (intervalo de CMI_{90}: 0,03-0,06 mg/l), frente a *Bacillus anthracis* y frente a microorganismos grampositivos anaerobios como *Clostridium* spp., incluyendo *C. perfringens* y *C. difficile,* y frente a *Peptococcus anaerobius* (intervalo de CMI_{90}: 0,12-1 mg/l).[52,54-56]

En un estudio reciente que ha analizado la actividad de la telavancina frente a 15.480 grampositivos recogidos durante 2012 en 89 instituciones en Estados Unidos, Europa, la región Asia-Pacífico y Latinoamérica, este antibiótico fue activo frente a *S. aureus* ($CMI_{50/90} = 0,12/0,25$ mg/l), *E. faecalis* sensibles a la vancomicina ($CMI_{50/90} = 0,5/0,5$ mg/l), estreptococos beta hemolíticos ($CMI_{50/90} = 0,06/0,12$ mg/l) y estreptococos del grupo *viridans* ($CMI_{50/90} = 0,03/0,06$ mg/l).[57]

La telavancina ha demostrado eficacia y seguridad en ensayos clínicos en el tratamiento de infecciones complicadas de la piel y los tejidos blandos, y de la neumonía nosocomial, causadas por microorganismos grampositivos. En las infecciones de la piel y los tejidos blandos, las tasas de curación fueron del 77 % para telavancina y del 75,3 % para vancomicina. En los pacientes infectados por SARM, la tasa de respuesta clínica fue del 90,7 % para telavancina y del 87,1 % para vancomicina. En la neumonía nosocomial, la tasa de curación clínica para telavancina fue del 82,7 %, en comparación con el 80,9 % para vancomicina. En los pacientes infectados por SARM, las tasas de curación fueron superiores con telavancina (82 %) que con vancomicina (74 %).[58,59]

En definitiva, la telavancina presenta unas mayores potencia y actividad bactericida que la vancomicina frente a microorganismos grampositivos multirresistentes, lo que puede suponer una ventaja en el tratamiento de las infecciones graves, en especial de las producidas por SARM, para las que constituye una importante contribución al arsenal terapéutico actual. La actividad bactericida de la telavancina representa asimismo una posible ventaja sobre el linezolid y la tigeciclina, que son bacteriostáticos. Además, la telavancina también puede utilizarse para el tratamiento de la neumonía, lo que representa una ventaja respecto a la daptomicina.

6 Oritavancina

La oritavancina es un lipoglucopéptido semisintético análogo de la vancomicina que tiene actividad frente a microorganismos grampositivos multirresistentes, incluyendo SARM y enterococos resistentes a la vancomicina (fenotipos VanA y VanB). Su acción sobre grampositivos se debe al menos a tres mecanismos conocidos: *1)* inhibición de la transglucosilación, y por tanto de la síntesis de la pared celular, por la unión a los terminales D-Ala-D-Ala del mismo modo que lo hace la vancomicina, pero más fuertemente, y también por unión a los depsipéptidos D-Ala-D-Lac (a diferencia de la vancomicina, que no se une a ellos), lo que facilita la inhibición de la síntesis de la pared celular incluso en microorganismos que presentan el tipo de resistencia VanA y que producen estos depsipéptidos; *2)* inhibición de la transpeptidación por unión a un sitio secundario en el peptidoglucano, en lo que también se diferencia de la vancomicina; y *3)* interacción con la membrana celular, produciendo su despolarización y la alteración de su integridad y su permeabilidad, lo que conduce a una rápida muerte celular. Estos diversos mecanismos de acción de la oritavancina le confieren una actividad rápidamente bactericida, dependiente de la concentración, frente a grampositivos sensibles y resistentes a la vancomicina, en fase de crecimiento exponencial, en fase estacionaria y en biopelículas. La oritavancina está actualmente en las últimas fases de desarrollo clínico para el tratamiento de las infecciones de la piel y de los tejidos blandos, incluyendo las producidas por SARM. Se administra por vía parenteral en dosis única de 1.200 mg. Puesto que su semivida es de 393 horas (dos semanas), podría utilizarse para el tratamiento ambulatorio de infecciones graves y reducir los costes hospitalarios.[60]

6.1 Actividad antimicrobiana

La oritavancina presenta una excelente actividad *in vitro* frente a estafilococos y enterococos, incluyendo *S. aureus* sensible y resistente a la meticilina, *S. aureus* con resistencia intermedia o total a la vancomicina, *S. aureus* con sensibilidad disminuida a la daptomicina y enterococos resistentes a la vancomicina. Mantiene la actividad frente a cepas de *S. aureus* y de enterococos resistentes a la vancomicina porque es capaz de unirse a los terminales D-Ala-D-Lac que se producen en estas cepas, y la vancomicina no.[60] En un estudio de vigilancia de la resistencia, que analizó su actividad frente a una colección de 12.367 patógenos grampositivos, la oritavancina inhibió a todos los aislados a una concentración $\leq 0,25$ mg/l. Asimismo, presentó una potencia similar frente a *S. aureus* y estafilococos coagulasa negativos ($CMI_{50/90} = 0,03/0,06$ mg/l), frente a enterococcos sensibles y resistentes a la vancomicina (intervalo de CMI_{90}: $\leq 0,008-0,5$ mg/ml), y frente a estreptococos (intervalo de CMI_{90}: $\leq 0,008-0,12$ mg/ml). Por su mecanismo de acción, presentó una potente actividad frente a cepas de *E. faecium* y *E. faecalis* tanto sensibles como resistentes a la vancomicina con los fenotipos VanA y VanB. No obstante, las CMI de oritavancina frente a cepas de *E. faecium* y *E. faecalis* con el fenotipo VanA fueron más altas (intervalo de CMI_{90}: $0,12-0,5$ mg/l) que las obtenidas frente a las cepas sensibles a la vancomicina (intervalo de CMI_{90}: $\leq 0,008-0,03$ mg/l). La oritavancina también presentó una buena actividad frente a los estreptococos, inhibiendo cepas de *S. pneumoniae*, estreptococos del grupo *viridans* y estreptococos beta hemolíticos, y su actividad no disminuyó frente a cepas resistentes a la penicilina o a la eritromicina. Asimismo, presentó una mayor actividad frente a cepas de estreptococos beta hemolíticos del serogrupo F ($CMI_{90} \leq 0,008$ mg/l) que frente a cepas de los serogrupos A, B, C o G ($CMI_{90} = 0,12$ mg/l).[61] Además, la oritavancina es activa frente a una amplia variedad de microorganismos grampositivos aerobios y anaerobios, incluyendo *C. jeikeium* ($CMI_{50/90} = 0,12/0,12$ mg/l), *Bacillus cereus* ($CMI_{50} = 0,5$ mg/l), *C. difficile* ($CMI_{90} = 1$ mg/l), *C. perfringens* ($CMI_{50/90} = 0,5/1$ mg/l), *Peptostreptococcus* spp. ($CMI_{50/90} = 0,25/0,5$ mg/l), *Propionibacterium acnes* ($CMI_{50/90} = 0,12/0,25$ mg/l) y *Listeria* spp. ($CMI_{50/90} \leq 0,03/0,06$ mg/l).[62-65]

La eficacia y la seguridad de la oritavancina se han estudiado en varios ensayos clínicos, y ha demostrado eficacia clínica en pacientes con infecciones de la piel y los tejidos blandos causadas por microorganismos grampositivos, incluyendo SARM. En estos ensayos se ha demostrado una no inferioridad en comparación con la vancomicina seguida de cefalexina oral (tasas de curación del 79 % en el grupo de oritavancina y del 76 % en el de vancomicina más cefalexina). En otros ensayos se ha observado que la oritavancina en dosis única de 1.200 mg es tan eficaz como en dosis de 200 mg al día, tanto frente a *S. aureus* como a SARM.[66]

Su excelente actividad frente a SARM y a los enterococos resistentes a la vancomicina, junto con su administración en dosis única, sugieren que en un futuro podría tener un importante papel en el tratamiento ambulatorio de las infecciones graves producidas por estos microorganismos.

7   Dalbavancina

La dalbavancina es un antibiótico lipoglucopéptido semisintético, derivado de un glucopéptido similar a la teicoplanina. Inhibe la síntesis de la pared celular mediante la unión al terminal C del péptido D-Ala-D-Ala, del mismo modo que la vancomicina, pero además se une mediante un anclaje lipófilo a la membrana celular bacteriana, lo que le confiere una actividad más potente *in vitro* que la que muestran la vancomicina y la teicoplanina, pero no es activa frente a enterococos resistentes a la vancomicina que presentan el fenotipo de resistencia VanA. Actualmente este antibiótico está en fase de desarrollo clínico para el tratamiento de las infecciones de la piel y de los tejidos blandos, y para el tratamiento de las bacteriemias relacionadas con catéteres causadas por microorganismos grampositivos, incluyendo SARM. La dalbavancina presenta una larga vida media, que oscila entre 149 y 250 horas, lo que permite la dosificación de una vez a la semana. Se administra por vía parenteral en dosis única de 1 g, seguida de una dosis de 500 mg una semana después, con lo cual podría permitir el tratamiento intravenoso extrahospitalario.[67]

7.1　Actividad antimicrobiana

La dalbavancina presenta un amplio espectro de actividad *in vitro* frente a prácticamente todos los microorganismos grampositivos de interés clínico, con la excepción de los enterococos resistentes a la vancomicina con el fenotipo VanA. Su espectro de actividad es similar al de otros glucopéptidos, pero es más potente que la vancomicina frente a la mayoría de los patógenos. En una serie publicada en 2004,[68] con 16.000 cepas clínicas de bacterias grampositivas recogidas en hospitales de todo el mundo, los valores de CMI oscilaron entre 0,015 y 32 mg/l. La CMI_{90} de la dalbavancina para *S. aureus* y estafilococos coagulasa negativos resistentes a diversos antimicrobianos fue de 0,06 mg/l. La dalbavancina tiene una potente actividad *in vitro* frente a cepas de *S. aureus* con sensibilidad intermedia a los glucopéptidos (CMI_{90} = 0,06-1 mg/l) y a cepas de *S. aureus* con sensibilidad disminuida al linezolid (CMI_{90} = 0,03-0,06 mg/l). Su actividad frente a *E. faecalis* y *E. faecium* sensibles a la vancomicina es similar a la de la teicoplanina, pero mayor que la de la vancomicina, y mantiene su actividad frente a cepas de enterococos resistentes a la vancomicina con los fenotipos VanB y VanC. Es muy activa frente a estreptococos del grupo *viridans* y *S. pneumoniae* sensible y no sensible a la penicilina, y tiene una excelente actividad frente a una variedad de especies grampositivas anaerobias, aerobios fastidiosos y especies de *Corynebacterium*, con las notables excepciones de *Clostridium clostridioforme* y determinadas especies de *Lactobacillus*. Es bactericida frente a *S. aureus* y estafilococos coagulasa negativos a una concentración cuatro veces superior a la CMI a las 24 horas.[67-70]

En ensayos clínicos se ha estudiado su eficacia al utilizarla en dos dosis, en comparación con la vancomicina, para el tratamiento de la bacteriemia asociada a catéter por estafilococos coagulasa negativos y por *S. aureus,* incluyendo SARM. Las tasas de curación fueron del 87 % y del 50 % para dalbavancina y vancomicina, respectivamente. También se ha comparado su eficacia con la de la vancomicina en las infecciones de la piel y los tejidos blandos, y se observó éxito clínico en el 94 % de los pacientes que recibieron dalbavancina, frente al 76 % de los que se trataron con vancomicina.[67]

En definitiva, la dalbavancina constituye una nueva prometedora contribución al arsenal terapéutico para el tratamiento de las infecciones por grampositivos multirresistentes. Su larga vida media permite su administración intravenosa una vez a la semana, lo cual podría disminuir los costes hospitalarios al utilizarla en régimen ambulatorio.

8 Ceftobiprol

El ceftobiprol es una nueva cefalosporina de amplio espectro con actividad bactericida frente a una amplia variedad de bacterias gramnegativas y grampositivas multirresistentes, incluyendo SARM y *S. pneumoniae,* y otros estreptococos sensibles y resistentes a la penicilina. Esta cefalosporina actúa inhibiendo la síntesis de la pared celular mediante una fuerte unión a la proteína fijadora de penicilina 2a (PBP2a), una peptidoglicano transpeptidasa implicada en la resistencia a la meticilina en los estafilococos. La inhibición de esta proteína por el ceftobiprol marca su actividad frente a SARM. Aunque se han realizado algunos ensayos clínicos que han demostrado la eficacia del ceftobiprol en las infecciones complicadas de la piel y de los tejidos blandos, en comparación con vancomicina, con tasas de curación similares (93,3 % y 93,5 %, respectivamente), sólo se ha aprobado su uso en Canadá y actualmente está en proceso de revisión por las agencias reguladoras en Estados Unidos y Europa. El ceftobiprol se administra por vía parenteral como la prodroga ceftobiprol medocaril, que tras su administración se convierte inmediatamente en la forma activa. Las dosis recomendadas son de 500 mg cada 8 horas en infusión intravenosa de 2 horas, o en infusión durante 1 hora cada 12 horas. Esta nueva cefalosporina tiene una semivida de 3 a 4 horas.[71]

8.1 Actividad antimicrobiana

El ceftobiprol presenta buena actividad *in vitro* frente a microorganismos grampositivos, y tiene bajo potencial de desarrollo de resistencias. Es especialmente notable su actividad frente a SARM, neumococos y otros estreptococos resistentes a la penicilina, así como frente a *S. aureus* con heterorresistencia o con sensibilidad intermedia a la vancomicina, frente a los que también es bactericida. Como ya se ha indicado, la actividad del ceftobiprol frente a estos microorganismos radica en su capacidad para fijarse a las PBP asociadas con resistencia en ciertos patógenos, como la PBP2a en *S. aureus* y en los estafilococos coagulasa negativos, y las PBP2x, PBP1a y PBP2b en *S. pneumoniae.* Su amplio espectro también se atribuye a su capacidad para resistir la acción hidrolítica de determinadas betalactamasas, como las producidas por los estafilococos. Por el contrario, el ceftobiprol no se une suficientemente a la PBP5 de *E. faecium*, lo que explica su baja actividad frente a este patógeno (CMI_{90} > 32 mg/l). En diferentes estudios,[72-74] la CMI_{90} para *S. aureus* sensible a la meticilina ha oscilado entre 0,5 y 1 mg/l, y frente a SARM entre 1 y 4 mg/l. En el caso de *S. aureus* con sensibilidad intermedia a la vancomicina, la CMI_{90} es ≤ 2 mg/l, y frente a estafilococos coagulasa negativos sensibles y resistentes a la meticilina los valores son de 0,25 mg/l y 1-2 mg/l, respectivamente. Para los neumococos sensibles a la penicilina, la CMI_{90} es ≤ 0,015 mg/l, y en los neumococos y otros estreptococos del grupo *viridans* resistentes a la penicilina los valores oscilan entre 0,25 y 2 mg/l. Los estreptococos beta hemolíticos son muy sensibles (intervalo de CMI_{90}: ≤ 0,015-0,06 mg/l), y frente a *E. faecalis* la CMI_{90} oscila entre 2 y 4 mg/l, aunque en algunas cepas la CMI puede alcanzar hasta > 32 mg/l.[74]

9 Ceftarolina

La ceftarolina es una nueva cefalosporina parenteral de amplio espectro con actividad bactericida frente a bacterias grampositivas multirresistentes, incluyendo SARM y cepas con sensibilidad reducida a la vancomicina, así como *S. pneumoniae* con sensibilidad reducida o resistencia a la penicilina, la eritromicina y las fluoroquinolonas. Su actividad antibacteriana se debe a la unión a las PBP, inhibiendo la síntesis de la pared celular. La ceftarolina se une las PBP 1 a 4, y tiene una especialmente alta afinidad por la PBP2a (asociada con resistencia a la meticilina). Esta afinidad por la PBP2a hace que sea activa frente a SARM y estafilococos coagulasa negativos resistentes a la meticilina. También se une a las seis PBP de *S. pneumoniae* (1A, 1B, 2x, 2A/B y 3), y además es activa frente a las enterobacterias. La ceftarolina es el metabolito activo de un profármaco, la ceftarolina fosamil, que tras su administración parenteral se convierte con rapidez en ceftarolina mediante las fosfatasas del torrente sanguíneo. En Estados Unidos se ha aprobado para el tratamiento de las infecciones bacterianas agudas de la piel y de los tejidos blandos, y para la neumonía bacteriana adquirida en la comunidad. En España actualmente está en proceso de aprobación para el tratamiento de la neumonía comunitaria. Se administra por vía parenteral a dosis de 600 mg cada 12 horas y alcanza una C_{max} de 20 mg/l. También presenta una excelente biodisponibilidad cuando se administra por vía intramuscular. Se excreta por vía renal y, por tanto, requiere ajuste de dosis en caso de insuficiencia renal.[75]

9.1 Actividad antimicrobiana

La ceftarolina tiene actividad bactericida *in vitro* frente a microorganismos grampositivos multirresistentes, incluyendo *S. aureus* y estafilococos coagulasa negativos sensibles y resistentes a la meticilina, con sensibilidad reducida o con resistencia a la vancomicina, con resistencia al linezolid y con sensibilidad disminuida a la daptomicina. También presenta una gran actividad *in vitro* frente a estreptococos beta hemolíticos y, tal como se ha demostrado en diferentes estudios realizados en Estados Unidos y en Europa,[76,77] frente a *S. pneumoniae* multirresistentes y aquellos resistentes a la penicilina, la amoxicilina y cefalosporinas parenterales como la ceftriaxona y la cefotaxima. La CMI de la ceftarolina frente a los neumococos resistentes a la cefotaxima (CMI > 4 mg/l) es de 0,5 mg/l. Aunque los estudios de actividad *in vitro* sugieren que puede ser eficaz frente a *E. faecalis* resistente a la vancomicina (no frente a *E. faecium*), no hay suficiente experiencia clínica que sustente la eficacia *in vivo* de la ceftarolina frente a estas cepas. Tiene una actividad frente a las bacterias grampositivas anaerobias similar a la de la amoxicilina-ácido clavulánico, y de cuatro a ocho veces mayor que la de la ceftriaxona. También es activa frente a cepas de bacterias anaerobias betalactamasa negativas, incluyendo *Actinomyces* spp., *Proprionibacterium* spp., *Eubacterium* spp., *C. perfringens*, *Clostridium ramosum* y *Clostridium innocuum*.[78]

Diversos ensayos clínicos han demostrado la no inferioridad de la ceftarolina, en comparación con el tratamiento estándar, en infecciones bacterianas agudas de la piel y de los tejidos blandos (tasas de curación del 96,7 % en el grupo de ceftarolina y del 88,9 % en el de tratamiento estándar).[75] Del mismo modo, también se ha mostrado no inferior, en comparación con la ceftriaxona, en el tratamiento de la neumonía bacteriana adquirida en la comunidad (tasas de curación del 86,6 % y del 78,2 % en los grupos de ceftarolina y ceftriaxona, respectivamente).[75]

En definitiva, la ceftarolina representa la primera cefalosporina con actividad bactericida frente a SARM que ha sido aprobada para el tratamiento de las infecciones agudas de la piel y los tejidos blandos, y de la neumonía comunitaria. El potencial para el desarrollo de resistencia en SARM se determinará con el tiempo y con su utilización.

10   Iclaprim

El iclaprim es una diaminopirimidina que inhibe selectivamente la enzima dihidrofolato reductasa bacteriana (una enzima muy importante en la vía de la síntesis del ácido fólico bacteriano), del mismo modo que la trimetoprima, pero con una mayor afinidad por ella y una inhibición más potente, por lo que también mantiene cierta actividad frente a las cepas resistentes a la trimetoprima. Tiene una potente actividad bactericida frente a los microorganismos sensibles a la trimetoprima, y en general es activo frente a microorganismos grampositivos, incluyendo SARM, con un bajo potencial de desarrollo de resistencia, incluso cuando se utiliza en monoterapia sin asociarse a una sulfonamida. Actualmente está en fase de desarrollo para el tratamiento de las infecciones complicadas de la piel y los tejidos blandos por grampositivos. Se administra por vía parenteral a dosis de 60 mg cada 12 horas (o de 0,8 mg/kg), y está en estudio una formulación oral para tratamiento secuencial.[79]

10.1 Actividad antimicrobiana

El iclaprim es activo frente a *S. aureus*, SARM, enterococos y estreptococos (incluyendo neumococos y estreptococos beta hemolíticos). En un estudio que evaluó su potencia y su actividad bactericida frente a 5.937 cepas recogidas de muestras clínicas significativas en Estados Unidos, Europa y Oriente Medio, entre 2004 y 2006, fue muy activo frente a *S. aureus* sensible y resistente a la meticilina (CMI_{50}/CMI_{90} = 0,06/0,12 mg/l para ambos). El 98,7 % de las cepas de *S. aureus* sensibles a la meticilina y el 94,6 % de las cepas de SARM se inhibieron con una CMI de iclaprim de ≤ 2 mg/l. Además, tuvo actividad bactericida frente a todas las cepas de *S. aureus* analizadas (4.516), incluyendo SARM (3.003). El iclaprim inhibió también el 100 % de las cepas de *S. pyog*enes con una CMI ≤ 0,12 mg/l (CMI_{50}/CMI_{90} = 0,015/0,03 mg/l) y fue bactericida frente al 45 % de ellas. Presentó muy buena actividad frente a *S. agalactiae* (CMI_{50}/CMI_{90} = 0,12/0,25 mg/l) y fue bactericida frente al 65 % de las cepas. Demostró buena actividad frente a *E. faecalis* (CMI_{50}/CMI_{90} = 0,015/4 mg/l), y aproximadamente el 72 % y el 97 % de las cepas se inhibieron con CMI ≤ 2 mg/l y ≤ 4 mg/l, respectivamente. También fue activo frente a *E. faecium* (CMI_{50}/CMI_{90} = 2/> 8 mg/l) incluyendo cepas resistentes a la vancomicina; aproximadamente el 58 % y el 75 % de las cepas se inhibieron con CMI ≤ 2 mg/l y ≤ 4 mg/l, respectivamente, y demostró actividad bactericida frente a cinco cepas de *E. faecalis* y *E. faecium*.[79] En otro estudio que analizó la actividad del iclaprim frente a 785 aislados clínicos de *S. pneumoniae*, recogidos en un programa de vigilancia en Canadá, el iclaprim inhibió el 90 % de las cepas a la concentración de 1 mg/l. La CMI_{90} del iclaprim frente a las cepas sensibles a trimetoprima-sulfametoxazol (n = 670; CMI_{90} = 0,06 mg/l) fue siete veces más baja que frente a las cepas resistentes a dicha asociación (n = 115; CMI_{90} > 8 mg/l), y en general no fue activo frente a cepas resistentes a la trimetoprima-sulfametoxazol.[80]

El iclaprim ha demostrado no inferioridad respecto a la vancomicina en el tratamiento de las infecciones complicadas de la piel y de los tejidos blandos por microorganismos grampositivos, incluyendo SARM (tasas de curación del 92 % en ambos grupos).[81]

La potente actividad bactericida del iclaprim frente a *S. aureus*, incluyendo SARM, junto con su buena actividad frente a los estreptococos beta hemolíticos y los enterococos, confirma a este antimicrobiano como una importante y prometedora contribución a los tratamientos actualmente existentes. En las infecciones por *S. pneumoniae,* su utilidad clínica dependerá de la prevalencia de las cepas resistentes a la trimetoprima-sulfametoxazol, por la escasa actividad del iclaprim frente a ellas.

Bibliografía

1. McDonald LC. Trends in antimicrobial resistance in health care-associated pathogens and effect of treatment. Clin Infect Dis. 2006; 42: S65-71.
2. Nathwani D. Health economic issues in the treatment of drug-resistant serious Gram-positive infections. J Infect. 2009; 59 (Suppl 1): S40-50.
3. Lowy FD. Staphylococcus aureus infections. N Engl J Med. 1998; 339: 520-32.
4. Murray BE. The life and times of the Enterococcus. Clin Microbiol Rev. 1990; 3: 46-65.
5. Fenoll A, Granizo JJ, Aguilar L,Giménez MJ, Aragoneses-Fenoll L, Hanquet G, *et al*. Temporal trends of invasive Streptococcus pneumoniae serotypes and antimicrobial resistance patterns in Spain from 1979 to 2007. Antimicrob Agents Chemother. 2009; 47: 1012-20.
6. Oppenheim BA. The changing pattern of infection in neutropenic patients. J Antimicrob Chemother. 1998; 41: 7-11.
7. Pfaller MA, Herwaldt LA. Laboratory, clinical and epidemiological aspects of coagulase-negative staphylococci. Clin Microbiol Rev. 1988; 1: 281-99.
8. Cuevas O, Cercenado E, Goyanes MJ, Vindel A, Trincado P, Boquete T, *et al*. Staphylococcus spp. en España: situación actual y evolución de la resistencia a antimicrobianos (1986-2006). Enferm Infecc Microbiol Clin. 2008; 26: 269-77.
9. Cercenado E. Enterococcus: resistencias fenotípicas y genotípicas y epidemiología en España. Enferm Infecc Microbiol Clin. 2011; 29 (Supl 5): 59-65.
10. Cercenado E. Actualización en las resistencias de las bacterias grampositivas. Med Clin (Barc). 2010; 135 (Supl 3): 10-5.
11. Barton E, MacGowan A. Future treatment options for Gram-positive infections – looking ahead. Clin Microbiol Infect. 2009; 15 (Suppl 6): 17-25.
12. Micek ST. Alternatives to vancomycin for the treatment of methicillin-resistant Staphylococcus aureus infections. Clin Infect Dis. 2007; 45: S184-90.
13. Moellering RC. Linezolid: the first oxazolidinone antimicrobial. Ann Intern Med. 2003; 138: 135-42.
14. Perry M, Jarvis B. Linezolid. Drugs. 2001; 61: 525-52.
15. Flamm RK, Farrell DJ, Mendes RE, Ross JE, Sader HS, Jones RN. LEADER surveillance program results for 2010: an activity and spectrum analysis of linezolid using 6801 clinical isolates from the United States (61 medical centers). Diagn Microbiol Infect Dis. 2012; 74: 54-61.
16. Herrero IA, Issa NC, Patel R. Nosocomial spread of linezolid-resistant vancomycin-resistant Enterococcus faecium. N Engl J Med. 2002; 346: 867-9.
17. Morales G, Picazo JJ, Baos E, Candel FJ, Arribi A, Peláez B, *et al*. Resistance to linezolid is mediated by the cfr gene in the first report of an outbreak of linezolid-resistant Staphylococcus aureus. Clin Infect Dis. 2010; 50: 821-5.
18. Cercenado E, Marín M, Insa R, Bouza E. Emerging linezolid resistance: dissemination of the cfr gene among Staphylococcus aureus, Staphylococcus epidermidis, Enterococcus faecium and Enterococcus faecalis and inability of the Etest method for detection. 50th Interscience Conference on Antimicrobial Agents and Chemotherapy. Boston, MA, USA. American Society for Microbiology; 2010. Abstr. C2-1490.
19. Meka VG, Gold HS. Antimicrobial resistance to linezolid. Clin Infect Dis. 2004; 39: 1010-5.
20. Shaw KJ, Barbachyn MR. The oxazolidinones: past, present, and future. Ann N Y Acad Sci. 2011; 1241: 48-70.
21. Biedenbach DJ, Farell DJ, Mendes RE, Ross JE, Jones RN. Stability of linezolid activity in an era of mobile oxazolidinone resistance determinants: results from the 2009 Zyvox® Annual Appraisal of Potency and Spectrum program. Diagn Microbiol Infect Dis. 2010; 68: 459-67.
22. Picazo JJ, Betriu C, Rodríguez-Avial I, Culebras E, López F, Gómez M y Grupo VIRA. Actividad comparativa de la daptomicina frente a Staphylococcus aureus resistente a meticilina y frente a estafilococos coagulasa negativa. Enferm Infecc Microbiol Clin. 2010; 28: 13-6.
23. Cercenado E, Cuevas O, Gama B, Vindel A, Marín M, Bouza E, and the Staphylococcus Study Group. Present situation of antimicrobial resistance of Staphylococcus in Spain (2010): seventh nationwide prevalence study and emerging resistance to linezolid. 21st Eu-

ropean Congress of Clinical Microbiology and Infectious Diseases. Milán, Italia; 2011. Abstr. P-1060.

24. Gómez-Gil R, Romero-Gómez MP, García-Arias A, Gallego-Ubeda M, Sota Busselo M, Cisterna R, *et al*. Nosocomial outbreak of linezolid-resistant Enterococcus faecalis infection in a tertiary care hospital. Diagn Microbiol Infect Dis. 2009; 65: 175-9.

25. Almirante B, Miró JM. Retos en el tratamiento antimicrobiano de la endocarditis infecciosa. Papel de la daptomicina. Enferm Infecc Microbiol Clin. 2012; 30 (Supl 1): 26-32.

26. Carpenter CF, Chambers HF. Daptomycin: another novel agent for treating infections due to drug-resistant Gram-positive pathogens. Clin Infect Dis. 2004; 38: 994-1000.

27. Silverman JA, Mortin LI, Vanpraagh AD, Li T, Alder J. Inhibition of daptomycin by pulmonary surfactant: in vitro modeling and clinical impact. J Infect Dis. 2005; 191: 2149-52.

28. Boucher HW, Sakoulas G. Perspectives on daptomycin resistance, with emphasis on resistance in Staphylococcus aureus. Clin Infect Dis. 2007; 45: 601-8.

29. Sader HS, Jones RN. Antimicrobial susceptibility of Gram-positive bacteria isolated from US medical centers: results of the daptomycin surveillance program (2007-2008). Diagn Microbiol Infect Dis. 2009; 65: 158-62.

30. Sader HS, Farrell DJ, Jones RN. Antimicrobial activity of daptomycin tested against Gram-positive strains collected in European hospitals: results from 7 years of resistance surveillance (2003-2009). J Chemother. 2011; 23: 200-6.

31. Cui L, Tominaga E, Neoh HM, Hiramatsu K. Correlation between reduced daptomycin susceptibility and vancomycin resistance in vancomycin-intermediate Staphylococcus aureus. Antimicrob Agents Chemother. 2006; 50: 1079-82.

32. Patel JB, Jevitt LA, Hageman J, MacDonald LC, Tenover FC. An association between reduced susceptibility to daptomycin and reduced susceptibility to vancomycin in Staphylococcus aureus. Clin Infect Dis. 2006; 42: 1652-3.

33. Kelesidis T, Humphries R, Uslan DZ, Pegues DA. Daptomycin nonsusceptible enterococci: an emerging challenge for clinicians. Clin Infect Dis. 2011; 52: 228-34.

34. Schoen C, Unzicker C, Stuhler G, Elias J, Einsele H, Ulrich Grigoleit G, *et al*. Life-threate-

ning infection caused by daptomycin-resistant Corynebacterium jeikeium in a neutropenic patient. J Clin Microbiol. 2009; 47: 2328-31.

35. Cercenado E. Tigecycline: a new antimicrobial agent against multiresistant bacteria. Therapy. 2007; 4: 255-70.

36. Cercenado E, Marín M, Sánchez-Martínez M, Cuevas O, Martínez-Alarcón J, Bouza E. In vitro activities of tigecycline and eight other antimicrobials against different Nocardia species identified by molecular methods. Antimicrob Agents Chemother. 2007; 51: 1102-4.

37. Biedenbach DJ, Beach ML, Jones RN. In vitro antimicrobial activity of GAR-936 tested against antibiotic-resistant Gram-positive blood stream infection isolates and strains producing extended-spectrum beta-lactamases. Diagn Microbiol Infect Dis. 2001; 40: 173-7.

38. Betriu C, Rodríguez-Avial I, Sánchez BA, Gómez M, Álvarez J, Picazo JJ. In vitro activities of tigecycline (GAR-936) against recently isolated clinical bacteria in Spain. Antimicrob Agents Chemother. 2002; 46: 892-5.

39. Edlund C, Nord CE. In-vitro susceptibility of anaerobic bacteria to GAR-936, a new glycylcycline. Clin Microbiol Infect. 2000; 6: 158-63.

40. Fritsche TR, Sader HS, Kirby JT, Jones RN. In vitro activity of the glycylcycline tigecycline tested against a worldwide collection of 10,127 contemporary staphylococci, streptococci and enterococci. Clin Microbiol Infect. 2004; 10 (Suppl. 3): 246-7.

41. Cercenado E, Cercenado S, Gómez JA, Bouza E. In vitro activity of tigecycline (GAR-936), a novel glycylcycline, against vancomycin-resistant enterococci and staphylococci with diminished susceptibility to glycopeptides. J Antimicrob Chemother. 2003; 52: 138-9.

42. Boucher HW, Wennersten CB, Eliopoulos GM. In vitro activities of the glycylcycline GAR-936 against Gram-positive bacteria. Antimicrob Agents Chemother. 2000; 44: 2225-9.

43. McAleese F, Peterson P, Ruzin A, Dunmun PM, Murphy E, Projan SJ, *et al*. A novel MATE family efflux pump contributes to the reduced susceptibility of laboratory derived Staphylococcus aureus mutants to tigecyclin. Antimicrob Agents Chemother. 2005; 49: 1865-71.

44. Eliopoulos GM. Quinupristin-dalfopristin and linezolid: evidence and opinion. Clin Infect Dis. 2003; 36: 473-81.

45. Jones RN, Ballow CH, Biedenbach DJ, Deinhart JA, Schentag JJ. Antimicrobial activity of quinupristin-dalfopristin (RP 59500, Synercid) tested against over 28,000 recent clinical isolates from 200 medical centers in the United States and Canada. Diagn Microbiol Infect Dis. 1998; 31: 437-51.

46. Schmitz FJ, Verhoef J, Fluit AC, and the Sentry Participants Group. Prevalence of resistance to MLS antibiotics in 20 European university hospitals participating in the European SENTRY surveillance programme. J Antimicrob Chemother. 1999; 43: 783-92.

47. Werner G, Cuny C, Schmitz FJ, Witte W. Methicillin-resistant, quinupristin-dalfopristin-resistant Staphylococcus aureus with reduced sensitivity to glycopeptides. J Clin Microbiol. 2001; 39: 3586-90.

48. Cohen MA, Huband MD. Activity of clinafloxacin, trovafloxacin, quinupristin/dalfopristin, and other antimicrobial agents versus Staphylococcus aureus isolates with reduced susceptibility to vancomycin. Diagn Microbiol Infect Dis. 1999; 33: 43-6.

49. Gordon KA, Beach ML, Biedenbach DJ, Jones RN, Rhomberg PR, Mutnick AH. Antimicrobial susceptibility patterns of β-hemolytic and viridans group streptococci: report from the SENTRY antimicrobial surveillance program (1997-2000). Diagn Microbiol Infect Dis. 2002; 43: 157-62.

50. Eliopoulos GM, Wennersten CB, Gold HS, Schülin T, Souli M, Farris MG, *et al.* Characterization of vancomycin-resistant Enterococcus faecium isolates from the United States and their susceptibility in vitro to dalfopristin-quinupristin. Antimicrob Agents Chemother. 1998; 42: 1088-92.

51. Cercenado E, Coque MT. Epidemiología de la resistencia a los antimicrobianos en micoorganismos grampositivos. Enferm Infecc Microbiol Clin. Monogr. 2006; 5: 14-26.

52. Saravolatz LD, Stein GE, Johnson LB. Telavancin: a novel lipoglycopeptide. Clin Infect Dis. 2009; 49: 1908-14.

53. Higgins DL, Chang R, Debabov DV, Leung J, Wu T, Krause KM, *et al.* Telavancin, a multifunctional lipoglycopeptide, disrupts both cell wall synthesis and cell membrane integrity in methicillin-resistant Staphylococcus aureus. Antimicrob Agents Chemother. 2005; 49: 1127-34.

54. Draghi DC, Benton BM, Krause KM, Thornsberry C, Pillar C, Sahm DF. Comparative surveillance study of telavancin activity against recently collected Gram-positive clinical isolates from across the United States. Antimicrob Agents Chemother. 2008; 52: 2383-8.

55. Leuthner KD, Cheung CM, Rybak MJ. Comparative activity of the new lipoglycopeptide telavancin in the presence and absence of serum against 50 glycopeptide non-susceptible staphylococci and three vancomycin-resistant Staphylococcus aureus. J Antimicrob Chemother. 2006; 58: 338-43.

56. Kaniga K, Blosser RS, Karloswsky JA, Sahm DF. In vitro activity of telavancin (TD-6424) against Bacillus anthracis. 44th Interscience Conference on Antimicrobial Agents and Chemotherapy. Washington, DC, USA. American Society for Microbiology; 2004. Abstr. E-2010.

57. Mendes RE, Sader HS, Farrell DJ, Jones RN. Worldwide appraisal and update (2010) of telavancin activity tested against a collection of Gram-positive clinical pathogens from five continents. Antimicrob Agents Chemother. 2012; 56: 3999-4004.

58. Stryjewski ME, Graham DR, Wilson SE, O'Riordan W, Young D, Lentnek A, *et al.* Assessment of telavancin in complicated skin and skin structure infections study. Clin Infect Dis. 2008; 46: 1683-93.

59. Rubinstein E, Corey GR, Boucher HW, Niederman MS, Shorr AF, Torres A, *et al.* Telavancin for the treatment of hospital-acquired pneumonia in severely ill and older patients: the ATTAIN studies. 48th Interscience Conference on Antimicrobial Agents and Chemotherapy and 46th Infectious Diseases Society of America. Washington, DC, USA. American Society for Microbiology; 2008. Abstr. K-529.

60. Zhanel GG, Schweizer F, Karlowsky JA. Oritavancin: mechanism of action. Clin Infect Dis. 2012; 54 (Suppl 3): S214-9.

61. Mendes RE, Farrell DJ, Sader HS, Jones RN. Oritavancin microbiologic features and activity results from the surveillance program in the United States. Clin Infect Dis. 2012; 54 (Suppl 3): S203-13.

62. Jones RN, Barrett MS, Erwin ME. In vitro activity and spectrum of LY333328, a novel glycopeptide derivative. Antimicrob Agents Chemother. 1997; 41: 488-93.

63. Biavasco F, Vignaroli C, Lupidi R, Manso E, Facinelli B, Varaldo PE. In vitro antibacterial activity of LY333328, a new semisynthetic glycopeptide. Antimicrob Agents Chemother. 1997; 41: 2165-72.

64. O'Connor R, Baines SD, Freeman J, Wilcox MH. In vitro susceptibility of genotypically distinct and clonal Clostridium difficile strains to oritavancin. J Antimicrob Chemother. 2008; 62: 762-5.

65. Citron DM, Kwok YY, Appleman MD. In vitro activity of oritavancin (LY333328), vancomycin, clindamycin, and metronidazole against Clostridium perfringens, Propionibacterium acnes, and anaerobic grampositive cocci. Anaerobe. 2005; 11: 93-5.

66. Bouza E, Burillo A. Oritavancin: a novel lipoglycopeptide active against Gram-positive pathogens including multiresistant strains. Int J Antimicrob Agents. 2010; 36: 401-7.

67. Billeter M, Zervos MJ, Chen AY, Dalovisio JR, Kurukularatne C. Dalbavancin: a novel once-weekly lipoglycopeptide antibiotic. Clin Infect Dis. 2008; 46: 577-83.

68. Streit JM, Fritsche TR, Sader H, Jones RN. Worldwide assessment of dalbavancin activity and spectrum against over 6,000 clinical isolates. Diagn Microbiol Infect Dis. 2004; 48: 137-43.

69. Goldstein BP, Draghi DC, Sheehan DJ, Hogan P, Sahm DF. Bactericidal activity and resistance development profiling of dalbavancin. Antimicrob Agents Chemother. 2007; 51: 1150-4.

70. Streit JM, Sader HS, Fritsche T, Jones RN. Dalbavancin activity against selected populations of antimicrobial-resistant Gram-positive pathogens. Diagn Microbiol Infect Dis. 2005; 53: 307-10.

71. Barbour A, Schmidt S, Rand KH, Derendorf H. Ceftobiprole: a novel cephalosporin with activity against Gram-positive and Gram-negative pathogens, including methicillin-resistant Staphylococcus aureus (MRSA). Intern J Antimicrob Agents. 2009; 34: 1-7.

72. Rouse MS, Steckelberg JM, Patel R. In vitro activity of ceftobiprole, daptomycin, linezolid, and vancomycin against methicillin-resistant staphylococci associated with endocarditis and bone and joint infection. Diagn Microbiol Infect Dis. 2007; 58: 363-5.

73. Jones RN, Deshpande LM, Mutnick AH, Biedenbach DJ. In vitro evaluation of BAL9141, a novel parenteral cephalosporin active against oxacillin-resistant staphylococci. J Antimicrob Chemother. 2002; 50: 915-32.

74. Fritsche TR, Sader HS, Jones RN. Antimicrobial activity of ceftobiprole, a novel anti-methicillin-resistant Staphylococcus aureus cephalosporin, tested against contemporary pathogens: results from the SENTRY Antimicrobial Surveillance Program (2005-2006). Diagn Microbiol Infect Dis. 2008; 61: 86-95.

75. Saravolatz LD, Stein GE, Johnson LB. Ceftaroline: a novel cephalosporin with activity against methicillin-resistant Staphylococcus aureus. Clin Infect Dis. 2011; 52: 1156-63.

76. Saravolatz L, Pawlak J, Johnson L. In vitro acitivity of ceftaroline against community-associated methicillin-resistant, vancomycin intermediate, vancomycin-resistant and daptomycin-nonsusceptilbe Staphylococcus aureus isolates. Antimicrob Agents Chemother. 2010; 54: 3027-30.

77. Fenoll A, Aguilar L, Robledo O, Giménez MJ, Granizo JJ, Biek D, *et al.* In vitro activity of ceftaroline against Streptococcus pneumoniae isolates exhibiting resistance to penicillin, amoxicillin, and cefotaxime. Antimicrob Agents Chemother. 2008; 52: 4209-10.

78. Citron D, Tyrrell K, Merriam C, Goldstein E. In vitro activity ceftaroline against 623 diverse strains of anaerobic bacteria. Antimicrob Agents Chemother. 2010; 54: 1627-32.

79. Sader HS, Fritsche TR, Jones RN. Potency and bactericidal activity of iclaprim against recent clinical Gram-positive isolates. Antimicrob Agents Chemother. 2009; 53: 2171-5.

80. Zhanel GG, Karlowsky JA. In vitro activity of iclaprim against respiratory and bacteremic isolates of Streptococcus pneumoniae. Antimicrob Agents Chemother. 2009; 53: 1690-2.

81. Krievins D, Brandt R, Hawser S, Hadvary P, Islam K. Multicenter, randomized study of the efficacy and safety of intravenous iclaprim in complicated skin and skin structure infections. Antimicrob Agents Chemother. 2009; 53: 2834-40.

Capítulo 4

Diagnóstico microbiológico de las infecciones relacionadas con catéteres vasculares

F. Marco,[1] C. Pitart,[1] J. Mensa[2]

[1] **Servicio de Microbiología**
  Centro de Investigación en Salud Internacional
    de Barcelona (CRESIB)
  Hospital Clínic
  Universitat de Barcelona
  Barcelona

[2] **Servicio de Enfermedades Infecciosas**
  Hospital Clínic
  Universitat de Barcelona
  Barcelona

Correspondencia:
Dr. Francesc Marco
fmarco@clinic.ub.es

Sinopsis

El diagnóstico de las infecciones relacionadas con catéteres vasculares requiere una correcta evaluación de las manifestaciones clínicas del paciente y una confirmación microbiológica. Antes de retirar el catéter y de iniciar el tratamiento antimicrobiano, deben efectuarse hemocultivos de sangre extraída a través del catéter y de una vena periférica. El catéter se cultiva mediante un método semicuantitativo o cuantitativo. El diagnóstico de infección relacionada con el catéter se establece cuando el microorganismo recuperado de la punta del catéter coincide con el de los hemocultivos.

Introducción

La atención sanitaria de los pacientes ingresados en centros hospitalarios no se entendería si no se emplearan catéteres intravasculares.[1] En la actividad asistencial diaria, los ejemplos más evidentes son los pacientes en situación muy grave atendidos en unidades de cuidados intensivos (UCI), los que presentan una enfermedad aguda o crónica grave y los que precisan hemodiálisis.[1,2] Sin embargo, el uso de catéteres comporta un riesgo inevitable de infecciones que se asocian a unas altas morbilidad y mortalidad.[3] Las infecciones relacionadas con catéteres intravasculares representan la principal causa de bacteriemia nosocomial, con una mortalidad atribuible del 12 % al 25 % en los pacientes graves,[4] y su diagnóstico antes de retirar el catéter sigue siendo un problema no resuelto tanto desde el punto de vista clínico como del microbiológico.

1   Tipos de catéteres

Existen diversos tipos de catéteres intravasculares, con diferentes técnicas de inserción, tamaños y materiales.[2,5-7] Los catéteres arteriales periféricos y los arteriales pulmonares se emplean durante períodos cortos de tiempo y suelen estar heparinizados, por lo que tienen poco riesgo de causar problemas trombóticos y colonización bacteriana. Los catéteres venosos periféricos son los más utilizados, pero producen escasas complicaciones infecciosas. Los catéteres venosos centrales son los causantes de la mayoría de las infecciones relacionadas con catéteres, y en este capítulo se describirán los diferentes métodos que se emplean para diagnosticarlas. Estos catéteres pueden ser de una o varias luces (de dos a cinco). Los no tunelizados son de silicona o poliuretano, y se insertan en las venas subclavia, yugular o femoral hasta llegar a la vena cava superior. En general son catéteres de corta duración y pueden cambiarse a través de una guía. En cambio, los tunelizados (tipo *Hickman*® o *Broviac*®, entre otros) son de larga duración y se implantan quirúrgicamente. Disponen de un manguito de *Dacron*® en el punto de salida que permite fijarlos y al mismo tiempo impide la entrada de microorganismos. Una variante de este tipo de catéter *(Groshong*®) es el que termina en una punta redondeada con una válvula que permanece cerrada si no se está utilizando. Los catéteres venosos centrales insertados por vía periférica constituyen una alternativa a los anteriores y son cada vez más utilizados, ya que permiten disponer de un acceso venoso durante largo tiempo (de seis semanas a seis meses). Pueden incorporar o no una válvula, y el extremo del catéter se sitúa en la vena cava superior. Los reservorios implantados se colocan en el tejido subcutáneo y disponen de una membrana que permite el acceso con una aguja desde el exterior.

2   Diagnóstico microbiológico de las infecciones relacionadas con catéteres

El diagnóstico de las infecciones relacionadas con catéteres constituye un auténtico reto. En la tabla 1 se citan las recomendaciones de la Infectious Diseases Society of America (IDSA) para su diagnóstico.[8] La fiebre y los escalofríos, frecuentes en este tipo de infecciones, no son síntomas específicos. La inflamación local en la zona de inserción del catéter tiene una sensibilidad igual o inferior al 3 %,[9] pues pueden objetivarse inflamación local

Cómo y cuándo deben cultivarse los catéteres y cómo realizar los hemocultivos	Nivel de evidencia-Recomendación
A. Cultivo de catéteres endovenosos	
A.1. Aspectos generales	
1. El cultivo debe realizarse cuando se retira un catéter ante la sospecha de una bacteriemia relacionada con él. No están indicados los cultivos sistemáticos de vigilancia	A-II
2. No deben realizarse cultivos cualitativos de catéteres	A-II
3. En los catéteres venosos centrales se cultivará preferiblemente la punta del catéter antes que el segmento subcutáneo	B-II
4. Si se cultivan catéteres impregnados con soluciones antimicrobianas, debe añadirse al medio de cultivo inhibidores específicos	A-II
5. El crecimiento de ≥ 15 UFC en la punta del catéter (5 cm) por el método semicuantitativo de Maki, o el crecimiento de $> 10^2$ UFC en un catéter cultivado por un método cuantitativo (sonicación), indican colonización del catéter	A-I
6. Si se sospecha una infección del catéter y hay un exudado en la zona de inserción, recoger una muestra para cultivo y tinción de Gram	B-II
A.2. Catéteres de corta duración, incluidos catéteres arteriales	
7. El método recomendado para el cultivo de la punta del catéter es el semicuantitativo de Maki	A-II
8. Si se sospecha infección del catéter arterial pulmonar, debe cultivarse el introductor	A-II
A.3. Catéteres de larga duración	
9. El crecimiento en las placas de cultivo de < 15 UFC del mismo microorganismo, tanto de la zona de inserción como de la conexión, es altamente sugestivo de que el catéter no es el origen de la infección	A-II
10. Si se retira un reservorio subcutáneo por sospecha de infección relacionada con el catéter, debe enviarse al laboratorio de microbiología para cultivo cualitativo junto con la punta del catéter	B-II
B. Hemocultivos	
11. Realizar los hemocultivos antes de iniciar el tratamiento antibiótico	A-I
12. Si es posible, la extracción de sangre debe hacerla personal especializado (equipo de extracciones)	A-II

Continúa

Continuación

Cómo y cuándo deben cultivarse los catéteres y cómo realizar los hemocultivos	Nivel de evidencia-Recomendación
13. La preparación de la zona de la piel en que se efectuará la extracción de sangre debe ser muy cuidadosa. Se empleará alcohol, tintura de yodo o una solución de alcohol-clorhexidina (> 0,5 %) en lugar de povidona yodada. Dejar actuar el tiempo suficiente para disminuir las probabilidades de contaminación	A-I
14. Si va a extraerse sangre por el catéter, limpiar la conexión del catéter con alcohol, tintura de yodo o una solución de alcohol-clorhexidina (> 0,5 %). Dejar actuar el tiempo suficiente para disminuir las probabilidades de contaminación	A-I
15. En los casos de sospecha de infección relacionada con un catéter se realizarán los hemocultivos de sangre periférica y obtenida a través del catéter antes de iniciar el tratamiento antibiótico. Los frascos de hemocultivo se marcarán de modo adecuado para conocer con precisión el origen de la muestra	A-II
16. Si no puede obtenerse sangre de una vena periférica, es recomendable realizar dos o más hemocultivos de sangre obtenida de diferentes luces del catéter	B-III
17. No está claro si en la anterior circunstancia los hemocultivos deben realizarse de sangre obtenida a través de todas las luces del catéter	C-III

UFC: unidades formadoras de colonias.

Tabla 1. Resumen de las recomendaciones de la IDSA para el diagnóstico de las infecciones relacionadas con catéteres.

y flebitis en ausencia de infección. También es posible que haya una infección relacionada con el catéter sin signos locales, como se ha observado en catéteres centrales de inserción periférica.[10] Por ello, para establecer el diagnóstico de certeza es imprescindible recurrir a técnicas microbiológicas. Además, hay que tener en cuenta que, en determinados pacientes, la retirada del catéter puede ser una decisión comprometida, y que sólo en un 15 % a un 25 % de los catéteres venosos centrales retirados por sospecha de infección que se cultivan con un método cuantitativo se confirma la infección relacionada.[11]

El diagnóstico microbiológico de una infección localizada, como por ejemplo en el punto de inserción, requiere cultivar en medios adecuados el material purulento de la secreción. La muestra ha de recogerse preferentemente con dos escobillones o, si es posible, se aspirará con una jeringa. De esta forma se obtiene suficiente material patológico. Si se emplean dos escobillones, uno puede destinarse a realizar una tinción de Gram, que permite visualizar los microorganismos presentes, y el otro para el cultivo. La presencia de una infección localizada puede asociarse con una bacteriemia relacionada con el catéter, pero por sí sola no sirve para identificarla o predecirla, ya que puede existir de forma independiente de una infección sistémica.[10]

El diagnóstico microbiológico de las infecciones relacionadas con catéteres puede hacerse empleando métodos que no requieren la retirada del catéter o métodos en los que es imprescindible retirarlo (véase la tabla 2).

	Criterio diagnóstico	Desventajas
Técnicas que no requieren retirar el catéter		
Hemocultivos cuantitativos simultáneos	Recuento de colonias en la sangre extraída del catéter ≥ 5 veces el obtenido con la sangre de una vena periférica	Carga de trabajo importante Coste económico
Hemocultivo cuantitativo de sangre extraída del catéter	Recuento ≥ 100 UFC/ml	No permite distinguir entre bacteriemia relacionada con el catéter y bacteriemia de alto grado
Diferencia en el tiempo de positividad de los hemocultivos	Crecimiento más rápido en hemocultivo de sangre extraída del catéter (≥ 2 h)	Difícil de interpretar si se administran antibióticos por el catéter
Tinción con naranja de acridina (+ Gram) de la sangre extraída del catéter	Observación de microorganismos	Poco utilizado, falta experiencia
Cepillado endoluminal	Recuento > 100 UFC/ml	Inducción de bacteriemia, arritmia, embolización
Frotis piel, conexión	Recuento ≥ 15 UFC	Variabilidad de los resultados Probable contaminación de la superficie
Técnicas que requieren retirar el catéter		
Cultivo semicuantitativo	Recuento ≥ 15 UFC /placa	No detecta microorganismos de la luz endoluminal
Cultivo cuantitativo	Recuento ≥ 10^3 UFC	No está bien definido el punto de corte (≥ 10^3 o ≥ 10^2 UFC)
Tinción del catéter (Gram, naranja de acridina)	Observación de microorganismos	Poco práctico No puede hacerse en todos los catéteres Carga de trabajo importante

UFC: unidades formadoras de colonias.

Tabla 2. Resumen de los métodos diagnósticos microbiológicos.

2.1   Métodos diagnósticos que no requieren retirar el catéter

Están destinados a evitar la retirada injustificada de un catéter venoso central y soslayar los riesgos asociados a la colocación de un nuevo catéter en otro emplazamiento. Han de ser la primera opción a considerar.

2.1.1   Hemocultivos cuantitativos simultáneos

El objetivo de este método es demostrar un mayor número de colonias del microorganismo causante de la infección en el cultivo de la sangre extraída a través del catéter venoso central que de la obtenida de una vena periférica. Para efectuar estos hemocultivos se necesita un sistema de cultivo diferente al utilizado normalmente en los laboratorios de microbiología. El más utilizado es el de lisis-centrifugación (*Isolator 10*®, Wampole, Granbury, NJ, USA).[12,13] El procedimiento consiste en inocular 10 ml de sangre (catéter venoso central y vena periférica) en este tipo de tubo, que permite lisar la sangre, y después de su centrifugación se siembra el sedimento en diferentes medios de cultivo que se incubarán en atmósferas adecuadas. A las 24-48 horas de incubación puede cuantificarse el número de colonias presentes. Cuando en el cultivo de la sangre obtenida a través del catéter se observa un recuento de colonias que es varias veces superior al de la sangre extraída de forma simultánea en la vena periférica, se considera que el resultado es predictivo de bacteriemia relacionada con el catéter. El valor utilizado para establecer el diagnóstico varía según los estudios publicados.[13-16] En general, las cifras propuestas oscilan en recuentos de microorganismos de dos a diez veces superiores en la sangre obtenida del catéter que en la procedente de la extracción venosa. La IDSA considera que el valor indicativo de bacteriemia relacionada con el catéter es un recuento de colonias en la sangre del catéter igual o superior a cinco veces ($\geq 5{:}1$) el obtenido en la sangre procedente de la punción de la vena periférica[5]. En un metaanálisis que analizó los diferentes métodos diagnósticos empleados en diversos estudios, el resultado de los cultivos cuantitativos realizados de forma simultánea fue el más preciso para establecer el diagnóstico de bacteriemia relacionada con el catéter, sobre todo en comparación con el cultivo cuantitativo del catéter considerado como método de referencia.[17] Los resultados agrupados de sensibilidad y especificidad para los catéteres de corta duración fueron del 75 % y el 97 %, respectivamente, y para los catéteres de larga duración del 93 % y el 100 %. Sin embargo, esta metodología tiene una utilidad limitada. El sistema de lisis-centrifugación, además de tener un mayor coste, no está disponible en la mayoría de los laboratorios de microbiología de nuestro entorno, ya que desde un punto de vista económico no pueden optar a tener dos sistemas de hemocultivo diferentes. Además, el procesamiento de la sangre comporta una carga de trabajo importante que no todos los laboratorios pueden asumir.

2.1.2 Hemocultivo cuantitativo a través del catéter

Una aproximación más conservadora en cuanto al número de hemocultivos practicados para diagnosticar una bacteriemia relacionada con el catéter es realizar una sola extracción de sangre a través del catéter, sin extraer sangre de una vena periférica, y procesarla de manera cuantitativa. El umbral a partir del cual se establece un diagnóstico positivo es de al menos 100 unidades formadoras de colonias (UFC)/ml.[18,19] Este método tiene el inconveniente de que no permite distinguir entre una bacteriemia relacionada con el catéter y una bacteriemia de alto grado, sobre todo en los pacientes inmunodeprimidos o esplenectomizados con sepsis grave.

2.1.3 Diferencia en el tiempo de positividad de los hemocultivos

Los actuales sistemas de hemocultivo permiten conocer el tiempo que tardan los microorganismos en multiplicarse en el interior de los frascos hasta alcanzar el umbral de positividad. Ello es posible porque cada 15 minutos analizan los cambios en la fluorescencia que se producen en el interior de los frascos según el crecimiento de los microorganismos. Esta capacidad puede utilizarse para comparar el tiempo de crecimiento de los microorganismos en los hemocultivos obtenidos de forma simultánea de una vena periférica y a través del catéter. Diversos estudios han analizado su utilidad para el diagnóstico de las infecciones relacionadas con catéteres.[20-23] El diagnóstico definitivo de bacteriemia relacionada con el catéter se establece cuando el hemocultivo de la sangre obtenida a través del catéter es positivo al menos 2 horas antes que el de la sangre procedente de una vena periférica. En el mismo metaanálisis citado previamente,[17] la sensibilidad y la especificidad para el diagnóstico de bacteriemia relacionada con catéteres de corta duración fueron del 89 % y el 87 %, respectivamente, y para los de larga duración del 90 % y el 72 %.

Puesto que la mayoría de los laboratorios de microbiología emplean los sistemas radiométricos de hemocultivo que permiten monitorizar el crecimiento de los microorganismos, parece lógico que deba considerarse emplearlos para intentar establecer el diagnóstico de las infecciones relacionadas con catéteres. Para mejorar el diagnóstico tendría que obtenerse la misma cantidad de sangre en las dos extracciones, remitir al laboratorio lo más pronto posible los frascos de hemocultivo e identificar correctamente la procedencia de la sangre de cada uno de ellos. Asimismo, han de tenerse en cuenta diversos aspectos relacionados con el número de muestras de sangre para hemocultivo tomadas a través de las luces del catéter y de una vena periférica. En un estudio[24] se demostró que es necesario efectuar extracciones de sangre a través de todas las luces del catéter para establecer el diagnóstico definitivo, o se corre el riesgo de no detectar un número sustancial de casos. Esta opción tiene como principal inconveniente la posibilidad de contribuir al desarrollo de una anemia nosocomial, sobre todo en los pacientes ingresados en las UCI.[25] Por ello, algunos autores recomiendan que en estos casos se practiquen dos hemocultivos, y si son positivos en ausencia de otro foco aparente, retirar el catéter venoso central.[26,27]

En la valoración del tiempo de positividad ha de considerarse la posibilidad de que el paciente esté recibiendo tratamiento antimicrobiano a través de la luz del catéter que se utiliza para extraer la sangre. En esta situación es posible que se obtenga un resultado falsamente negativo en catéteres colonizados o relacionados con infección clínica.[28]

2.1.4   *Tinción con naranja de acridina de la sangre extraída del catéter*

Es un método de diagnóstico rápido, que puede realizarse en unos 30 minutos. Su objetivo es detectar los microorganismos que se encuentran en la luz del catéter origen de la supuesta infección. La sangre extraída a través del catéter es lisada con solución salina hipotónica para eliminar los hematíes. A continuación se toma una alícuota para preparar una capa de leucocitos en un portaobjetos mediante una citocentrífuga, que se tiñe con naranja de acridina y después se observa al microscopio de fluorescencia.[29,30] La presencia de microorganismos implica un diagnóstico positivo. En el primer estudio que empleó esta técnica, realizado en población pediátrica, los autores observaron una sensibilidad y una especificidad del 87 % y el 94 %, respectivamente.[29] Estudios posteriores, en población adulta, han encontrado valores semejantes.[30] Se ha descrito que la sensibilidad aumenta hasta un 96 % si después de la tinción con naranja de acridina se efectúa una tinción de Gram de otro portaobjetos, ya que facilita la identificación morfológica de los microorganismos con una especificidad del 92 %, un valor predictivo positivo (VPP) del 91 % y un valor predictivo negativo (VPN) del 97 %.[31] Sin embargo, es una técnica que no se ha generalizado aunque es relativamente sencilla de realizar y tiene un coste razonable.

2.1.5   *Cepillado endoluminal*

Esta técnica diagnóstica consiste en introducir en la luz del catéter, a través del conector, una guía de acero que termina en un cepillo de nailon, con el fin de arrastrar la biocapa de la luz del catéter. Una vez efectuado el cepillado endoluminal, se retira y se coloca en un recipiente adecuado con un medio líquido (tampón fosfato salino). A continuación se somete a sonicación y agitación, para desprender los microorganismos adheridos, y se siembra la suspensión en placas de agar sangre. Esta técnica se fundamenta en el hecho de que las bacterias se adhieren a la vaina de fibrina de la superficie interna de los catéteres, y al introducir el cepillo se arrastra esta fibrina. En el estudio de Kite *et al.*[32] se consideraron positivos los recuentos mayores de 100 UFC/ml, con una sensibilidad del 95 % y una especificidad del 84 %. Esta técnica tiene diversos inconvenientes, entre ellos ser poco práctica y no estar exenta de efectos secundarios potencialmente graves, como embolización o desarrollo de bacteriemia por fragmentación de la biopelícula.[17,33]

2.1.6   Cultivos de muestras superficiales y de la conexión

Los cultivos cutáneos superficiales pretenden conocer el grado de colonización extraluminal de los catéteres. La muestra se toma con una torunda frotando la zona de piel alrededor de la entrada del catéter (1-2 cm de radio) y se siembra en una placa de agar sangre. Se considera que el catéter está colonizado o puede ser origen de la infección clínica cuando el número de microorganismos de una especie determinada es ≥ 15 UFC.[34-36] También puede emplearse una torunda de menor tamaño (de alginato) para frotar el interior de la conexión con el propósito de detectar microorganismos que puedan dar lugar a una progresión endoluminal. Este frotis se siembra igualmente en agar sangre y se valora del mismo modo que el cultivo cutáneo. El interés de este método radica en su alta sensibilidad (80 % a >90 %) y su VPN (97 %) cuando ambos cultivos son negativos o positivos, por lo que deben usarse para excluir el diagnóstico de infección relacionada con un catéter.[35,37] En un trabajo[38] se intentó mejorar el VPP y la especificidad de estos cultivos añadiendo otro cultivo del primer segmento subcutáneo del catéter tras retirarlo unos 2 cm. La especificidad y el VPP del segmento subcutáneo (94 % y 68 %, respectivamente) fueron mejores que los de la piel, por lo que los autores recomiendan realizar el cultivo de la conexión y de los 2 cm subcutáneos del catéter. En un estudio realizado en pacientes admitidos en una UCI cardíaca se demostró que la realización sistemática de cultivos de muestras superficiales (piel y conexión) fue útil para identificar a los pacientes que podían beneficiarse de medidas preventivas o de descontaminación, así como para establecer el posible origen de las infecciones relacionadas con catéteres.[36]

2.2   Métodos diagnósticos que requieren retirar el catéter

2.2.1   Cultivo cualitativo de la punta del catéter

Es una técnica obsoleta que no debe utilizarse para el diagnóstico de la infección relacionada con el catéter.[5,7] Consiste en introducir asépticamente el extremo distal del catéter (4-5 cm) en un tubo con medio de cultivo líquido. El principal inconveniente de este método es que no permite cuantificar el número de UFC, y un cultivo positivo tras una incubación de 20 a 24 horas puede deberse a un único microorganismo, lo que no permite diferenciar una colonización significativa de una contaminación accidental.

2.2.2   Cultivo semicuantitativo de la punta del catéter

Es una técnica sencilla de realizar y es la más empleada en los laboratorios de microbiología. Consiste en hacer rodar el extremo distal del catéter (4-5 cm) al menos cuatro veces por la superficie de una placa de agar sangre, que a continuación se incuba durante 24 a 48 horas. Descrita por Maki *et al.*,[39] se la considera el método de referencia y se ha convertido en la técnica diagnóstica más estudiada. Si en el cultivo se obtienen al menos 15 UFC se considera que el catéter está colonizado. El diagnóstico de bacteriemia relacionada con el catéter sólo puede establecerse si se recupera el mismo microorganismo en un hemocultivo realizado con sangre procedente de una vena periférica. La decisión de establecer el punto de corte en ≥ 15 UFC se debe a que, en el estudio inicial, la mayoría de los pacientes con bacteriemia tenían recuentos superiores a 15 con una especificidad del 76 %. Es posible que en los casos de sepsis originada en un catéter el recuento de colonias sea inferior al valor propuesto o incluso negativo (cuando la infección se origine de manera exclusiva de la luz del catéter), pero si se considera positivo un recuento ≤ 5 UFC disminuye la especificidad, aunque puede mejorar la sensibilidad. La limitación más clara de este método es que sólo detecta colonización de la superficie externa del catéter, sin aportar información de la colonización endoluminal. Este aspecto ha de tenerse en cuenta en catéteres de larga duración, en los cuales la colonización endoluminal puede ser la causa del desarrollo de bacteriemias, y en aquellos que están impregnados de sustancias antisépticas sólo en su superficie externa. En estudios que han analizado la sensibilidad de esta técnica para diagnosticar la bacteriemia relacionada con catéteres de larga duración (más de 30 días) se ha encontrado que oscila entre el 45 % y el 75 %.[40,41] En un análisis que valora los resultados del cultivo semicuantitativo en 14 estudios que evaluaron catéteres de corta duración, los resultados agrupados de sensibilidad y especificidad fueron del 84 % y el 85 %, respectivamente.[17] En un estudio de Bouza *et al.*,[42] la sensibilidad y la especificidad de esta técnica fueron superiores al 90 % para los catéteres venosos centrales tanto de corta como de larga duración, pero entre estos últimos se incluyeron catéteres con un tiempo de implantación de 7 días o más.

2.2.3   *Cultivos cuantitativos de la punta del catéter*

Se han descrito diversos métodos para cuantificar el número de microorganismos presentes en las superficies interna y externa del catéter. El método de Cleri *et al.*[43] consiste en introducir el segmento distal del catéter en 2 ml de caldo de cultivo y lavar un mínimo de tres veces la luz del catéter con la ayuda de una jeringa y una aguja. A continuación se efectúan diluciones del caldo de cultivo inicial y se siembran 100 μl de cada dilución en placas de agar sangre. Con esta técnica puede estudiarse y cuantificarse la colonización global del catéter, ya que se analizan ambas superficies (interna y externa). Los autores establecieron que un catéter estaba colonizado cuando el recuento de microorganismos era ≥ 10^3 UFC por segmento, puesto que todos los catéteres con este valor se asociaron con bacteriemia. Con el empleo de este valor, la sensibilidad y la especificidad en los casos de bacteriemia fueron del 100 % y el 92,5 %, respectivamente. Sin embargo, este método tiene un inconveniente importante, que es la carga de trabajo y tiempo que comporta para los laboratorios de microbiología.

Unos años más tarde se propuso una modificación de la técnica que evitaba manipular el catéter.[44] Para ello se introduce el segmento distal del catéter en un tubo con 1 ml de agua destilada y se agita durante un minuto con la ayuda de un vórtex. A continuación se siembran 0,1 ml de la suspensión en una placa de agar sangre, que se incuba durante 24 a 48 horas. En el estudio inicial se empleó como punto de corte > 10^3 UFC/ml y se observaron una sensibilidad del 97,5 % y una especificidad del 88 % para los catéteres de pacientes con signos clínicos de infección. Si sólo se analizaba el subgrupo de catéteres que producían bacteriemia, las cifras subían al 100 %.[44]

Otra opción es la propuesta por Sherertz *et al.,*[45] que consiste en introducir la punta del catéter en 10 ml de caldo de tripticasa-soja, sonicarlo durante un minuto y a continuación agitarlo con un vórtex durante 15 segundos. Después se siembran 0,1 ml del caldo original y de las diluciones 1:10 y 1:100 en placas de agar sangre, para cuantificar el grado de colonización. Los datos del estudio indican que, con un punto de corte de ≥ 100 UFC/ml, puede distinguirse entre origen de la infección y colonización. El empleo de sonicación seguido de agitación tiene la ventaja de permitir desprender los microorganismos tanto de la superficie interna del catéter como de la externa. La sensibilidad y la especificidad son similares a las del método semicuantitativo para el diagnóstico de la bacteriemia relacionada con catéteres de corta duración.[42] Sin embargo, en los catéteres de larga duración el método de sonicación ha demostrado una mayor sensibilidad que el método de Cleri[41]. En el estudio de Bouza *et al.*[42] que analizó la utilidad de tres métodos (semicuantitativo, agitación con vórtex y sonicación) para el diagnóstico de la colonización de catéteres, se encontró que la probabilidad de detectarla fue similar con todos. Cuando se compararon los resultados según el tipo de catéter (corta o larga duración), el método de Maki fue igualmente eficaz para detectar colonización o bacteriemia relacionada con el catéter. Los autores concluyen que la sencillez y la rapidez de este método lo convierten en la primera elección en la labor diaria del laboratorio de microbiología. Según el metaanálisis de Safdar *et al.,*[17] los datos agrupados de sensibilidad y especificidad de los cultivos cuantitativos de los catéteres de corta duración fueron del 82 % y el 89 %, respectivamente, y para los de larga duración del 83 % y el 97 %.

Liñares *et al.*[46] propusieron una modificación del método de Cleri para diferenciar la colonización endoluminal de la colonización de la superficie exterior. Para ello se lava la superficie interna del catéter con 2 ml de caldo de cultivo, y se siembran 100 µl del caldo y de las diluciones 1:10 y 1:100 en placas de agar sangre para contabilizar los microorganismos presentes en la luz del catéter. A continuación se realiza el método de Maki, que permite conocer el grado de colonización de la superficie externa. El empleo conjunto de ambas técnicas tiene una excelente sensibilidad para las infecciones y la bacteriemia relacionadas con catéteres, pero es demasiado laborioso como para realizarlo sistemáticamente en los laboratorios de microbiología.

2.2.4 *Tinción de la punta del catéter*

Algunos autores han descrito el empleo de tinciones de la punta del catéter (una vez retirado), como la de Gram[47] o la de naranja de acridina,[48] con la finalidad de identificar los microorganismos causantes de la infección. La especificidad y la sensibilidad son variables según los estudios, pero la técnica ha demostrado su utilidad en el diagnóstico de las infecciones relacionadas con catéteres. Sin embargo, no suelen usarse porque representan una carga de trabajo importante para el laboratorio, no pueden emplearse en todos los catéteres y se requieren microscopios especiales.

2.2.5 *Técnicas diagnósticas moleculares*

Warwick *et al.*[49] emplearon la reacción en cadena de la polimerasa cuantitativa para detectar DNA bacteriano en la sangre extraída del catéter en pacientes con nutrición parenteral. Aunque es una técnica sensible y específica, que puede contribuir a reducir el número de catéteres retirados, son pocos los laboratorios que pueden utilizarla y no se ha extendido su uso, ya que la carga de trabajo no es despreciable si se quiere tener el resultado lo más pronto posible.

2.2.6 *Identificación de los microorganismos detectados*

Los microorganismos detectados en los diferentes cultivos han de identificarse para conocer si son el mismo, y así poder establecer un diagnóstico de certeza de la infección.

Lo primero a realizar en el laboratorio de microbiología es la identificación bioquímica y el estudio de sensibilidad a los antibióticos. La identificación también puede hacerse mediante el sistema MALDI-TOF MS *(matrix-assisted laser desorption/ ionization time of flight mass spectrometry)*,[50] que analiza el perfil proteico (sobre todo proteínas ribosómicas) del microorganismo y lo compara con una completa base de datos para establecer la identificación en cuanto a género y especie. El resultado se obtiene en pocos minutos, pero esta opción está al alcance de pocos laboratorios. La identificación bioquímica y el resultado de la sensibilidad tienen ciertas limitaciones, según sea el microorganismo aislado, ya que son técnicas fenotípicas. Si los microorganismos no forman parte de la flora cutánea habitual, estas técnicas probablemente son suficientes para establecer el diagnóstico definitivo, pero si el agente causante es un estafilococo coagulasa negativo pueden plantearse muchas dudas. Una posible aproximación, en general reservada para casos concretos y de investigación, sería recurrir a métodos moleculares como el análisis del perfil generado tras una electroforesis en campo pulsado del DNA cromosómico digerido con enzimas de restricción.

3   Conclusión

No existe un método ideal para realizar el diagnóstico microbiológico de las infecciones relacionadas con catéteres. Si hay signos locales evidentes de infección debe retirarse el catéter y obtener una muestra para tinción de Gram y cultivo. No se retirarán los catéteres de aquellos pacientes con fiebre cuya situación clínica no sea grave y que no tengan signos de infección en el punto de inserción. Hay que intentar establecer el diagnóstico de infección relacionada con el catéter antes de retirarlo. Con los nuevos sistemas de hemocultivo disponibles en los laboratorios de microbiología, la primera opción es analizar la diferencia en el tiempo de positividad entre los hemocultivos realizados con sangre obtenida a través del catéter y de una vía periférica. Los cultivos de muestras superficiales de la zona de inserción y de la conexión pueden ayudar al diagnóstico por su alto VPN. Si se retira el catéter, se cultivará su punta de manera semicuantitativa, según la técnica de Maki. Un método cuantitativo con agitación también es útil y no representa una gran carga de trabajo para el laboratorio.

Bibliografía

1. Raad II, Hanna HA. Intravascular catheter-related infections: new horizons and recent advances. Arch Intern Med. 2002; 162: 871-8.
2. Raad I, Hanna H, Maki D. Intravascular catheter-related infections: advances in diagnosis, prevention, and management. Lancet Infect Dis. 2007; 10: 645-57.
3. Wenzel RP, Edmond MB. The impact of hospital-acquired bloodstream infections. Emerging Infect Dis. 2001; 7: 174-7.
4. O'Grady NP, Alexander M, Dellinger EP, Gerberding JL, Heard SO, Maki DG, et al. Guidelines for the prevention of intravascular catheter-related infections. Centers for Disease Control and Prevention. MMWR Recomm Rep. 2002; 51(RR-10): 1-29.
5. Mermel LA, Allon M, Bouza E, Craven DE, Flynn P, O'Grady NP, et al. Clinical practice guidelines for the diagnosis and management of intravascular catheter-related infection: 2009 update by the Infectious Diseases Society of America. Clin Infect Dis. 2009; 49: 1-45.
6. León C, Ariza J, SEIMC, SEMICYUC. Guías para el tratamiento de las infecciones relacionadas con catéteres intravasculares de corta permanencia en adultos: conferencia de consenso SEIMC-SEMICYUC. Enferm Infecc Microbiol Clin. 2004; 22: 92-101.
7. Bouza E, Liñares J, Pascual A. Diagnóstico microbiológico de las infecciones asociadas a catéteres intravasculares. Procedimientos en Microbiología Clínica. N.º 15. SEIMC; 2004: 1-23.
8. Mermel LA, Farr BM, Sherertz RJ, Raad II, O'Grady N, Harris JS, et al. Guidelines for the management of intravascular catheter-related infections. Clin Infect Dis. 2001; 32: 1249-72.
9. Safdar N, Maki DG. Inflammation at the insertion site is not predictive of catheter-related bloodstream infection with short-term, noncuffed central venous catheters. Crit Care Med. 2002; 30: 2632-5.
10. Walshe LJ, Malak SF, Eagan J, Sepkowitz KA. Complication rates among cancer patients with peripherally inserted central catheters. J Clin Oncol. 2002; 20: 3276-81.
11. Raad II, Bodey GP. Infectious complications of indwelling vascular catheters. Clin Infect Dis. 1992; 15: 197-210.
12. Dorn GL, Land GA, Wilson GE. Improved blood culture technique based on centrifugation: clinical evaluation. J Clin Microbiol. 1979; 9: 391-6.
13. Mosca R, Curtas S, Forbes B, Meguid MM. The benefits of Isolator cultures in the management of suspected catheter sepsis. Surgery. 1987; 102: 718-23.
14. Chatzinikolaou I, Hanna H, Hachem R, Alakech B, Tarrand J, Raad I. Differential quantitative blood cultures for the diagnosis of catheter-related bloodstream infections associated with short- and long-term catheters: a prospective study. Diagn Microbiol Infect Dis. 2004; 50: 167-72.
15. Douard MC, Arlet G, Longuet P, Troje C, Rouveau M, Ponscarme D, et al. Diagnosis

of venous access port-related infections. Clin Infect Dis. 1999; 29: 1197-202.

16. Flynn PM, Shenep JL, Barrett FF. Differential quantitation with a commercial blood culture tube for diagnosis of catheter-related infection. J Clin Microbiol. 1988; 26: 1045-6.

17. Safdar N, Fine JP, Maki DG. Meta-analysis: methods for diagnosing intravascular device-related bloodstream infection. Ann Intern Med. 2005; 142: 451-66.

18. Capdevila JA, Planes AM, Palomar M, Gasser I, Almirante B, Pahissa A, *et al.* Value of differential quantitative blood cultures in the diagnosis of catheter-related sepsis. Eur J Clin Microbiol Infect Dis. 1992; 11: 403-7.

19. Siegman-Igra Y, Anglim AM, Shapiro DE, Adal KA, Strain BA, Farr BM. Diagnosis of vascular catheter-related bloodstream infection: a meta-analysis. J Clin Microbiol. 1997; 35: 928-36.

20. Blot F, Schmidt E, Nitenberg G, Tancrède C, Leclercq B, Laplanche A, *et al.* Earlier positivity of central-venous- versus peripheral-blood cultures is highly predictive of catheter-related sepsis. J Clin Microbiol. 1998; 36: 105-9.

21. Blot F, Nitenberg G, Chachaty E, Raynard B, Germann N, Antoun S, *et al.* Diagnosis of catheter-related bacteraemia: a prospective comparison of the time to positivity of hub-blood versus peripheral-blood cultures. Lancet. 1999; 354: 1071-7.

22. Malgrange VB, Escande MC, Theobald S. Validity of earlier positivity of central venous blood cultures in comparison with peripheral blood cultures for diagnosing catheter-related bacteremia in cancer patients. J Clin Microbiol. 2001; 39: 274-8.

23. Gaur AH, Flynn PM, Giannini MA, Shenep JL, Hayden RT. Difference in time to detection: a simple method to differentiate catheter-related from non-catheter-related bloodstream infection in immunocompromised pediatric patients. Clin Infect Dis. 2003; 37: 469-75.

24. Guembe M, Rodríguez-Creixems M, Sánchez Carrillo C, Pérez Parra A, Martín Rabadán P, Bouza E. How many lumens should be cultured in the conservative diagnosis of catheter-related bloodstream infections? Clin Infect Dis. 2010; 50: 1575-9.

25. DesJardin JA, Falagas ME, Ruthazer R, Griffith J, Wawrose D, Schenkein D, *et al.* Clinical utility of blood cultures drawn from indwelling central venous catheters in hospitalized patients with cancer. Ann Intern Med. 1999; 131: 641-7.

26. Rello J, Ochagavia A, Sabanes E, Roque M, Mariscal D, Reynaga E, *et al.* Evaluation of outcome of intravenous catheter-related infections in critically ill patients. Am J Respir Crit Care Med. 2000; 162: 1027-30.

27. Blot SI, Depuydt P, Annemans L, Benoit D, Hoste E, De Waele JJ, *et al.* Clinical and economic outcomes in critically ill patients with nosocomial catheter-related bloodstream infections. Clin Infect Dis. 2005; 41: 1591-8.

28. Raad I, Hanna HA, Alakech B, Chatzinikolaou I, Johnson MM, Torrand J. Differential time to positivity: a useful method for diagnosing catheter-related bloodstream infections. Ann Intern Med. 2004; 104: 18-25.

29. Rushforth JA, Hoy CM, Kite P, Puntis JW. Rapid diagnosis of central venous catheter sepsis. Lancet. 1993; 342: 402-3.

30. Bong J, Kite P, Ammori B, Wilcox M, McMahon M. The use of a rapid in situ test in the detection of central venous catheter-related bloodstream infection: a prospective study. J Parenter Enteral Nutr. 2003; 27: 146-50.

31. Kite P, Dobbins BM, Wilcox MH, McMahon MJ. Rapid diagnosis of central-venous-catheter-related bloodstream infection without catheter removal. Lancet. 1999; 354: 1504-7.

32. Kite P, Dobbins BM, Wilcox MH, Fawley WN, Kindon AJ, Thomas D, *et al.* Evaluation of a novel endoluminal brush method for in situ diagnosis of catheter related sepsis. J Clin Pathol. 1997; 50: 278-82.

33. Bouza E, Burillo A, Muñoz P. Catheter-related infections: diagnosis and intravascular treatment. Clin Microbiol Infect. 2002; 8: 265-74.

34. Snydman DR, Gorbea HF, Pober BR, Majka JA, Murray SA, Perry LK. Predictive value of surveillance skin cultures in total-parenteral-nutrition-related infection. Lancet. 1982; 2: 1385-8.

35. Cercenado E, Ena J, Rodríguez-Creixems M, Romero I, Bouza E. A conservative procedure for the diagnosis of catheter-related infections. Arch Intern Med. 1990; 150: 1417-20.

36. Bouza E, Muñoz P, Burillo A, López-Rodríguez J, Fernández-Pérez C, Pérez MJ, *et al.* The challenge of anticipating catheter tip colonization in major heart surgery patients in the

intensive care unit: are surface cultures useful? Crit Care Med. 2005; 33: 1953-60.

37. Fan ST, Teoh-Chan CH, Lau KF, Chu KW, Kwan AK, Wong KK. Predictive value of surveillance skin and hub cultures in central venous catheters sepsis. J Hosp Infect. 1988; 12: 191-8.

38. Fortún JJ, Pérez-Molina JAJ, Asensio AA, Calderón CC, Casado JLJ, Mir NN, *et al.* Semiquantitative culture of subcutaneous segment for conservative diagnosis of intravascular catheter-related infection. J Parenter Enteral Nutr. 2000; 24: 210-4.

39. Maki DG, Weise CE, Sarafin HW. A semiquantitative culture method for identifiying intravenous catheter related infection. N Engl J Med. 1977; 296: 1305-9.

40. Rello J, Gatell JM, Almirall J, Campistol JM, González J, Puig de la Bellacasa J. Evaluation of culture techniques for identification of catheter-related infection in hemodialysis patient. Eur J Clin Microbiol Infect Dis. 1989; 8: 620-2.

41. Raad I, Costerton W, Sabharwal U, Sacilowski M, Anaissie E, Bodey GP. Ultrastructural analysis of indwelling catheters: a quantitative relationship between luminal colonization and duration of placement. J Infect Dis. 1993; 168: 400-7.

42. Bouza E, Alvarado N, Alcalá L, Sánchez-Conde M, Pérez MJ, Muñoz P, *et al.* A prospective, randomized, and comparative study of 3 different methods for the diagnosis of intravascular catheter colonization. Clin Infect Dis. 2005; 40: 1096-100.

43. Cleri DJ, Corrado ML, Seligman SJ. Quantitative culture of intravenous catheters and others intravascular inserts. J Infect Dis. 1980; 141: 781-6.

44. Brun-Bruisson C, Abrouk F, Legran P, Huet Y, Larabi S, Rapin M. Diagnosis of central venous catheter-related sepsis. Critical level of quantitative tip cultures. Arch Intern Med. 1987; 147: 873-7.

45. Sherertz RJ, Raad II, Belani A, Koo LC, Rand KH, Pickett DL, *et al.* Three-year experience with sonicated vascular catheter cultures in a clinical microbiology laboratory. J Clin Microbiol. 1990; 28: 76-82.

46. Liñares J, Sitges-Serra A, Garau J, Pérez JL, Martín R. Pathogenesis of catheter sepsis: a prospective study with quantitative and semiquantitative cultures of catheter hub and segments. J Clin Microbiol. 1985; 21: 357-60.

47. Cooper GL, Hopkins CC. Rapid diagnosis of intravascular catheter-associated infection by direct Gram staining of catheter segments. N Engl J Med. 1985; 312: 1142-7.

48. Zufferey J, Rime B, Francioli P, Bille J. Simple method for rapid diagnosis of catheter-associated infection by direct acridine orange staining of catheter tips. J Clin Microbiol. 1988; 26: 175-7.

49. Warwick S, Wilks M, Hennessy E, Powell-Tuck J, Small M, Sharp J, *et al.* Use of quantitative 16S ribosomal DNA detection for diagnosis of central vascular catheter-associated bacterial infection. J Clin Microbiol. 2004; 42: 1402-8.

50. Carbonnelle E, Grohs P, Jacquier H, Day N, Tenza S, Dewailly A, *et al.* Robustness of two MALDI-TOF mass spectrometry systems for bacterial identification. J Microbiol Methods. 2012; 89: 133-6.

Capítulo 5

Epidemiología actual de las infecciones relacionadas con catéteres vasculares

J. Fortún

**Servicio de Enfermedades Infecciosas
Hospital Universitario Ramón y Cajal
Madrid**

Correspondencia:
Dr. Jesús Fortún
fortunabete@gmail.com

Introducción

Son muchos los pacientes hospitalizados que son sometidos a algún tipo de cateterización intravenosa, y en muchas ocasiones esta necesidad supone el criterio de ingreso. Además, la utilización de catéteres vasculares es esencial para el tratamiento de enfermos graves, oncológicos y en hemodiálisis.

La infección es la principal complicación de la cateterización intravascular y constituye la causa más habitual de bacteriemia nosocomial. Ésta se asocia con mucha mayor frecuencia a los catéteres centrales que a los periféricos, y es especialmente relevante en los pacientes ingresados en las unidades de cuidados intensivos (UCI). Aunque habitualmente tiene una baja mortalidad, datos de Estados Unidos estiman la mortalidad atribuible a la bacteriemia asociada a catéter en un 12 % a un 25 %, y un sobrecoste por episodio que oscila entre 3.000 y 50.000 dólares.[1]

Se calcula que cada año, en un país como Estados Unidos, se colocan más de mil millones de dispositivos intravasculares para la administración de fluidos intravenosos, hemoderivados, nutrición parenteral total (NPT) o hemodiálisis.[2]

Son muy numerosos los tipos de catéteres vasculares utilizados. La tabla 1 recoge la descripción detallada de los más empleados en la práctica clínica.

Tipo de catéter	Lugar de inserción	Tamaño	Comentarios
Catéter venoso periférico	Venas de antebrazo o manos	5-7 cm	Flebitis tras uso prolongado Rara vez produce bacteriemia
Catéter arterial periférico	Habitualmente en la arteria radial Puede implantarse en las arterias femoral, axilar, braquial y tibial posterior	5-7 cm	Bajo riesgo de infección Rara vez produce bacteriemia
Catéter intermedio *(midline)*	Vena basílica o cefálica, sin alcanzar las venas centrales	6-20 cm	Menor riesgo de flebitis que con el catéter venoso periférico
Catéter venoso central no tunelizado	Inserción percutánea en una vena central (subclavia, yugular interna o femoral)	>8 cm, según el tamaño del paciente	Causante de la mayoría de las bacteriemias relacionadas con catéteres
Catéter arterial pulmonar	Implantado mediante un introductor de *Teflon®* en una vena central (subclavia, yugular interna o femoral)	>30 cm, según el tamaño del paciente	Habitualmente impregnado de heparina Frecuencia de bacteriemia similar a la del catéter venoso central no tunelizado
Catéter venoso central de inserción periférica	Implantado a través de la vena basílica, cefálica o braquial, accede a la vena cava	>20 cm, según el tamaño del paciente	Frecuencia de bacteriemia inferior a la del catéter venoso central no tunelizado
Catéter venoso central tunelizado (tipo *Hickman®* o *Broviac®*)	Vena subclavia, yugular interna o femoral	>8 cm, según el tamaño del paciente	La vaina almohadillada exterior impide la migración bacteriana periluminal Frecuencia de bacteriemia inferior a la del catéter venoso central no tunelizado
Reservorio subcutáneo totalmente implantable (tipo *Port-a-cath®*)	Implantación completa subcutánea Acceso al reservorio mediante aguja percutánea Implantación en la vena subclavia o yugular interna	>8 cm, según el tamaño del paciente	Las tasas más bajas de bacteriemia Mejor tolerancia cosmética por el paciente
Catéter umbilical	Vena o arteria umbilicales	<6 cm, según el tamaño del paciente	Similar riesgo de bacteriemia en la arteria y la vena umbilicales

Tabla 1. Tipos de catéteres vasculares.

1   Tipos de infecciones asociadas a los catéteres vasculares

Aunque la complicación infecciosa más relevante es la bacteriemia relacionada con el catéter, existen diversas situaciones clínicas asociadas al catéter: la flebitis es la presencia de signos inflamatorios en la vena cateterizada; la infección de la puerta de entrada es la presencia de signos inflamatorios o exudado en los 2 cm de piel circundante a la inserción del catéter; tunelitis es la presencia de eritema o induración de más de 2 cm en el trayecto subcutáneo de un catéter tunelizado (tipo *Hickman®* o *Broviac®*); infección del reservorio es la presencia de signos inflamatorios o exudado en el lecho subcutáneo adyacente al reservorio de los catéteres implantados (tipo *Port-a-cath®*); y con independencia de la presencia de síntomas locales o sistémicos (incluida la bacteriemia), se considera como colonización del catéter el crecimiento significativo de microorganismos en los cultivos (> 15 unidades formadoras de colonias [UFC] en cultivo semicuantitativo o > 100 UFC en cultivo cuantitativo del extremo distal del catéter).[2]

La mayoría de los datos epidemiológicos se centran en los casos de bacteriemia relacionada con un catéter, y existe menos información sobre el resto de las complicaciones infecciosas en ausencia de ésta.[2]

2   Factores de riesgo y estimación de la frecuencia de la bacteriemia relacionada con un catéter

Desde un punto de vista epidemiológico, la unidad más utilizada para estimar la bacteriemia relacionada con el catéter es la densidad de incidencia o tasa de incidencia, que se expresa como el número de casos de bacteriemia por mil días de cateterización.[3] Otro parámetro utilizado con frecuencia es la incidencia acumulada, que es una proporción y se expresa como el número de bacteriemias relacionadas con catéteres por cien pacientes portadores de un catéter vascular.[3]

La mayoría de las bacteriemias relacionadas con el catéter tienen su origen en la zona de inserción, la conexión o ambas.[4] La conexión es la principal fuente de infección en los catéteres de larga duración.[5]

El riesgo de bacteriemia varía según el tipo de catéter, su forma de uso, el lugar de inserción, la experiencia y la sensibilización del equipo clínico que lo utiliza, la frecuencia de administración de fármacos o de otras sustancias a su través, la duración de la cateterización, las características del paciente y las medidas de prevención o profilaxis que se lleven a cabo.[2]

Se ha demostrado que la aplicación combinada de una serie de medidas básicas, como el lavado de manos, el uso de guantes estériles para manipularlo y la utilización de clorhexidina durante la inserción y el mantenimento del catéter, reduce el riesgo de infección.[6] Se dispone de numerosas estrategias para disminuir las complicaciones infecciosas, como la aplicación de programas de formación, la incorporación de diferentes medidas funcionales durante la inserción (denominadas lista de comprobación), la retirada precoz de los catéteres, la sustitución de catéteres multilumen por otros con menos luces, la retirada precoz de las soluciones lipídicas, la protección de las conexiones y la incorporación de antisépticos y de antibióticos a los catéteres vasculares.[6]

En los últimos años se ha observado una especial sensibilización en los centros hospitalarios de todo el mundo hacia el cuidado de la bacteriemia relacionada con catéteres. Peter Pronovost introdujo, en las UCI del estado americano de Michigan, un protocolo basado en el adecuado cumplimiento de una serie de prácticas bien conocidas para el correcto manejo de los catéteres vasculares. En 2003, el estudio llamado *Keystone Initiative* redujo la tasa de incidencia de bacteriemia relacionada con catéteres en las UCI del estado de Michigan, en tres meses, de 2,7 por mil días de cateterización a ninguna.[7] Se estimó que esta iniciativa, que posteriormente se generalizó a otros estados americanos, salvó en 18 meses 1.500 vidas y ahorró 100 millones de dólares. En los últimos años esta estrategia ha tenido una gran implantación en muchos países y ha favorecido diversos proyectos nacionales e internacionales, como el llevado a cabo en España bajo la denominación de *Bacteriemia Zero,* coordinado por la Sociedad Española de Medicina Intensiva, Crítica y Unidades Coronarias (SEMICYUC).[8]

3   Cambios en la epidemiología de los agentes productores de bacteriemia relacionada con catéteres

Los microorganismos que con más frecuencia producen infecciones y bacteriemia relacionadas con catéteres no tunelizados son los estafilococos coagulasa negativos y *Staphylococcus aureus,* que ocasionan las dos terceras partes de los episodios; el resto están producidas por bacilos gramnegativos (10 % a 20 %), *Candida* spp. (5 % a 10 %) y *Enterococcus* spp. (5 % a 10 %), con una muy limitada participación de otros microorganismos.[9]

Según datos de los Centers for Disease Control and Prevention y el Surveillance and Control of Pathogens of Epidemiological Importance de EE.UU., en los últimos años los bacilos gramnegativos son causa de más del 20 % de las bacteriemias relacionadas con catéteres.[9,10] Este incremento epidemiológico de los bacilos gramnegativos también ha sido destacado en otros países, incluido España. Un trabajo realizado en el Hospital Clínic de Barcelona confirmó este progresivo aumento, coincidiendo con el incremento general de la frecuencia de las bacteriemias relacionadas con catéteres, que en dicho centro pasaron de 0,10 episodios por mil días de uso de catéteres en los años 1991-1992 a 0,31 episodios en 2007-2008.[11] La participación de los bacilos gramnegativos en las bacteriemias relacionadas con catéteres pasó del 4,7 % en los años 1991-1992 al 40,2 % en 2007-2008, con el consiguiente descenso de las producidas por bacterias grampositivas. El análisis multivariado relacionó este incremento con los trasplantes de órgano sólido, el uso previo de penicilinas y las estancias hospitalarias de más de once días. Por el contrario, la cirrosis, la diabetes y el uso de quinolonas se asociaron de forma independiente con las bacteriemias relacionadas con catéteres producidas por bacterias grampositivas.[11]

El tratamiento empírico de las bacteriemias relacionadas con catéteres debe cubrir las bacterias grampositivas y, según las recientes guías de práctica clínica, el tratamiento adicional de las bacterias gramnegativas debe reservarse para los pacientes graves, con neutropenia o portadores de catéteres femorales.[2] No está claro si tras el mayor protagonismo que están adquiriendo los bacilos gramnegativos esta estrategia tendrá que ser ampliada.

En los catéteres de implantación quirúrgica y los insertados periféricamente, los agentes que con más frecuencia producen infección son los mismos que en los catéteres centrales no tunelizados. Un problema añadido es la participación de microorganismos resistentes, fundamentalmente en las UCI. En muchos centros, *Staphylococcus aureus* resistente a la meticilina está presente en la mitad de las bacteriemias relacionadas con catéteres detectadas en estas unidades, aunque en los últimos años su incidencia ha descendido como consecuencia de las medidas de control aplicadas.[12] El progresivo aumento de la resistencia a las cefalosporinas de tercera generación en *Klebsiella* spp. y en *Escherichia coli,* y la resistencia a la ceftazidima y los carbapenémicos en *Pseudomonas aeruginosa,* han complicado esta situación.[10] Por último, también se ha producido un incremento porcentual de las cepas de especies de *Candida* diferentes a *C. albicans* que pueden mostrar una tasa más alta de resistencia al fluconazol.

4 Epidemiología de las infecciones relacionadas con catéteres en las unidades de cuidados intensivos

En torno al 80 % de las bacteriemias en los pacientes ingresados en la UCI se relacionan con catéteres vasculares.[13] La bacteriemia, primaria o asociada a un catéter vascular, es la segunda complicación infecciosa adquirida en la UCI después de la neumonía relacionada con la ventilación mecánica.[14] En las UCI americanas se estima que se producen anualmente 180.000 bacteriemias relacionadas con catéteres.[15] Los datos sobre la mortalidad en estos pacientes no son fáciles de obtener, debido a la participación conjunta de otros importantes factores de morbilidad en ellos, pero algunos trabajos la sitúan entre el 12 % y el 17 %.[16,17]

Recientemente se ha publicado un estudio sobre la epidemiología de las bacteriemias primarias y relacionadas con catéteres vasculares que incluyó 46.930 pacientes ingresados durante los años 2005 a 2008 en 120 UCI de más de 100 hospitales españoles.[3] Se utilizó la información incluida en el registro ENVIN-HELICS. Durante el periodo de estudio, 1.415 pacientes (3 %) desarrollaron bacteriemia primaria o asociada a un catéter vascular. La densidad de incidencia disminuyó de 7,49 bacteriemias por mil días de uso del catéter en 2005 a 4,89 en 2008. La tabla 2 recoge los agentes causantes observados en el último año del estudio (2008). Destaca la presencia de bacterias grampositivas,

Nº total de bacteriemias relacionadas con catéteres	446	
Cocos grampositivos	292	65,5%
Staphylococcus epidermidis	103	23,1%
Otros estafilococos coagulasa negativos	85	19,1%
Enterococcus faecalis	35	7,9%
Staphylococcus aureus sensible a meticilina	11	2,5%
Staphylococcus aureus resistente a meticilina	7	1,6%
Enterococcus faecium	4	0,9%
Enterococcus spp.	2	0,5%
Bacilos gramnegativos	123	27,6%
Pseudomonas aeruginosa	22	4,9%
Escherichia coli	18	4,0%
Enterobacter cloacae	14	3,1%
Klebsiella pneumoniae	12	2,7%
Serratia marcescens	12	2,7%
Acinetobacter baumannii	11	2,5%
Proteus mirabilis	6	1,4%
Hongos	27	6,1%
Candida albicans	15	3,4%
Candida parapsilosis	7	1,6%
Otros	4	0,9%

Tabla 2. *Agentes causantes de bacteriemia relacionada con un catéter en pacientes ingresados en 120 unidades de cuidados intensivos españolas en el año 2008.*[3]

en especial de *Staphylococcus epidermidis* y de otros cocos grampositivos, que superan el 60% del total de los patógenos identificados. La presencia de bacilos gramnegativos llegó al 27% de todos los aislados, en especial *P. aeruginosa* (5%). Finalmente, las levaduras, entre las que predominan *C. albicans* y *Candida parapsilosis,* han aumentado hasta suponer aproximadamente el 6% de todos los microorganismos implicados. El estudio de los patrones de multirresistencia de los agentes más prevalentes confirmó que la presencia de *S. epidermidis* y de estafilococos coagulasa negativos resistentes a la meticilina es superior al 80% en todos los años analizados. Se mantuvo una tendencia al descenso de *S. aureus* resistente a la meticilina en los dos últimos años, con una frecuencia inferior al 40%. Por el contrario, no se identificaron estafilococos resistentes a la vancomicina. Entre los bacilos gramnegativos, el 35% de las cepas de *P. aeruginosa* productoras de bacteriemias relacionadas con catéteres fueron resistentes al imipenem y el 50% al ciprofloxacino, y el 70% de las de *Acinetobacter baumannii* fueron resistentes al imipenem.[3]

Un estudio realizado en diferentes UCI en Europa muestra una importante oscilación, desde 1,23 episodios de bacteriemia relacionada con catéteres por mil días de cateterización en Francia hasta 4,2 en Reino Unido.[13] El ministerio de sanidad francés mantiene un sistema de vigilancia nacional de este tipo de infecciones desde 1990, denominado *Réseau d'Alerte, d'Investigation et de Surveillance des Infections Nosocomiales* (RAISIN). En 2001, más de 1.500 hospitales estaban incluidos en el programa.[13,14] Un análisis realizado en 2005, sobre más de 5.000 pacientes ingresados en UCI de 38 centros franceses durante más de 48 horas, estimó una duración media de la cateterización en estos pacientes de 11,7 días y una incidencia de bacteriemia relacionada con ella de 1,23 episodios por mil días de uso del catéter.[15] Otro estudio francés, también realizado en pacientes ingresados en la UCI, halló una incidencia similar de bacteriemia relacionada con catéteres (un episodio por mil días de uso del catéter) y una incidencia de colonización de cinco a seis episodios por mil días de uso del catéter.[16]

En Alemania, los datos epidemiológicos más relevantes sobre bacteriemias relacionadas con catéteres son los obtenidos por el sistema de vigilancia *Krankenhaus-Infektions-Surveillance-Systems* (KISS),[17] que confirman una incidencia en los pacientes ingresados en la UCI de 1,8 episodios por mil días de cateterización en 1997-2002, cifra que se redujo a 1,5 en 2005. En este país, los estudios que han analizado la prolongación de la estancia en la UCI de los pacientes con bacteriemia relacionada con el catéter la estiman en 4,8 a 7,2 días.[18]

En Italia, un estudio iniciado en 2005 por el Gruppo Italiano per la Valutazione Degli Interventi in Terapia Intensiva (GIVITI) confirmó en 2007, en una población de más de 37.000 pacientes ingresados en 124 UCI, una incidencia de bacteriemia relacionada con catéteres de dos episodios por mil días de uso del catéter (intervalo de confianza del 95 % [IC95 %]: 1,9-2,2), con una media de cateterización de 8,6 días.[19] Un estudio realizado por el ministerio de sanidad italiano confirmó una media de prolongación de la estancia en la UCI de los pacientes con bacteriemia relacionada con el catéter de 12,7 días.[20]

En Reino Unido no hay propiamente un sistema de vigilancia de bacteriemias relacionadas con catéteres en las UCI. El estudio más reciente lo realizó el departamento de salud escocés durante 2005 en seis UCI de cinco hospitales.[21] En él, la incidencia de bacteriemia relacionada con un catéter fue de 4,2 episodios por mil días de cateterización (IC95 %: 1,4-9,8), y la permanencia en la UCI de los pacientes con este tipo de bacteriemia se alargó cuatro días.[22]

5 Epidemiología de las infecciones relacionadas con catéteres en los pacientes que reciben nutrición parenteral

La NPT se utiliza como alternativa a la alimentación oral. En la mayoría de las ocasiones es una práctica limitada a un corto período de tiempo, por la imposibilidad de utilizar la alimentación oral o por intolerancia a ésta, lo cual es frecuente en los pacientes hospitalizados tanto en las UCI como en las plantas quirúrgicas. Por el contrario, en un reducido número de pacientes, normalmente con problemas de malabsorción crónica, la NPT es permanente y se lleva a cabo en el domicilio.

Debido a la alta osmolaridad de la NPT, ha de administrarse a través de catéteres venosos centrales. Cuando es domiciliaria, habitualmente se realiza con catéteres tunelizados o de implantación subcutánea.[23] La utilización de catéteres centrales con inserción periférica suele reservarse para los pacientes con NPT limitada a 12-18 meses.[24]

Un hospital de tercer nivel irlandés ha analizado la epidemiología de las bacteriemias relacionadas con catéteres en pacientes con NPT entre los años 1997 y 2008.[25] La densidad de incidencia global de estas bacteriemias en los pacientes que la recibieron fue de 14,4 episodios por mil días de uso del catéter, y su distribución etiológica incluyó estafilococos coagulasa negativos (69,4 %), *S. aureus* sensible a la meticilina (14,4 %), *Candida* spp. (5 %), enterobacterias (5 %), *S. aureus* resistente a la meticilina (3,2 %), bacilos gramnegativos no fermentadores (2,3 %) y enterococos (0,9 %).

La epidemiología de las infecciones y de las bacteriemias relacionadas con catéteres en los pacientes que reciben NPT en el domicilio tiene algunos aspectos diferenciales. Un trabajo revisó 39 estudios publicados en 14 países entre 1970 y 2012,[23] y halló una densidad de incidencia de estas bacteriemias entre 0,38 y 4,58 episodios por mil días de cateterización, con una media de 1,31. Sin embargo, esta densidad varió según la enfermedad de base de los pacientes. En los estudios que incluían más de un 50 % de pacientes con enfermedades benignas, la densidad de incidencia de bacteriemia relacionada con el catéter oscilaba entre 0,19 y 2,41 episodios (media de 0,82) por mil días de uso del catéter; sin embargo, era de 1,9 a 6,8 episodios (media de 2,71) en los que incluían más de un 50 % de pacientes con neoplasias. La distribución de los agentes causantes en el mencionado estudio[23] incluyó bacterias grampositivas (61 %) y gramnegativas (23 %), hongos (8 %), infecciones polimicrobianas (4 %) y otros agentes (4 %).

El análisis de los factores de riesgo de infección en estos pacientes halló una asociación con:

- El tipo de catéteres: el calibre del catéter (> 2 mm),[26] el número de luces (doble luz)[27] y la canalización yugular[26] se asociaron de forma significativa (p < 0,01) con una mayor frecuencia de bacteriemia relacionada con el catéter. La utilización de catéteres centrales de inserción periférica también se asoció con una mayor frecuencia de infección que los otros catéteres centrales.[28] Algunos estudios han comunicado una mayor frecuencia de infección con los catéteres subcutáneos respecto a los tunelizados, pero otros no lo han confirmado.[23] El uso de taurolidina redujo significativamente el riesgo de infección;[29,30] por el contrario, el sellado con heparina produjo más infecciones que la utilización de solución salina o heparina con etanol (p = 0,026).[26]

- El cuidado del catéter y factores educativos: para el mantenimiento del catéter es necesaria una apropiada educación de los pacientes sobre su uso y cuidados. Disponer de personal especializado en los centros que tratan a este tipo de pacientes tiene un impacto beneficioso.[23]

- La enfermedad de base: además del ya mencionado aumento del riesgo en los pacientes con neoplasias, otras situaciones también se asocian a un mayor riesgo de infección, como la enfermedad de Crohn,[31] la utilización de morfina o sedantes,[32] y la existencia de trastornos motores.[33]

6 Epidemiología de las infecciones relacionadas con catéteres en los pacientes con cáncer. Trombosis e infección

La utilización de catéteres centrales de larga duración es frecuente en los pacientes oncológicos, ya que puede mejorar la calidad de vida, reduce la frecuencia de venopunciones y permite la administración de quimioterapia, NPT y otros tratamientos intravenosos.[34]

Un aspecto diferencial de la cateterización de los pacientes con cáncer es la frecuencia de trombosis y la relación de ésta con la infección o la bacteriemia relacionadas con el catéter. Desde el punto de vista patogénico, la trombosis se ha implicado como un paso previo a la infección, por lo que aquellas circunstancias que se han relacionado con un mayor riesgo de trombosis del catéter indirectamente se han relacionado con un riesgo aumentado de infección.

Diversos estudios observacionales han descrito situaciones asociadas a un mayor riesgo de trombosis, pero su carácter retrospectivo y su diseño hacen que muchas de sus conclusiones sean cuestionables. Algunos de los factores asociados con un menor riesgo de trombosis en los pacientes oncológicos portadores de catéteres son la implantación subcutánea (en relación con los catéteres tunelizados y los insertados periféricamente),[35] ser de silicona o poliuretano (frente a los de polietileno o polivinilo),[36] tener una sola luz (comparados con los de varias luces)[37] y el acceso en la yugular o la subclavia (respecto al acceso femoral).[38]

Las estrategias dirigidas a la prevención de la trombosis y de la infección de los catéteres son cuestión de amplio debate. Los sellados con heparina han sido la práctica habitual, pero algunos estudios recientes han cuestionado su eficacia y además la han relacionado con un aumento del riesgo de trombopenia.[39] Diferentes metaanálisis han analizado la eficacia de la profilaxis con anticoagulantes para prevenir la trombosis del catéter en los pacientes con cáncer. En una revisión Cochrane sistemática publicada en 2011, que incluía 12 estudios y 36.000 pacientes con cáncer, el uso de heparina no fraccionada o de heparinas de bajo peso molecular no se asoció a una reducción significativa de la trombosis, a sangrado ni a infección.[40]

7 Epidemiología de las infecciones relacionadas con catéteres venosos periféricos

Está bien aceptado que, en el ámbito hospitalario, los catéteres venosos centrales comportan un mayor riesgo de bacteriemia relacionada con el catéter que los venosos periféricos.[41] Sin embargo, el enorme uso de este tipo de catéteres en la práctica clínica habitual se asocia con un importante incremento del número de flebitis, trombosis y bacteriemias relacionadas con el catéter.[42]

Un estudio realizado en Barcelona entre 2001 y 2003 confirmó que los catéteres venosos periféricos justificaban el 51 % de las bacteriemias relacionadas con catéteres de su hospital, frente al 49 % que produjeron los catéteres venosos centrales. Lo excepcional de este estudio, en relación a otros, es que las densidades de incidencia también fueron similares: 0,19 y 0,18 episodios de bacteriemia relacionada con el catéter por mil días de cateterización, respectivamente. Comparados con los catéteres venosos centrales, los periféricos produjeron bacteriemia con más frecuencia si habían sido colocados en el servicio de urgencias (0 % frente a 42 %), llevaban menos tiempo insertados cuando se desarrolló la bacteriemia (5 frente a 15 días) y se detectó *S. aureus* con más frecuencia (53 % frente a 33 %). Las bacteriemias asociadas a catéteres venosos periféricos producidas por *S. aureus* tuvieron una mayor frecuencia de complicaciones (7 %) y una mayor mortalidad (27 %) que las causadas por otros agentes (0 % y 11 %, respectivamente).[43]

8 Epidemiología de las infecciones relacionadas con catéteres en pacientes sometidos a hemodiálisis

Las infecciones constituyen la segunda causa de muerte en los pacientes sometidos a hemodiálisis.[44,45] Antes de disponer de una fístula venosa, el 80 % de los pacientes son dializados mediante catéteres venosos centrales. La bacteriemia relacionada con el catéter constituye la primera sospecha en caso de fiebre en estos pacientes; sin embargo, otras infecciones no relacionadas con los accesos venosos también son importantes.[45,46]

Un estudio realizado en Alabama, con 500 pacientes en hemodiálisis durante 1,5 años, observó que fue necesaria antibioticoterapia por algún proceso infeccioso en 305 (61 %).[45] Se confirmó una bacteriemia relacionada con el catéter en 184 de las 305 infecciones (60 %). La densidad de incidencia de la infección global fue de 4,6 por mil días de uso del catéter, y la de bacteriemia relacionada con el catéter fue de 3,2 por mil días de uso del catéter. Aproximadamente dos tercios de las infecciones se trataron de manera ambulatoria y el resto requirió ingreso hospitalario. Esta decisión dependió del agente causante, y destaca que precisaron ingreso el 53 % de las bacteriemias relacionadas con catéteres producidas por *S. aureus*. Sin embargo, la necesidad de hospitalización no se asoció a otros factores como la edad (> 65 años), el sexo o la diabetes.

Otro estudio realizado en Israel sobre 433 pacientes, con un seguimiento más largo (9 años) y con mayor tiempo utilizando una fístula venosa, obtuvo resultados muy similares.[46] La densidad de la infección global fue de 5,7 episodios por mil días de uso del catéter. Las infecciones relacionadas con la cateterización supusieron el 20 % del total de los episodios, pero también fueron relevantes las infecciones del pie (19 %), las neumonías (13 %) y otras infecciones de piel y partes blandas (9 %). En este caso, la diabetes sí se asoció a un significativo aumento de las infecciones, pero mayoritariamente en las no relacionadas con la cateterización.[46]

Hay diversas circunstancias que pueden hacer diferente el tratamiento de la bacteriemia relacionada con el catéter en los pacientes en hemodiálisis (véase la tabla 3). En estos pacientes, las bacteriemias debidas al catéter están producidas en su mayoría por estafilococos, con una especial relevancia de *S. aureus,* tanto sensible como resistente a la meticilina.[2] En lo posible, la selección de la antibioticoterapia ha de basarse en aspectos farmacocinéticos que permitan dosificaciones adecuadas tras la diálisis (p. ej., vancomicina, cefazolina o ceftazidima), o que no se modifiquen con ella (p. ej., ceftriaxona). Aunque la mayoría de las bacterias gramnegativas que producen bacteriemia relacionada con el catéter en estos pacientes suelen ser sensibles a los aminoglucósidos, éstos tienen un alto riesgo de ototoxicidad[47] y, por ello, son preferibles las cefalosporinas.

En los pacientes en hemodiálisis que presentan una bacteriemia relacionada con el catéter hay que considerar que, aunque el catéter es la fuente de infección, también es su herramienta terapéutica para realizar la hemodiálisis. El tratamiento antibiótico sistémico aislado se asocia (como en el resto de los pacientes con este tipo de bacteriemia) con un riesgo de recidiva cinco veces mayor que si además se retira el catéter.[48] Si tras instaurar la antibioticoterapia sistémica el paciente permanece afebril y no hay focos metastásicos, el cambio mediante guía tiene una frecuencia de éxito similar a la conseguida con la retirada inmediata y la colocación demorada de un nuevo catéter.[49,50] Las bacteriemias relacionadas con catéteres producidas por estafilococos coagulasa negativos o por bacterias gramnegativas pueden tratarse con éxito con sellado antibiótico durante dos a tres semanas, o con un cambio mediante guía diferido hasta la defervescencia tras 48 horas.[51,52] Sin embargo, estas prácticas no suelen ser eficaces frente a *S. aureus*, para el que se recomienda la retirada inmediata.[51,53]

Según los datos obtenidos en el *United States Renal Data System* (USRDS), la hospitalización por infección de los pacientes en hemodiálisis se incrementó un 34 % entre

- Tratamiento ambulatorio de muchas infecciones.
- Posibilidad de administración de los antibióticos en las sesiones de hemodiálisis.
- Unidades de hemodiálisis a veces geográficamente distantes.
- Resultados microbiológicos y concentraciones de antibióticos demorados debido a la distancia del laboratorio.
- Dificultades logísticas para realizar y procesar los hemocultivos diferenciales.
- Accesos venosos periféricos no disponibles y que pueden invalidar nuevos accesos venosos.
- La retirada del catéter infectado implica una limitación en ausencia de otra vía venosa para la diálisis.
- Preferencia por antibióticos que puedan administrarse durante la diálisis.

Tabla 3. Aspectos diferenciales de las bacteriemias asociadas a catéteres en los pacientes sometidos a hemodiálisis.

los años 1993 y 2006.[54] Aunque en EE.UU. no se conoce el número de bacteriemias relacionadas con catéteres en los pacientes en hemodiálisis, se estima que puede ser próximo a 50.000 por año.[55] En 2006, los ingresos por esta causa fueron 103 por cada mil pacientes en hemodiálisis y año.[54] La incidencia de hospitalizaciones fue mayor que la de las producidas por neumonía (76 ingresos por mil pacientes y año) o celulitis (26 ingresos por mil pacientes y año). Son especialmente destacables las complicaciones asociadas a las bacteriemias relacionadas con catéteres causadas por *S. aureus,* que suelen asociarse a una media de prolongación de la estancia hospitalaria de 9 a 13 días, y algunas series confirman un riesgo de desarrollo de endocarditis o de osteomielitis del 21 % y el 31 %, respectivamente.[56,57] Se ha estimado que el coste medio de un paciente en hemodiálisis con bacteriemia relacionada con el catéter por *S. aureus* es de 24.000 dolares (17.000 dólares para las no complicadas y 32.000 dólares para las complicadas), y que la mortalidad asociada es del 19 %, similar a la comunicada en otras series.[56]

El riesgo de bacteriemia relacionada con el catéter es diferente según el tipo de acceso venoso. En 2006, la *National Healthcare Safety Network* americana comunicó una incidencia de bacteriemia en portadores de catéteres venosos centrales temporales (no tunelizados) de 27,1 episodios por cien pacientes y mes, de 4,2 en los pacientes con catéteres venosos permanentes (tunelizados), de 0,9 en los pacientes con injertos arteriovenosos y de 0,5 en los pacientes con fístulas arteriovenosas.[58] Otro estudio anterior, realizado en diez hospitales americanos, confirmó una incidencia de bacteriemia de 3,5 episodios por cien pacientes y mes en los portadores de catéteres venosos centrales y de 0,13 en los portadores de fístulas o injertos arteriovenosos.[59]

9 Epidemiología de las infecciones relacionadas con catéteres en niños y neonatos

En los niños, la frecuencia de bacteriemia relacionada con el catéter varía según la enfermedad de base, el tipo de catéter, la localización anatómica y el tipo de infusión.[60,61] Entre los prematuros, el riesgo de infección es inversamente proporcional al peso del niño, y es muy alto en aquellos con un peso al nacimiento de 1.000 a 1.500 gramos.[62] La mayoría de las infecciones nosocomiales en los neonatos están relacionadas con la cateterización vascular,[63] y en los ingresados en la UCI la incidencia de bacteriemia relacionada con ella puede ser tan alta como de 18 episodios por mil días de uso del catéter.[64] La mayoría de estas bacteriemias están producidas por estafilococos coagulasa negativos (34 %), seguidos de *S. aureus* (25 %).[65] En los neonatos, los estafilococos coagulasa negativos son causa del 50 % de las bacteriemias relacionadas con catéteres, seguidos de *Candida* spp. (que es especialmente prevalente en este tipo de pacientes),[66] enterococos y bacterias gramnegativas.[67] Es muy alta la participación de bacilos gramnegativos en niños con síndrome del intestino corto.[68] El menor volumen de sangre extraída en los niños y los neonatos hace que el valor predictivo positivo y la sensibilidad de los hemocultivos para el diagnóstico sean menores que en los adultos.

10 Programas de vigilancia multicéntricos para el estudio de las bacteriemias relacionadas con catéteres

La mayoría de los estudios sobre bacteriemias relacionadas con catéteres se centran en poblaciones específicas de pacientes o en determinadas situaciones clínicas, pero también son interesantes otros estudios que analizan las tasas de infección general en una institución y que permiten análisis comparativos entre diferentes hospitales.

Recientemente se han comunicado los datos sobre bacteriemias relacionadas con catéteres del programa VINCat, programa institucional de vigilancia de las infecciones nosocomiales desarrollado en Cataluña.[69,70] Este programa se basa en la vigilancia sistemática y continuada de este tipo de bacteriemias en los centros participantes. La detección de los casos se realiza mediante evaluación diaria de todos los hemocultivos positivos comunicados por los laboratorios de microbiología. Debido a las características del estudio, las tasas de incidencia no se dan por días de cateterización sino por días de hospitalización, lo cual subestima las tasas de bacteriemia relacionada con catéteres porque los pacientes no los portan durante todos los días que permanecen ingresados, pero permite analizar un gran número de episodios en un programa multiinstitucional. En este estudio se analizaron 2.977 episodios de bacteriemia relacionada con catéteres durante los años 2007 a 2010 en 40 hospitales catalanes. La densidad de su incidencia (por mil días de hospitalización) fue de 0,26 episodios, y resultó significativamente mayor en los hospitales de más de 500 camas (0,36 episodios) en comparación con los hospitales de 200 a 500 camas (0,17 episodios) y los de menos de 200 camas (0,09) (véase la tabla 4). Estas diferencias fueron más marcadas en la bacteriemia por un catéter venoso central, que supuso el 75 % de todas las bacteriemias relacionadas con catéteres, frente al 4,7 % en los portadores de un catéter central insertado periféricamente y el 18,8 % en aquellos con catéteres venosos periféricos. En 740 casos (25 %) la bacteriemia se produjo

Tamaño del hospital	Bacteriemia relacionada con catéteres, global (± DE)	Bacteriemia relacionada con catéter venoso central (± DE)	Bacteriemia relacionada con catéter central de inserción periférica (± DE)	Bacteriemia relacionada con catéter venoso periférico (± DE)
500 camas	0,38 ± 0,18	0,29 ± 0,15	0,04 ± 0,03	0,05 ± 0,04
200-500 camas	0,18 ± 1,10	0,14 ± 0,08	0,01 ± 0,01	0,04 ± 0,04
< 200 camas	0,10 ± 0,07	0,05 ± 0,05	0,01 ± 0,03	0,04 ± 0,05
Centros especializados	0,50 ± 0,56	0,32 ± 0,37	0,03 ± 0,04	0,15 ± 0,17

DE: desviación estándar.

Tabla 4. Bacteriemias relacionadas con catéteres (por mil días de hospitalización, según el tamaño del hospital y el tipo de catéter). Estudio VINCat.[70] Años 2007-2010.

en pacientes con NPT. En este subgrupo sí se estimó la bacteriemia relacionada con el catéter por mil días de cateterización, y se halló una tasa de 1,57 episodios por mil días de cateterización. El 34 % de las bacteriemias relacionadas con catéteres ocurrieron en la UCI, el 36 % en plantas de hospitalización médica y el 30 % en plantas quirúrgicas. La distribución por agentes fue similar a la de otras series: estafilococos coagulasa negativos (50 %), *S. aureus* (22 %), grupo *Klebsiella/Enterobacter/Serratia* (18 %), *Candida* spp. (8 %), *P. aeruginosa* (7 %) y miscelánea (10 %).

La vigilancia de las bacteriemias relacionadas con catéteres desempeña un papel muy importante en los programas de control de la infección hospitalaria, tanto en los que se realizan en una sola institución como en los multicéntricos. Este tipo de programas permite disponer de valores estándar y posibilita la implantación de estrategias de intervención dirigidas a reducir y prevenir las infecciones nosocomiales.

Bibliografía

1. Raad I, Hanna H, Maki D. Intravascular catheter-related infections: advances in diagnosis, prevention, and management. Lancet Infect Dis. 2007; 7: 645-57.

2. Mermel LA, Allon M, Bouza E, Craven DE, Flynn P, O'Grady NP, et al. Clinical practice guidelines for the diagnosis and management of intravascular catheter-related infection: 2009 update by the Infectious Diseases Society of America. Clin Infect Dis. 2009; 49: 1-45.

3. Álvarez Lerma F, Olaechea Astigarraga P, Palomar Martínez M, Insausti Ordeñana J, López Pueyo MJ; Grupo de Estudio ENVIN--HELICS. Epidemiología de las bacteriemias primarias y relacionadas con catéteres vasculares en pacientes críticos ingresados en servicios de medicina intensiva. Med Intensiva. 2010; 34: 437-45.

4. Maki DG, Stolz SM, Wheeler S, Mermel LA. Prevention of central venous catheter-related bloodstream infection by use of an antiseptic impregnated catheter: a randomized, controlled trial. Ann Intern Med. 1997; 127: 257-66.

5. Raad I, Costerton W, Sabharwal U, Sacilowski M, Anaissie E, Bodey GP. Ultrastructural analysis of indwelling vascular catheters: a quantitative relationship between luminal colonization and duration of placement. J Infect Dis. 1993; 168: 400-7.

6. O'Grady NP, Alexander M, Burns LA, Dellinger EP, Garland J, Heard SO, et al.; Healthcare Infection Control Practices Advisory Committee (HICPAC). Guidelines for the prevention of intravascular catheter-related infections. Clin Infect Dis. 2011; 52: e162-93.

7. Pronovost P, Needham D, Berenholtz S, Sinopoli D, Chu H, Cosgrove S, et al. An intervention to decrease catheter-related bloodstream infections in the ICU. N Engl J Med. 2006; 355: 2725-32.

8. Módulo de formación Bacteriemia Zero. Disponible en: http: //hws.vhebron.net/formacion-BZero/index.html

9. Wisplinghoff H, Bischoff T, Tallent SM, Seifert H, Wenzel RP, Edmond MB. Nosocomial bloodstream infections in US hospitals: analysis of 24,179 cases from a prospective nationwide surveillance study. Clin Infect Dis. 2004; 39: 309-17.

10. Gaynes R, Edwards JR. Overview of nosocomial infections caused by Gram-negative bacilli. Clin Infect Dis. 2005; 41: 848-54.

11. Marcos M, Soriano A, Iñurrieta A, Martínez JA, Romero A, Cobos N, et al. Changing epidemiology of central venous catheter-related bloodstream infections: increasing prevalence of Gram-negative pathogens. J Antimicrob Chemother. 2011; 66: 2119-25.

12. Burton DC, Edwards JR, Horan TC, Jernigan JA, Fridkin SK. Methicillin-resistant Staphylococcus aureus central line-associated bloodstream infections in US intensive care units, 1997–2007. JAMA. 2009; 301: 727-36.

13. Tacconelli E, Smith G, Hieke K, Lafuma A, Bastide P. Epidemiology, medical outcomes and costs of catheter-related bloodstream infections in intensive care units of four European countries: literature and registry-based estimates. J Hosp Infect. 2009; 72: 97-103.

14. National Nosocomial Infections Surveillance (NNIS) System Report, data summary from January 1992 through June 2004, issued October 2004. Am J Infect Control. 2004; 32: 470-85.

15. Mermel LA. Prevention of intravascular catheter-related infections. Ann Intern Med. 2000; 132: 391-402.

16. Endimiani A, Tamborini A, Luzzaro F, Lombardi G, Toniolo A. A two-year analysis of risk factors and outcome in patients with bloodstream infection. Jpn J Infect Dis. 2003; 56: e1-e7.

17. Orsi GB, Di Stefano L, Noah N. Hospital-acquired, laboratory-confirmed bloodstream infection: increased hospital stay and direct costs. Infect Control Hosp Epidemiol. 2002; 23: e190-e197.

14. RAISIN, Réseau d'Alerte, d'Investigation et de Surveillance des Infections Nosocomiales. Enquete de Prevalence Nationale 2001 Resultats. Saint Maurice: Institut National de Veille Sanitaire; 2003. p. 1-40.

15. Hospital in Europe Link for Infection Control through Surveillance. Surveillance of nosocomial infections in intensive care units, protocol, version 6.1. Lyon, France: HELICS; 2004. p. 1-52.

16. Merrer J. Epidemiology of catheter-related infections in intensive care unit. Ann Fr Anesth Reanim. 2005; 24: 278-81.

17. KISS, Krankenhaus-Infektions-Surveillance-System. Modul ITS-KISS Referenzdaten Berechnungszeitraum: Januar 1997 bis Juni 2005. Berlin: Nationales Referenzzentrum für Surveillance von Nosokomialen Infektionen; 2005. p. 1-9.

18. Gastmeier P, Weist K, Ruden H. Catheter--associated primary bloodstream infections: epidemiology and preventive methods. Infection. 1999; 27(Suppl. 1): S1-S6.

19. GiViTI, Gruppo italiano per la Valutazione degli interventi in Terapia Intensiva. Rapporto Petalo Sorveglianza Infezioni anno 2007. Milano: Istituto Mario Negri; 2007. p. 1-16.

20. Ministero della Salute. Servizio Informativo Sanitario e Dipartimento della Programmazione. Schede di Dimissione Ospedaliera e anno 2003; Ministero della Salute. Roma: Servizio Informativo Sanitario; 2005.

21. Scottish Executive Health Department. Surveillance of intensive care unit associated infection. Pilot report. Glasgow: Health Protection Scotland; 2005. p. 1-30.

22. Plowman R, Graves N, Griffin MAS, Roberts JA, Swan AV, Cookson B, *et al.* The rate and cost of hospital acquired infections occurring in patients admitted to selected specialities of a district general hospital in England and the national burden imposed. J Hosp Infect. 2001; 47: 198-209.

23. Dreesen M, Foulon V, Spriet I, Goossens GA, Hiele M, De Pourcq L, *et al.* Epidemiology of catheter-related infections in adult patients receiving home parenteral nutrition: a systematic review. Clin Nutr. 2013; 32: 16-26.

24. Gillanders L, Angstmann K, Ball P, Chapman-Kiddell C, Hardy G, Hope J, *et al.* Australasian Society of Parenteral and Enteral Nutrition. AuSPEN clinical practice guidelines for home parenteral nutrition patients in Australia and New Zealand. Nutrition. 2008; 24: e988-1012.

25. Collins CJ, Fraher MH, Bourke J, Phelan D, Lynch M. Epidemiology of catheter-related bloodstream infections in patients receiving total parenteral nutrition. Clin Infect Dis. 2009; 49: 1769-70.

26. Bozzetti F, Mariani L, Bertinet DB, Chiavenna G, Crose N, De Cicco M, *et al.* Central venous catheter complications in 447 patients on home parenteral nutrition: an analysis over 100.000 catheter days. Clin Nutr. 2002; 21: e475-85.

27. Raman M, Gramlich L, Whittaker S, Allard JP. Canadian home total parenteral nutrition registry: preliminary data on the patient population. Can J Gastroenterol. 2007; 21: e643-8.

28. Delegge MH, Borak G, Moore N. Central venous access in the home parenteral nutrition population-you PICC. J Parenter Enteral Nutr. 2005; 29: e425-8.

29. Bisseling TM, Willems MC, Versleijen MW, Hendriks JC, Vissers RK, Wanten GJ. Taurolidine lock is higly effective in preventing catheter-related bloodstream infections in patients on home parenteral nutrition: a heparin-controlled prospective study. Clin Nutr. 2010; 29: e464-8.

30. Touré A, Lauverjat M, Peraldi C, Boncompain-Gerard M, Gelas P, Barnoud D, *et al*. Taurolidine lock solution in the secondary prevention of central venous catheter-associated bloodstream infection in home parenteral nutrition patients. Clin Nutr. 2012; 31: 567-70.

31. O'Keefe SJ, Burners JU, Thompson RL. Recurrent sepsis in home parenteral nutrition patients: an analysis of risk factors. J Parenter Enteral Nutr. 1994; 18: e256-63.

32. Richards DM, Scott NA, Shaffer JL, Irving M. Opiate and sedative dependence predicts a poor outcome for patients receiving home parenteral nutrition. J Parenter Enteral Nutr. 1997; 21: e336-8.

33. Reimund JM, Arondel Y, Finck G, Zimmermann F, Duclos B, Baumann R. Catheter--related infection in patients on home parenteral nutrition: results of a prospective study. Clin Nutr. 2002; 21: e33-8.

34. Lee AY, Kamphuisen PW. Epidemiology and prevention of catheter-related thrombosis in patients with cancer. J Thromb Haemost. 2012; 10: 1491-9.

35. Saber W, Moua T, Williams EC, Verso M, Agnelli G, Couban S, *et al*. Risk factors for catheter-related thrombosis (CRT) in cancer patients: a patient-level data (IPD) meta-analysis of clinical trials and prospective studies. J Thromb Haemost. 2011; 9: 312-9.

36. Gallieni M, Pittiruti M, Biffi R. Vascular access in oncology patients. CA Cancer J Clin. 2008; 58: 323-46.

37. Evans RS, Sharp JH, Linford LH, Lloyd JF, Tripp JS, Jones JP, *et al*. Risk of symptomatic DVT associated with peripherally inserted central catheters. Chest. 2010; 138: 803-10.

38. Hamilton HC, Foxcroft DR. Central venous access sites for the prevention of venous thrombosis, stenosis and infection in patients requiring long-term intravenous therapy. Cochrane Database Syst Rev. 2007; (3): CD004084.

39. Schallom ME, Prentice D, Sona C, Micek ST, Skrupky LP. Heparin or 0.9 % sodium chloride to maintain central venous catheter patency: a randomized trial. Crit Care Med. 2012; 40: 1820-6.

40. Akl EA, Vasireddi SR, Gunukula S, Yosuico VE, Barba M, Sperati F, *et al*. Anticoagulation for patients with cancer and central venous catheters. Cochrane Database Syst Rev. 2011; (4): CD006468.

41. Vomberg RP, Behnke M, Geffers C, Sohr D, Ruden H, Dettenkofer M, *et al*. Device-associated infection rates for non-intensive care unit patients. Infect Control Hosp Epidemiol. 2006; 27: e357-61.

42. Tagalakis V, Kahn SR, Libman M, Blostein M. The epidemiology of peripheral vein infusion thrombophlebitis: a critical review. Am J Med. 2002; 113: e146-51.

43. Pujol M, Hornero A, Saballs M, Argerich MJ, Verdaguer R, Cisnal M, *et al*. Clinical epidemiology and outcomes of peripheral venous catheter-related bloodstream infections at a university-affiliated hospital. J Hosp Infect. 2007; 67: 22-9.

44. Allon M, Depner TA, Radeva M, Bailey J, Beddhu S, Butterly D, *et al*.; HEMO Study Group. Impact of dialysis dose and membrane on infection-related hospitalization and death: results of the HEMO Study. J Am Soc Nephrol. 2003; 14: 1863-70.

45. Allon M, Radeva M, Bailey J, Beddhu S, Butterly D, Coyne DW, *et al*.; HEMO Study Group. The spectrum of infection-related morbidity in hospitalized haemodialysis patients. Nephrol Dial Transplant. 2005; 20: 1180-6.

46. Berman SJ, Johnson EW, Nakatsu C, Alkan M, Chen R, LeDuc J. Burden of infection in patients with end-stage renal disease requiring long-term dialysis. Clin Infect Dis. 2004; 39: 1747-53.

47. Ali MZ, Goetz MB. A meta-analysis of the relative efficacy and toxicity of single daily dosing versus multiple daily dosing of aminoglycosides. Clin Infect Dis. 1997; 24: 796-809.

48. Mokrzycki MH, Zhang M, Cohen H, Golestaneh L, Laut JM, Rosenberg SO. Tunnelled haemodialysis catheter bacteraemia: risk factors for bacteraemia recurrence, infectious complications and mortality. Nephrol Dial Transplant. 2006; 21: 1024-31.

49. Tanriover B, Carlton D, Saddekni S, Hamrick K, Oser R, Westfall AO, *et al*. Bacteremia associated with tunneled dialysis catheters: comparison of two treatment strategies. Kidney Int. 2000; 57: 2151-5.

50. Beathard GA. Management of bacteremia associated with tunnelled cuffed hemodialysis catheters. J Am Soc Nephrol. 1999; 10: 1045-9.

51. Fernández-Hidalgo N, Almirante B, Calleja R, Ruiz I, Planes AM, Rodríguez D, *et al*.

Antibiotic-lock therapy for long-term intravascular catheter-related bacteraemia: results of an open, non-comparative study. J Antimicrob Chemother. 2006; 57: 1172-80.

52. Fortún J, Grill F, Martín-Dávila P, Blázquez J, Tato M, Sánchez-Corral J, *et al.* Treatment of long-term intravascular catheter-related bacteraemia with antibiotic-lock therapy. J Antimicrob Chemother. 2006; 58: 816-21.

53. Maya ID, Carlton D, Estrada E, Allon M. Treatment of dialysis catheter-related Staphylococcus aureus bacteremia with an antibiotic lock: a quality improvement report. Am J Kidney Dis. 2007; 50: 289-95.

54. US Renal Data System. USRDS 2008 annual data report: atlas of chronic kidney disease and end-stage renal disease in the United States. Bethesda, MD: National Institutes of Health, National Institute of Diabetes and Digestive and Kidney Diseases; 2008.

55. Tokars JI. Bloodstream infections in hemodialysis patients: getting some deserved attention. Infect Control Hosp Epidemiol. 2002; 23: 713-5.

56. Li Y, Friedman JY, O'Neal BF, Hohenboken MJ, Griffiths RI, Stryjewski ME, *et al.* Outcomes of Staphylococcus aureus infection in hemodialysis-dependent patients. Clin J Am Soc Nephrol. 2009; 4: 428-34.

57. Patel PR, Kallen AJ, Arduino MJ. Epidemiology, surveillance, and prevention of bloodstream infections in hemodialysis patients. Am J Kidney Dis. 2010; 56: 566-77.

58. Klevens RM, Edwards JR, Andrus ML, Peterson KD, Dudeck TC, Horan TC. Dialysis surveillance report: National Healthcare Safety Network - data summary for 2006. Semin Dial. 2008; 21: 24-8.

59. Dopirak M, Hill C, Oleksiw M, Dumigan D, Arvai J, English E, *et al.* Surveillance of hemodialysis-associated primary bloodstream infections: the experience of ten hospital-based centers. Infect Control Hosp Epidemiol. 2002; 23: 721-4.

60. Baltimore RS. Neonatal nosocomial infections. Semin Perinatol. 1998; 22: 25-32.

61. Almuneef MA, Memish ZA, Balkhy HH, Hijazi O, Cunningham G, Francis C. Rate, risk factors and outcomes of catheter-related bloodstream infection in a paediatric intensive care unit in Saudi Arabia. J Hosp Infect. 2006; 62: 207-13.

62. Gilad J, Borer A. Prevention of catheter-related bloodstream infections in the neonatal intensive care setting. Expert Rev Anti Infect Ther. 2006; 4: 861-73.

63. Jarvis WR, Edwards JR, Culver DH, Hughes JM, Horan T, Emori TG, *et al.* Nosocomial infection rates in adult and pediatric intensive care units in the United States. National Nosocomial Infections Surveillance System. Am J Med. 1991; 91: 185S-91S.

64. Garland JS, Alex CP, Henrickson KJ, McAuliffe TL, Maki DG. A vancomycin-heparin lock solution for prevention of nosocomial bloodstream infection in critically ill neonates with peripherally inserted central venous catheters: a prospective, randomized trial. Pediatrics. 2005; 116: e198-205.

65. Wiener ES, McGuire P, Stolar CJ, Rich RH, Albo VC, Ablin AR, *et al.* The CCSG prospective study of venous access devices: an analysis of insertions and causes for removal. J Pediatr Surg. 1992; 27: 155-63.

66. Almirante B, Rodríguez D, Cuenca-Estrella M, Almela M, Sánchez F, Ayats J, *et al.* Epidemiology, risk factors, and prognosis of Candida parapsilosis bloodstream infections: case-control population-based surveillance study of patients in Barcelona, Spain, from 2002 to 2003. J Clin Microbiol. 2006; 44: 1681-5.

67. Gaynes RP, Edwards JR, Jarvis WR, Culver DH, Tolson JS, Martone WJ. Nosocomial infections among neonates in high-risk nurseries in the United States. National Nosocomial Infections Surveillance System. Pediatrics. 1996; 98: 357-61.

68. Piedra PA, Dryja DM, LaScolea LJ, Jr. Incidence of catheter-associated Gram-negative bacteremia in children with short bowel syndrome. J Clin Microbiol. 1989; 27: 1317-9.

69. Almirante B, Limón E, Freixas N, Gudiol F; VINCat Program. Laboratory-based surveillance of hospital-acquired catheter-related bloodstream infections in Catalonia. Results of the VINCat Program (2007-2010). Enferm Infecc Microbiol Clin. 2012; 30(Suppl 3): 13-9.

70. Freixas N, Bella F, Limón E, Pujol M, Almirante B, Gudiol F. Impact of a multimodal intervention to reduce bloodstream infections related to vascular catheters in non-ICU wards: a multicentre study. Clin Microbiol Infect. 2012 Sep 20. doi: 10.1111/1469-0691.12049.

Capítulo 6

Clínica y complicaciones, locales y sistémicas, de las infecciones relacionadas con catéteres vasculares

M. Montero Alonso, M. Salavert Lletí

**Unidad de Enfermedades Infecciosas
Hospital Universitario y Politécnico La Fe
Valencia**

Correspondencia:
Dr. Miguel Salavert Lletí
salavert_mig@gva.es

Introducción

Los dispositivos de acceso vascular y los catéteres o cánulas intravasculares se utilizan cada vez más en el medio sanitario para la administración de fluidos, fármacos, nutrición, productos sanguíneos y hemoderivados, y para la monitorización hemodinámica y la hemodiálisis. Constituyen también una forma viable de mantener un tratamiento sistémico en los pacientes atendidos por unidades de hospitalización domiciliaria, en hospitales de día y en residencias de enfermos crónicos o de larga estancia. Gracias a ellos se consiguen muchos de los objetivos terapéuticos y un manejo adecuado del control y la prevención de todo tipo de enfermedades. Sin embargo, su uso no está exento de posibles incidentes, y se considera que más de un 15 % de los pacientes en quienes se implantan catéteres vasculares pueden sufrir complicaciones de algún tipo. Entre ellas destacan las de tipo mecánico (que ocurren en un 5-20 % de los casos e incluyen punción arterial, hematomas, hemotórax y neumotórax), las de tipo trombótico (2-26 %) y las de origen infeccioso (5-26 %).[1]

La bacteriemia relacionada con catéteres vasculares ha llegado a ser la principal causa de bacteriemia nosocomial, además de asociarse a una morbimortalidad importante, a un incremento en la duración de la estancia hospitalaria y, por ello, a un aumento de los costes sanitarios.[2,3] Aproximadamente tres de cada mil pacientes ingresados en el hospital padecerán una bacteriemia, y en casi un tercio de ellos será secundaria a una infección relacionada con un catéter vascular.[4]

En este capítulo se describen las principales manifestaciones clínicas que pueden aparecer y derivarse de las infecciones relacionadas con catéteres vasculares, y en especial las complicaciones, tanto locales como generalizadas, debidas a la propia colonización del dispositivo.

1   Definiciones de las infecciones asociadas a catéteres vasculares y sus complicaciones

Las complicaciones infecciosas de los catéteres vasculares pueden establecerse de forma locorregional o alcanzar una mayor extensión, o manifestarse a distancia del foco original (extravascular o intravascular) con carácter sistémico. No en pocas ocasiones coexisten manifestaciones locales y sistémicas. Las complicaciones locales ocurren en ausencia de una aparente bacteriemia, pueden estar asociadas al propio catéter y han sido definidas, entre otros organismos, por los Centers for Disease Control and Prevention de EE.UU.[5] Entre las definiciones para ambos tipos de complicaciones se incluyen las siguientes:

- Catéter colonizado: crecimiento de más de 15 unidades formadoras de colonias (UFC) en el cultivo semicuantitativo, o de más de 1.000 UFC en el cultivo con métodos cuantitativos, del segmento proximal o distal del catéter en ausencia de síntomas o signos clínicos acompañantes, y con hemocultivos de sangre extraída de una vía venosa periférica negativos.
- Flebitis: signos inflamatorios, no siempre de origen infeccioso, en una porción corta y limitada del trayecto vascular o alrededor del orificio de salida del catéter de implantación venosa.
- Infección del orificio o lugar de entrada: eritema, dolor, tumefacción o induración de carácter inflamatorio hasta en los dos últimos centímetros de piel y de tejidos blandos circundantes al punto de entrada del catéter vascular, que pueden asociarse a otros signos y síntomas de infección, como fiebre, exudación o supuración por el punto de entrada o salida del catéter, con o sin evidencia de bacteriemia acompañante.
- Infección del túnel subcutáneo o «tunelitis»: inflamación, eritema o induración de más de dos centímetros de diámetro en el orificio de entrada del catéter vascular y que sigue el trayecto subcutáneo de un catéter tunelizado, en ausencia de hemocultivos positivos.
- Infección de la bolsa del dispositivo o reservorio: infección del hueco o lecho subcutáneo de un dispositivo de implantación intravascular (p. ej., *Port-a-Cath*®), con frecuencia asociada a inflamación, eritema o induración del tejido de la bolsa. Pueden producirse una rotura espontánea y drenaje exudativo o francamente purulento, o bien necrosis de la piel que lo recubre. Puede ocurrir con o sin bacteriemia asociada.

- Bacteriemia relacionada con el catéter vascular: detección del mismo microorganismo (género, especie y antibiotipo) en el cultivo de la punta del catéter y al menos en un hemocultivo de sangre extraída de una vía vascular periférica, preferentemente por venopunción directa, en un paciente con semiología de bacteriemia y siempre que se excluyan otro diagnóstico etiológico alternativo a la bacteriemia y otro foco de origen. En ausencia de cultivo del catéter vascular o de confirmación microbiológica, como evidencia indirecta puede considerarse también el diagnóstico de «probable» bacteriemia relacionada con un catéter cuando el cuadro clínico desaparece en las 48 horas siguientes a la retirada del catéter.
- Bacteriemia relacionada con la infusión: crecimiento del mismo microorganismo en el líquido de infusión y en los hemocultivos de sangre obtenida por venopunción directa, sin otra fuente evidente de infección.
- Tromboflebitis séptica: infección del endotelio vascular y del trombo formado alrededor del catéter vascular con extensión por la vena canalizada. La bacteriemia o la fungemia se mantienen casi siempre aunque se retire el catéter.
- Complicaciones a distancia: implantaciones de inóculos microbianos infectantes en otros territorios distantes, por desprendimiento de porciones o fragmentos del foco de origen infeccioso relacionado con un catéter vascular y la consiguiente diseminación en forma de metástasis sépticas, que pueden dar lugar, entre otros, a procesos como endocarditis, abscesos micóticos vasculares cerebrales, endoftalmitis, neumonías nodulares cavitarias, implantes cutáneos y subcutáneos, artritis u osteomielitis.

Las infecciones relacionadas con catéteres vasculares reciben la categoría de verdaderamente complicadas si provocan fenómenos supurativos locales o tromboflebitis séptica, o complicaciones hematógenas a distancia (principalmente endocarditis, artritis séptica y espondilodiscitis).[6]

2   Fisiopatogenia de las complicaciones infecciosas locales y sistémicas

La infección relacionada con el uso de un catéter vascular se produce por uno de los siguientes cuatro mecanismos:

1) Por vía extraluminal, desde la piel y a través de la superficie externa del catéter, que es el origen más frecuente de la infección, sobre todo en los catéteres de corta duración (media de 7 a 9 días).[7-10] Los microorganismos que alcanzan la punta del catéter suelen proceder de la piel del paciente, pero también pueden llegar desde las manos del personal sanitario o desde elementos del entorno del paciente.
2) Por vía intraluminal, desde la conexión, debido a la contaminación existente entre el equipo de infusión y el catéter, en relación con su manipulación. Es una vía de

infección fundamental en las cateterizaciones prolongadas, sobre todo si están tunelizadas. Se asocia a bacteriemia con mayor frecuencia que la vía extraluminal.[10-14]

3) Por contaminación del líquido de infusión, que a su vez puede ser intrínseca, en el momento de su manufacturación (excepcional en la actualidad por las estrictas medidas de control durante la fabricación), o extrínseca, sobre todo por manipulación de sus componentes con diseminación endoluminal, y la conexión está contaminada en la mayoría de los casos.[13,15,16]

4) Por siembra hematógena, a partir de un foco séptico distante.[13]

Cabe mencionar una serie de importantes determinantes patogénicos de las infecciones asociadas a catéteres vasculares:

- Material con que está fabricado el dispositivo: los catéteres de silicona son los que presentan menor adherencia bacteriana; los de cloruro de polivinilo y polietileno ofrecen una mayor facilidad a la adhesión bacteriana que los de teflón, de elastómeros de silicona o de poliuretano.[17]
- Factores del huésped: ante la presencia del catéter se genera una biocapa rica en fibrina y fibronectina, sustancias muy adherentes para *Staphylococcus aureus* y *Candida* spp. Ambos producen coagulasas y se benefician del proceso de trombogénesis generado alrededor del catéter, adhiriéndose firmemente a la monocapa.[17]
- Factores de virulencia del microorganismo: la adhesión se mejora mediante la producción, por algunos microorganismos como los estafilococos coagulasa negativos, *S. aureus*, *Pseudomonas aeruginosa* y algunas especies de *Candida,* de una sustancia polimérica extracelular que forma una biopelícula microbiana.[18-21]
- Lugar de cateterización: se correlaciona con el microorganismo implicado en la infección. Así, *Staphylococcus* spp. son los más frecuentes en todas las localizaciones, fundamentalmente los coagulasa negativos, y los bacilos gramnegativos y las levaduras son causa de menos del 10 % de las infecciones de catéteres de vena subclavia o yugular, mientras que en los catéteres femorales alcanzan en algunas series el 39 % y el 17 %, respectivamente.[22]

3   Clínica: manifestaciones generales y propias de las complicaciones

Las manifestaciones clínicas de las infecciones relacionadas con catéteres vasculares pueden variar desde locales o locorregionales hasta formas sistémicas inespecíficas, sólo con fiebre, o más específicas, con bacteriemia que puede cumplir o no criterios de sepsis grave o de *shock* séptico.[2] En este apartado se describen con mayor amplitud, con el fin de dimensionar clínicamente cada una de ellas, algunas de las definiciones que antes se han enunciado (véase la tabla 1). El riesgo de complicaciones graves es mayor con determinados microorganismos, como *S. aureus*, *P. aeruginosa* y *Candida* spp., o con las infecciones polimicrobianas, y la

Locales o locorregionales	Generales	Sistémicas/a distancia
Infección del orificio de entrada	Fiebre	Endocarditis
Infección del túnel subcutáneo (tunelitis)	Quebrantamiento, malestar general	Embolias sépticas (endovasculares o viscerales y parenquimatosas: pulmonares, renales, etc.)
Infección del bolsillo del reservorio	Escalofríos	Osteomielitis/artritis
Flebitis	Estado de sepsis grave/*shock* séptico	Meningitis, abscesos del sistema nervioso central, aneurismas «micóticos»
Pseudoaneurismas		Abscesos hepatoesplénicos
Tromboflebitis séptica*		Piomiositis
		Endoftalmitis

*La tromboflebitis séptica puede considerarse una complicación tanto local como sistémica, dependiendo de la intensidad y la extensión de su forma de presentación y de las manifestaciones asociadas.

Tabla 1. Clasificación de las manifestaciones clínicas y de las complicaciones de las infecciones relacionadas con catéteres vasculares.

mayoría de las series y experiencias se refieren a catéteres vasculares de larga duración y en poblaciones seleccionadas de pacientes (graves, inmunosuprimidos o receptores de trasplantes).

3.1   Fiebre

Es uno de los síntomas o signos clínicos más frecuentes, asociada o no a escalofríos, como manifestación aislada o junto a clínica de síndrome tóxico o séptico, que supone la presencia de dos o más de los siguientes hallazgos: temperatura $> 38\,^{\circ}C$ o $< 36\,^{\circ}C$, frecuencia cardíaca > 90 latidos por minuto, frecuencia respiratoria > 20 respiraciones por minuto o $PaCO_2 < 32\,mmHg$, más de 12.000 o menos de 4.000 leucocitos por mililitro o $> 10\,\%$ de formas inmaduras sin foco aparente.[23,24]

3.2   Complicaciones locales

3.2.1   Infección localizada en el punto de inserción del catéter

Se caracteriza por la presencia de eritema, induración, edema, inflamación o sensibilidad aumentada, incluso con dolor, en un área menor de 2 cm desde la salida del catéter (véase la figura 1). También puede asociarse a otros signos y síntomas de infección, incluso con fiebre, bacteriemia y secreción purulenta por el punto de entrada. No obstante, no suele acompañarse de síntomas generales. Su frecuencia se ha estimado en un 7 % a un 35 %, según los autores, y suele aparecer entre los días primero y décimo de implantación del catéter.[25,26] Microbiológicamente cursará con o sin crecimiento de microorganismos en el exudado de la zona, y los hemocultivos pueden ser positivos. En el desarrollo de infección en el punto de inserción desempeña un papel relevante la sujeción del catéter, el calibre de éste, el tipo de apósito y los cuidados seguidos en las curas. Las causas más habituales de infección del orificio o sitio de salida son el cuidado deficiente del punto de entrada del catéter vascular y la técnica inadecuada en el cambio de los apósitos. Un catéter fijado de manera incorrecta y con un diámetro grande produce una gran lesión traumática cutánea que puede ser más fácilmente colonizada por los microorganismos presentes en la piel, acumulados bajo los apósitos. El tratamiento consiste en general en mejorar el cuidado y las prácticas de higiene y mantenimiento del sitio de salida, la administración de antibióticos o la retirada del catéter. Las infecciones en el sitio de salida pueden prevenirse evaluando esta zona con frecuencia, cuidándola adecuadamente y usando antisépticos para reducir el número de microorganismos en la piel.[27,28] Suelen solucionarse con la retirada del catéter y curas locales. En caso de catéteres vasculares de larga duración, pueden resolverse con tratamiento tópico. Sin embargo, la presencia de exudado purulento, sobre todo cuando se asocia a fiebre, requiere la retirada del catéter y a veces hasta una incisión local y antibioticoterapia adaptada si hay celulitis local asociada.

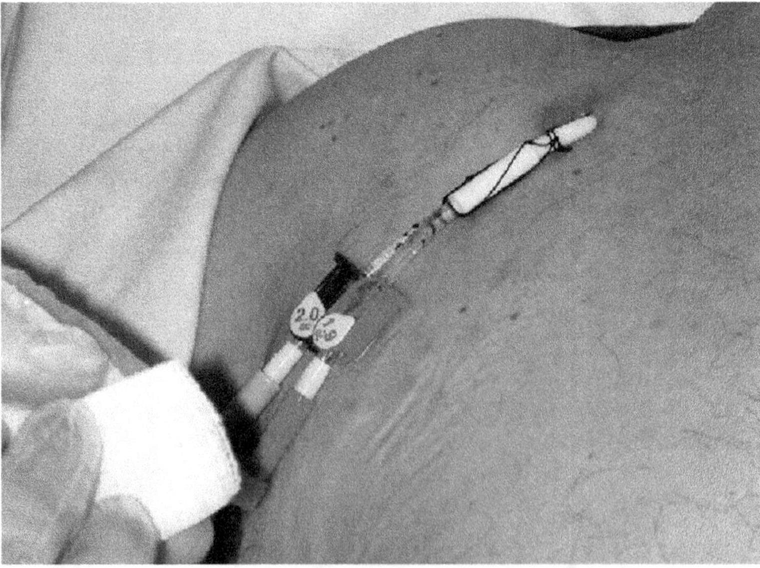

Figura 1. Eritema subcutáneo circundante al orificio de entrada de un catéter de Hickman® *en un episodio de infección local por* Staphylococcus aureus *en un paciente hematológico con leucemia aguda.*

3.2.2　*Infección del trayecto subcutáneo (túnel) del catéter o tunelitis*

Se caracteriza por inflamación, dolor, eritema o induración a más de 2 cm desde la salida de un catéter tunelizado (*Hickman®*, *Broviac®* o de hemodiálisis), es decir, del trayecto subcutáneo, con o sin infección concomitante del torrente sanguíneo, con o sin exudado purulento a la salida del túnel. Supone en torno a un 10 % del total de las infecciones relacionadas con catéteres vasculares y clínicamente resulta muy evidente por la presencia de un cordón enrojecido y doloroso a lo largo del trayecto subcutáneo del vaso sanguíneo. Con frecuencia obliga a retirar el catéter tunelizado, por el deficiente acceso de los antibióticos a la fascia y los tejidos circundantes. Debido al deficiente flujo sanguíneo de la fascia, los antibióticos no suelen erradicar la infección del túnel,[29] y este tipo de infección constituye una complicación de alto riesgo para generar estados de sepsis graves o de *shock*, así como manifestaciones sépticas metastásicas a distancia. En ocasiones la infección del túnel subcutáneo puede tratarse eficazmente manteniendo el catéter si no se extiende más allá de 2 cm desde el orificio de entrada, pero cualquier infección (con o sin supuración) que supere esta extensión requiere la retirada del catéter y, a veces, hasta un desbridamiento quirúrgico.

3.2.3　*Infección del bolsillo o del reservorio*

Se caracteriza por dolor, eritema o induración sobre el bolsillo que aloja el reservorio del dispositivo de acceso intravascular. Puede llegar a progresar hasta la erosión o la rotura de la piel que cubre el reservorio, con exudado purulento o incluso dejando áreas de necrosis, y también puede producirse la extrusión de parte del dispositivo. En ocasiones hay fiebre y bacteriemia asociadas. En situaciones no excesivamente complicadas y si la infección es leve, puede intentarse conservar el catéter mediante tratamiento local (sellado) y antibióticos sistémicos, cambiando el reservorio, pero si hay exudado purulento, necrosis y bacteriemia asociada será necesario retirar todo el sistema e instaurar tratamiento antibiótico sistémico.[30]

3.2.4　*Flebitis*

Consiste en la presencia de al menos dos de los siguientes signos inflamatorios locales: tumefacción o induración, eritema, calor o dolor alrededor del sitio de salida del catéter. Es muy similar a la infección del punto de inserción del catéter, pero habitualmente sin exudado purulento ni gran extensión en el trayecto de la vena afectada (cordón venoso palpable). Por lo general tiene carácter infeccioso, ligado a la colonización bacteriana, sobre todo en caso de falta de cuidados de mantenimiento de la vía, o de su no retirada tras el plazo de uso apropiado, pero en otras ocasiones tiene una naturaleza no necesariamente infecciosa y puede deberse a la reacción inflamatoria derivada de sustancias químicas irritantes o a la extravasación de algunos fármacos que pueden producir flogosis local, dando lugar a una flebitis irritativa química por micropartículas en suspensión, como es el caso de la vancomicina, la amfotericina B desoxicolato, el cloruro potásico, los citostáticos y otras sustancias infundidas en soluciones parenterales. De todas formas, es quizá la manifestación local más frecuente de infección asociada a un catéter vascular, aunque muchas investigaciones consideran que la flebitis se inicia primariamente como un fenómeno físico-químico que incrementa de manera notable el riesgo de colonización microbiana y el posterior desarrollo de infección. Puesto que un alto porcentaje de los catéteres vasculares se colocan en pacientes oncohematológicos o con otros factores de inmunosupresión, la presencia de signos inflamatorios no constituye un dato de gran sensibilidad ni especificidad para asegurar o descartar una infección relacionada con el catéter.

3.2.5 *Tromboflebitis séptica o supurada*

Aunque suele tener un componente sistémico, se abordará dentro de las manifestaciones locales de las infecciones relacionadas con catéteres vasculares. Supone la presencia de microorganismos que condicionan una inflamación de la pared de la vena y perivascular, con frecuencia junto con trombosis dentro de la luz que facilita la persistencia de la bacteriemia asociada. Puede afectar tanto a un catéter superficial-periférico como a uno venoso central. Actualmente, la forma superficial es muy poco frecuente y suele presentarse sobre todo como afectación de un catéter venoso central, en especial en pacientes con factores predisponentes, como cáncer,[31] tratamiento con corticosteroides o inmunosupresores,[32] grandes quemados y pacientes muy graves.[33,34] Predominan en los catéteres vasculares insertados en los miembros. La tromboflebitis séptica supone aproximadamente entre el 5 % y el 10 % de los distintos tipos de infección relacionada con un catéter. El mecanismo patogénico fundamental es la migración de microorganismos por vía extraluminal,[35] de manera que la infección desencadena una respuesta inflamatoria local que favorece el desarrollo de la trombosis. Sin embargo, en ocasiones acontece primero la trombosis, en la cual anidan los leucocitos y los microorganismos, que favorecen la infección local de la luz y del endotelio vascular y la posterior bacteriemia.[35] La tromboflebitis supurada es una complicación asociada principalmente con infecciones por *S. aureus*, pero se han comunicado pequeñas series[36-38] que incluyen también bacilos gramnegativos, como *Serratia marcescens*, y hongos, tanto especies de *Candida* como incluso algún caso excepcional por hongos filamentosos, como *Aspergillus* spp. Es una complicación que debe sospecharse siempre que, al retirar el catéter vascular y hacer un uso adecuado de los antimicrobianos, persista la bacteriemia y se manifieste con o sin signos de sepsis.[39] En más del 90 % de los casos se observan manifestaciones clínicas locales en forma de eritema, dolor a la palpación del trayecto venoso, engrosamiento de éste, presencia de exudado purulento en el punto de inserción, bien espontáneo o tras comprimir o drenar la vena, e incluso formación de un absceso local.[40] En ocasiones puede ser clínicamente poco o nada evidente, con escasos síntomas y signos locales de infección, inespecíficos o ausentes, y sólo cierta molestia o dolor en la base del cuello, la fosa supraclavicular o el hombro,[41] edema distal a la vena afectada o en el miembro,[33] o disfunción del catéter aparentemente mecánica. Además, si la trombosis no es completa puede ser del todo asintomática.[42] Se asocia a una gran morbimortalidad.[43] Suele presentarse como una bacteriemia con signos francos de sepsis, que persisten tras la retirada del catéter, pero en algunos casos puede acompañarse de infecciones metastásicas en diferentes localizaciones, con más frecuencia embolias sépticas en el parénquima pulmonar, que a veces constituyen su forma peculiar de presentación.[34,39] Si se trata de un catéter vascular periférico, pueden producirse un pseudoaneurisma localizado o complicaciones en forma de lesiones embolígenas distales en la mano.[44]

Se han identificado una serie de datos en la exploración física que orientan a la presencia de este proceso. Así, una diferencia $\geq 2\,cm$ en la circunferencia de los brazos medida 5 cm por encima del olécranon, una distensión venosa asimétrica visible en el tórax o en el brazo homolateral o contralateral, y la presencia de venas de la mano distendidas persistentemente tras la elevación del brazo homolateral o contralateral,[45] pueden ser indicadores de trombosis séptica asociada a un catéter venoso central. En ocasiones el diagnóstico se confirma al obtener pus tras comprimir y exprimir el vaso afectado. Algunas veces puede recurrirse a la ecografía Doppler vascular para confirmar la sospecha.

En cuanto al momento de aparición, se ha visto que en el caso de los catéteres periféricos la incidencia suele ser máxima tras el tercer día de cateterización, con una mediana de cuatro días (intervalo de 1-12 días),[46] y en los catéteres venosos centrales se ha descrito una mediana de 13 a 14 días (intervalo de 6-30 días).[31,47]

Es importante diferenciar este proceso de una bacteriemia relacionada con un catéter vascular en la que coexiste una trombosis, aunque no necesariamente séptica, que suele cursar con escasa repercusión clínica sistémica y con bastante buena respuesta a la retirada del dispositivo intravascular y al tratamiento antimicrobiano adecuado.[48] La trombosis asociada a un catéter venoso central se observa con más frecuencia cuando el catéter se encuentra en la vena yugular interna que cuando está en la vena subclavia.[49]

Ante la sospecha de trombosis séptica de un catéter vascular debe retirarse de inmediato el dispositivo y se administrarán de forma precoz antimicrobianos en dosis altas por vía intravenosa. En ocasiones se precisa cirugía para drenar los abscesos perivasculares y lograr un adecuado control del foco, sobre todo en caso de sepsis resistente al tratamiento convencional o de embolias persistentes.

En la trombosis supurativa asociada a un catéter vascular, con independencia del tipo de catéter y del microorganismo implicado, debe procederse a la pronta retirada del catéter sospechoso de haber iniciado el cuadro, como aconsejan todas las guías al uso. Si se trata de trombosis sépticas de localización más profunda, una intervención instrumental dirigida o un procedimiento quirúrgico estarían indicados sólo para el drenaje de colecciones perivasculares, o en caso de sepsis no controlada o de embolias pulmonares recidivantes. Muchos autores[32,50-53] han abogado por la ligadura y la resección de la vena afectada, si es necesario y técnicamente posible, pero este planteamiento terapéutico ha cambiado en las últimas décadas y en la actualidad un número considerable de tromboflebitis supuradas pueden resolverse de manera satisfactoria con la retirada del catéter, una antibioticoterapia apropiada y medidas más conservadoras. El tratamiento antibiótico debe prolongarse mucho más allá de 15 días en caso de afectación de grandes venas centrales, como en las endocarditis infecciosas y en otras infecciones endovasculares complicadas, y puede llegar hasta las cuatro a seis semanas en función del microorganismo implicado, de la extensión local del proceso y del grado de afectación sistémica. En las formas superficiales, el tratamiento antibiótico se mantendrá menos tiempo, de dos a tres semanas, excepto si el episodio tiene como agente implicado en el cuadro clínico de tromboflebitis supurativa a *S. aureus,* en cuyo caso deberá prolongarse hasta al menos cuatro semanas. En las formas locales leves podría plantearse inicialmente un tratamiento conservador con medidas locales, aplicación de calor y elevación del miembro afectado, junto con la administración de antimicrobianos sistémicos, evaluación en 24 horas y, si no se observa mejoría clínica, se produce deterioro o persiste la clínica de sepsis, proceder entonces a la resección de la vena afectada y de aquellas otras tributarias que también estén afectadas, y al drenaje de los abscesos periflebíticos asociados. Actualmente hay controversia respecto a la indicación o no de anticoagulación, y en general no se dispone de evidencia científica suficiente para indicarla de forma sistemática en todos los casos. En casos concretos, algunos autores[54,55] ha referido cierto beneficio con la heparinización o el uso de fibrinolíticos, siempre y cuando el problema no pueda abordarse quirúrgicamente.

3.3   *Complicaciones sistémicas*

Las manifestaciones generales de las infecciones relacionadas con catéteres vasculares son esencialmente las de toda infección endovascular. La fiebre, las manifestaciones de lesión en múltiples órganos y otras complicaciones propias de la bacteriemia son compartidas por la infección relacionada con un catéter. Estas manifestaciones sistémicas, y sus posibles complicaciones, pueden agruparse en cuatro grandes grupos de menor a mayor gravedad en cuanto a pronóstico: *1)* bacteriemia o fungemia relacionada con un catéter vascular no complicada; *2)* bacteriemia o fungemia relacionada con un catéter vascular complicada con sepsis grave o *shock* séptico; *3)* metástasis sépticas endovasculares; y *4)* implantes sépticos extravasculares que afectan a otros órganos o parénquimas. La incidencia de complicaciones hematógenas a distancia no está bien analizada en estudios prospectivos, excepto la bacteriemia relacionada con un catéter por *S. aureus,* pero pueden llegar a producirse lesiones focales supurativas hasta en casi el 20 % de los episodios, según las series.[50,56,57] Estas complicaciones ocurrieron, por ejemplo, en el 13 % de 324 pacientes consecutivos con un seguimiento de tres meses, y tuvieron la siguiente distribución: 9,5 % endocarditis, 3,4 % artritis séptica, 2,1 % espondilodiscitis, y 1,8 % dos o más de estas complicaciones a la vez.[50] La incidencia de espondilodiscitis hematógena nosocomial por *S. aureus* fue del 0,7 % en un estudio danés[58,59] que incluyó 5.222 pacientes con bacteriemia nosocomial por dicho microorganismo en un período de 10 años. En una tercera parte de las bacteriemias, el origen fue un catéter intravenoso.[58,59]

3.3.1   *Bacteriemia o fungemia asociadas a un catéter vascular*

La aparición de una infección hematógena diseminada por bacterias u hongos en un paciente portador de un catéter vascular depende de diversos factores, pero fundamentalmente del tipo de cánula, del microorganismo causal y de la enfermedad de base del sujeto o de la existencia de cirugía previa. Supone la presencia de manifestaciones clínicas de infección, con fiebre, escalofríos, afectación del estado general o hipotensión arterial, junto con uno o más hemocultivos de sangre periférica positivos, sin otra causa o foco de infección.[60] Además, es necesario que se cumpla al menos una de las siguientes condiciones:[61]

- Cultivo positivo de la punta del catéter (cultivo semicuantitativo por la técnica de Maki con ≥ 15 UFC o cuantitativo con ≥ 100 UFC) y hemocultivo de sangre periférica positivo, hallando el mismo microorganismo (igual especie y antibiograma).

- Hemocultivos cuantitativos de sangre extraída simultáneamente a través del catéter y de una vía periférica, que sean positivos con una razón ≥ 4:1 (sangre obtenida del catéter frente a sangre periférica).

- Hemocultivos de sangre extraída simultáneamente del catéter y de una vía periférica, ambos positivos con un tiempo de al menos dos horas entre el hemocultivo de sangre obtenida del catéter y el de la extraída de una vena periférica, lapso de tiempo medible sólo en los laboratorios de microbiología que disponen de sistemas automatizados de hemocultivo. La presencia de bacteriemia relacionada con un catéter vascular depende del tipo de acceso vascular; así, según los datos del estudio EPINE realizado en 2011,[51] la prevalencia de bacteriemia relacionada con un catéter vascular periférico fue del 0,85 %, con un catéter venoso central del 5,09 %, con un catéter central de inserción periférica del 3,92 %, con el uso de nutrición parenteral supuso un incremento de hasta el 6,25 %, y la coexistencia de inmunosupresión arrojaba una cifra del 2,06 %. La bacteriemia relacionada con un catéter es la cuarta infección nosocomial en orden de frecuencia, con una prevalencia de alrededor de dos episodios por cada cien pacientes con un catéter venoso central.[62] Los catéteres insertados en la vena yugular o femoral se colonizan con mayor rapidez que los colocados en la vena subclavia,[63] e incluso algunos estudios muestran un incremento de hasta cinco veces en las tasas de infección entre el acceso yugular y el subclavio.[64,65]

3.3.2 *Bacteriemia complicada con sepsis grave o* shock *séptico*

La infección asociada a un catéter, en especial si se trata de uno venoso central, puede presentarse como una forma grave de sepsis y evolucionar incluso a *shock* séptico,[66] hasta en un 30% a un 40% de los casos según diferentes series.[28,67-71] Deben cumplirse las definiciones y los criterios de sepsis, modificados en la conferencia de consenso de 1991,[66] según los cuales se considera síndrome de respuesta inflamatoria sistémica a la presencia de dos o más de los siguientes signos: temperatura $> 38\,°C$ o $< 36\,°C$, frecuencia cardíaca ≥ 90 l.p.m., taquipnea con una frecuencia respiratoria ≥ 20 r.p.m. o hiperventilación indicada por una $PaCO_2 \leq 32$ mmHg o necesidad de ventilación mecánica, leucocitosis ≥ 12.000 o leucocitopenia < 4.000 leucocitos/mm^3, o más de un 10% de neutrófilos no segmentados. A estos criterios pueden añadirse los siguientes biomarcadores de inflamación en los casos de origen infeccioso: proteína C reactiva elevada y procalcitonina elevada (ambas dos veces por encima del valor normal de referencia).

Cuando la causa de este síndrome es infecciosa se denomina síndrome séptico, y se clasifica en diferentes estadios de sepsis:

- Sepsis grave: se acompaña de disfunción de uno o más órganos (encefalopatía, acidosis láctica, daño pulmonar agudo, fallo renal, etc.), o de hipotensión e hipoperfusión tisular que remonta con la infusión de volumen.

- *Shock* séptico: sepsis grave con hipotensión mantenida debida a la infección, acompañada de alteraciones de la perfusión (acidosis metabólica o hiperlactacidemia) o disfunción de órganos, que no responde a la resucitación con fluidoterapia y persiste a pesar de la reposición adecuada de volumen, por lo que precisa fármacos vasoactivos.

3.3.3 *Metástasis sépticas endovasculares*

Las metástasis sépticas endovasculares incluyen las endocarditis y la infección relacionada con otros materiales protésicos endovasculares, como prótesis valvulares cardíacas, dispositivos cardiovasculares implantables, injertos vasculares y otros catéteres.

Algunos estudios recientes[72-74] han identificado el catéter venoso central, con o sin bacteriemia documentada, como la principal causa de la endocarditis asociada a los cuidados sanitarios, concepto que amplía la definición de endocarditis nosocomial a las manipulaciones diagnósticas o terapéuticas que se realizan de forma ambulatoria. Todas las series de endocarditis nosocomial hacen referencia a la cateterización endovascular como un factor de riesgo de infección. Esta complicación tendría que sospecharse siempre que una vez retirado el catéter vascular persista la bacteriemia, principalmente en los pacientes con una cardiopatía valvular conocida, cuando aparezcan metástasis sépticas y cuando el microorganismo causal sea *S. aureus*, *Enterococcus faecalis* o *Candida* spp. Los catéteres venosos centrales se consideran la causa de la endocarditis en el 39,8 % al 63 % de estos episodios.[72-74] Por otro lado, la endocarditis bacteriana, sobre todo con afectación de válvulas derechas, se asocia con una frecuencia del 2 % al 10 % al uso de un catéter venoso central.[75-76] El mecanismo de aparición de la endocarditis tiene un gran paralelismo con el modelo *in vivo* de endocarditis en el animal de experimentación. La patogenia de la lesión en los pacientes afectados se explica por el traumatismo causado sobre el endocardio por el extremo distal del catéter, en caso de ser venoso central. Incluso en períodos tan breves como una hora se produce inicialmente una endocarditis trombótica no bacteriana, que es una situación adecuada para la colonización por microorganismos. Respecto a las formas comunitarias de presentación de la endocarditis, las asociadas a la atención sanitaria se producen más en pacientes de edad avanzada y con más comorbilidad, y conllevan una mayor mortalidad hospitalaria.[72-74] Incluso estando relacionada con el antecedente de bacteriemia por catéteres vasculares, no siempre es necesaria la presencia del catéter en el interior de las cavidades para que se produzca la afectación cardíaca, puesto que predominan las endocarditis izquierdas sobre las derechas. El tratamiento no difiere mucho del de las endocarditis convencionales, con todos sus condicionamientos médicos y quirúrgicos.

3.3.4   *Metástasis sépticas extravasculares*

3.3.4.1   Osteoarticulares (osteomielitis, espondilodiscitis, artritis)

La osteomielitis secundaria a una infección relacionada con un catéter puede tener un origen local, como consecuencia del traumatismo por contigüidad del catéter vascular con el hueso, o un origen secundario debido a una infección metastásica a distancia por diseminación hematógena, de aparición más tardía (entre 1 y 12 meses). La afectación ósea o articular debida a la diseminación hematógena de un proceso infeccioso relacionado con un catéter vascular ha sido poco estudiada. No obstante, el enfoque diagnóstico y terapéutico no difiere del habitual en los casos de infección osteoarticular. Se ha observado que la localización más habitual es el raquis, y que las vértebras que con más frecuencia se afectan son las lumbares.[77] Los síntomas más comunes de presentación de la espondilitis o de la espondilodiscitis son dolor de espalda intenso, discapacidad funcional con posible debilidad para la sedestación y la bipedestación, o dificultad para la marcha, y ocasionalmente febrícula o fiebre de bajo grado (salvo que se asocie una afectación de los tejidos blandos, como una piomiositis de la musculatura retrosomática o del músculo psoas ilíaco), que por lo general pueden aparecer durante más de tres meses antes del diagnóstico definitivo. Las afecciones que se asocian con más frecuencia son la diabetes mellitus y la insuficiencia renal crónica.[78] La patogenia implica, en la mayoría de los casos, la existencia de una bacteriemia intermitente o mantenida, según la capacidad y la rapidez en controlar el foco endovascular septicémico en el catéter vascular. Los hemocultivos proporcionan el diagnóstico microbiológico de apoyo clínico en un 20 % a un 59 % de los casos.[79] Los datos obtenidos de estudios longitudinales realizados en los años 1990 y a principios de este nuevo siglo muestran que *S. aureus* constituye una causa cada vez mayor de osteomielitis vertebral hematógena, y que su resistencia a la meticilina ha aumentado en la última década,[58,80,81] si bien la emergencia de cepas de estafilococos coagulasa negativos como causa de espondilodiscitis es creciente, debido precisamente al uso cada vez mayor de catéteres vasculares en poblaciones de edad avanzada o con inmunodepresión que pueden complicarse con infección local y una posterior bacteriemia relacionada con el catéter.

3.3.4.2 Endoftalmitis

La endoftalmitis puede clasificarse patogénicamente como exógena o endógena, pero en cualquier caso es una emergencia oftalmológica. La forma exógena se debe principalmente a lesiones traumáticas penetrantes en el globo ocular o es secundaria a cirugía intraocular. La forma endógena o metastásica se produce por diseminación hematógena desde otro foco infeccioso a distancia. En este sentido, las infecciones endovasculares relacionadas con catéteres vasculares y las endocarditis, aparte de otros posibles focos no intravasculares, constituyen uno de los orígenes más habituales de endoftalmitis endógenas. Tienen una prevalencia baja, entre un 2 % y un 8 % de todos los casos de endoftalmitis. Suelen ser unilaterales y afectar sobre todo al ojo derecho, probablemente por un mayor flujo arterial desde la arteria carótida derecha. Se han identificado como comorbilidad asociada la diabetes mellitus, la insuficiencia renal crónica, el uso de drogas por vía parenteral y especialmente tener implantado un catéter venoso central. Los microorganismos patógenos más frecuentes en la endoftalmitis endógena son los relacionados con el foco de origen de la bacteriemia que la produce. Clínicamente suele cursar con dolor ocular acompañado de quemosis o enrojecimiento conjuntival y pérdida de la agudeza visual, y en ocasiones muestra manifestaciones clínicas sistémicas, con fiebre y afectación del estado general. A la exploración oftalmológica se evidencian pseudofaquia, hipopión, fenómeno de Tyndall positivo, presión intraocular normal pero infiltración vítrea y engrosamiento macular. Pueden asociarse, además, complicaciones locales como un absceso vítreo y desprendimiento de coroides o, en formas más avanzadas, de retina. Los hemocultivos pueden ser positivos hasta en un 71 % de los pacientes, mientras que entre el 61 % y el 70 % presentarán un cultivo positivo de humor vítreo o de otras muestras, como humor acuoso, pero no es infrecuente que los cultivos de muestras oculares sean negativos, sobre todo si el paciente ya recibe algún tipo de tratamiento antibiótico y según la rapidez y la idoneidad del transporte y el procesamiento de estas muestras.

El tratamiento incluye antibióticos por vía sistémica e intravítrea. La práctica de una vitrectomía a tiempo mejora los resultados visuales en las formas más graves. La duración de la antibioticoterapia tendrá que ser larga y está condicionada en parte por la causa subyacente de la bacteriemia que fue el origen del proceso ocular.[82,83]

3.3.4.3   Manifestaciones neurológicas

Los síndromes clínicos con afectación del sistema nervioso central pueden presentarse con manifestaciones similares a las de la endocarditis infecciosa, normalmente como lesiones embolígenas isquémicas (véase la figura 2) o como hemorragias secundarias en el contexto de embolias sépticas, tanto en forma de hemorragias subaracnoideas como intraparenquimatosas, estas últimas con menor frecuencia.

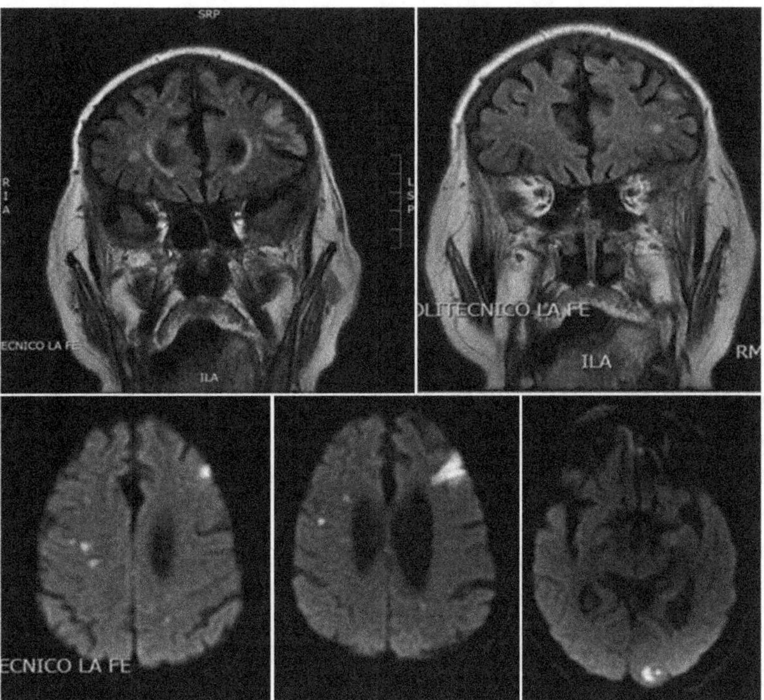

Figura 2. Absceso de músculo psoas ilíaco izquierdo conformando una piomiositis secundaria a sepsis y bacteriemia por Staphylococcus aureus *resistente a la meticilina, de origen en un catéter vascular central de inserción femoral, en un paciente con grandes quemaduras. Obsérvese la lesión hipodensa de márgenes bien definidos, en alguna de las imágenes con varios lóculos semitabicados, que produce un aumento de tamaño del músculo psoas izquierdo y franca asimetría respecto al derecho.*

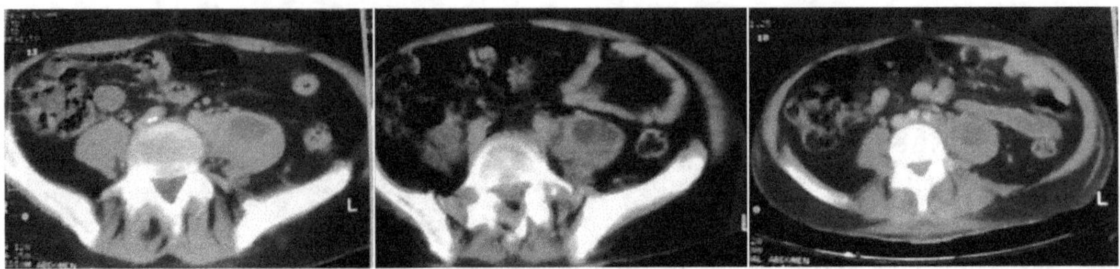

Figura 3. Imagen de resonancia magnética cerebral que muestra numerosos focos parenquimatosos compatibles con lesiones isquémicas de predominio cortical, frontal izquierdo, ambos centros semiovales y occipital bilateral, sin asociar componente hemorrágico, muy sugestivas de émbolos sépticos múltiples, en un paciente varón de 67 años de edad con insuficiencia renal crónica terminal y bacteriemia por Staphylococcus aureus *relacionada con el catéter vascular central de hemodiálisis.*

3.3.4.4   Manifestaciones musculares

La afectación muscular en la bacteriemia es muy infrecuente. En casos de sepsis de origen estafilocócico se produce en menos del 1 %, y es muy rara en las bacteriemias con endocarditis asociada. Se observa sobre todo en pacientes con endocarditis de cavidades izquierdas. *S. aureus* es la causa más frecuente y da lugar a afectaciones del tipo de la piomiositis en sus distintas fases (véase la figura 3).[84]

3.3.4.5   Abscesos pulmonares, hepatoesplénicos y renales

La aparición tardía de abscesos glandulares y parenquimatosos de órganos diana, como fenómeno de maduración de embolias sépticas previas, produce normalmente la reaparición o la no desaparición de la fiebre, manifestaciones locales en forma de dolor o molestias, y disfunción del órgano implicado, en mayor o menor grado. Todos ellos, dentro de su excepcionalidad, pueden ocurrir casi en cualquier tipo de órgano o víscera bien vascularizado, en relación al tipo de circulación (pulmonar o general) y de los vasos (venosos, arteriales) donde se origine la infección relacionada con un catéter, pero con bastante más frecuencia en el parénquima pulmonar, el hígado, el bazo y los riñones; son mucho más raras las colecciones purulentas de páncreas, suprarrenales, próstata, tiroides, parótidas y otras glándulas. Requieren una antibioticoterapia apropiada y a menudo también drenaje percutáneo o incluso cirugía para conseguir un control óptimo del foco. La retirada del origen de las metástasis sépticas, localizado en el catéter vascular, es un aspecto clave para evitar nuevas complicaciones de este tipo.[85,86]

Bibliografía

1. McGee DC, Gould MK. Preventing complications of central venous catheterization. N Engl J Med. 2003; 348: 1123-33.
2. O'Grady NP, Alexander M, Dellinger EP, Gerberding JL, Heard SO, Maki DG, *et al.* Guidelines for the prevention of intravascular catheter-related infections. Centers for Disease Control and Prevention. MMWR Recomm Rep. 2002; 51(RR-10): 1-29.
3. Eggimann P. Diagnosis of intravascular catheter infection. Curr Opin Infect Dis. 2007; 20: 353-9.
4. Pratt RJ, Pellowe CM, Wilson JA, Loveday HP, Harper PJ, Jones SR, *et al.* epic2: National evidence-based guidelines for preventing healthcare-associated infections in NHS hospitals in England. J Hosp Infect. 2007; 65 (Suppl 1): S1-164.
5. Mermel LA, Allon M, Bouza E, Craven DE, Flynn P, O'Grady NP, *et al.* Clinical practice guidelines for the diagnosis and management of intravascular catheter-related infection: 2009 update by the Infectious Diseases Society of America. Clin Infect Dis. 2009; 49: 1-45.
6. Fortún J. Infecciones asociadas a dispositivos intravasculares utilizados para la terapia de infusión. Enferm Infecc Microbiol Clin. 2008; 26: 168-74.
7. Maki DG, Weise CE, Sarafin HW. A semiquantitative culture method for identifying intravenous catheter related infection. N Engl J Med. 1977; 296: 1305-9.
8. Snydman DR, Gorbea HF, Pober BR, Majka JA, Murray SA. Predictive value of surveillance skin cultures in total parenteral nutrition related infection. Lancet. 1982; 2: 1385-8.
9. Cercenado E, Ena J, Rodríguez-Creixems M, Romero J, Bouza E. A conservative procedure for diagnosis of catheter related infections. Arch Intern Med. 1990; 150: 1417-20.
10. Raad I, Costerton W, Sabharwal U, Sacilowski M, Anaissie E, Bodey GP. Ultrastructural analysis of indwelling vascular catheters: a quantitative relationship between luminal colonization and duration of placement. J Infect Dis. 1993; 168: 400-7.
11. Miller JJ, Venus B, Mathru M. Comparison of the sterility of long-term central venous catheterizacion using single lumen, triple lumen, and pulmonary artery catheters. Crit Care Med. 1984; 12: 634-7.
12. Gil R, Kruse JA, Thill-Baharozian MC, Carlson RW. Triple vs single lumen central venous catheters. A prospective study in a critically ill population. Arch Intern Med. 1989; 149: 1139-43.
13. Liñares J, Sitges-Serra A, Garau J, Pérez JL, Martín R. Pathogenesis of catheter sepsis: a prospective study using quantitative and semiquantitative cultures of catheter hub and segments. J Clin Microbiol. 1985; 21: 357-60.
14. Sitges-Serra A, Liñares J, Garau J. Catheter sepsis: the clue is the hub. Surgery. 1985; 97: 355-7.
15. Collignon PJ, Soni N, Pearson IY, Woods WP, Munro R, Sorrell TC. Is semiquantitative culture of central vein catheter tips useful in the diagnosis of catheter associated bacteriemia? J Clin Microbiol. 1986; 24: 532-5.
16. León C, Sánchez MA, Lucena F. Infección por catéter: antes y después de la conferencia de consenso. Enferm Infecc Microbiol Clin. 1997; 15(Supl 3): 27-32.
17. Gandelman G, Frishman WH, Wiese C, Green-Gastwirth V, Hong S, Aronow WS, *et al.* Intravascular device infections: epidemiology, diagnosis, and management. Cardiol Rev. 2007; 15: 13-23.
18. McKenzie FE. Case mortality in polymicrobial bloodstream infections. J Clin Epidemiol. 2006; 59: 760-1.
19. Herrmann M, Vaudaux PE, Pittet D. Fibronectin, fibrinogen, and laminin act as mediators of adherence of clinical staphylococcal isolates to foreign material. J Infect Dis. 1988; 158: 693-701.
20. Branchini ML, Pfaller MA, Rhine-Chalberg J, Frempong T, Isenberg HD. Genotypic variation in slime production among blood and catheter isolates of Candida parapsilosis. J Clin Microbiol. 1994; 32: 452-6.
21. Lorente L, Jiménez A, Santana M, Iribarren JL, Jiménez JJ, Martín MM, *et al.* Microorganisms responsible for intravascular catheter-related bloodstream infection according to the catheter site. Crit Care Med. 2007; 35: 2424-7.
22. Mermel LA, Farr BM, Sherertz RJ, Raad II, O'Grady N, Harris JS, *et al.* Guidelines for the management of intravascular catheter-related infections. Clin Infect Dis. 2001; 32: 1249-72.
23. Levy MM, Fink MP, Marshall JC, Abraham E, Angus D, Cook D, *et al.* 2001 SCCM/

ESICM/ACCP/ATS/SIS International Sepsis Definitions Conference. Crit Care Med. 2003; 31: 1250-6.

24. Talan DA, Moran GJ, Abrahamian FM. Severe sepsis and septic shock in the emergency department. Infect Dis Clin N Am. 2008; 22: 1-31.

25. Tully JL, Friedland GH, Baldini MA, Goldman DA. Complications of intravenous therapy with needles and teflon catheters. Am J Med. 1981; 70: 702-6.

26. Righter J, Bishop LA, Hill B. Infections and pheripheral venous catheterization. Diagn Microbiol Infect Dis. 1983; 1: 89-93.

27. Hamilton HC, Foxcroft D. Central venous access sites for the prevention of venous thrombosis, stenosis and infection in patients requiring long-term intravenous therapy [review]. Cochrane Database Syst Rev 2007; 3: CD004084.

28. Maki DG, Kluger DM, Crnich CJ. The risk of bloodstream infection in adults with different intravascular devices; a systematic review of 200 published prospective studies. Mayo Clin Proc. 2006; 81: 1159-71.

29. Beathard GA, Urbanes A. Infection associated with tunneled hemodialysis catheters. Semin Dial. 2008; 21: 528-38.

30. Ingram J, Weitzman S, Greenberg ML, Parkin P, Filler R. Complications of indwelling venous access lines in the pediatric hematology patient: a prospective comparison of external venous catheters and subcutaneous ports. Am J Pediatr Hematol Oncol. 1991; 13: 130-6.

31. SEQ-AEHH-SEOM-SEMI. Tratamiento de las infecciones relacionadas con catéteres venosos de larga duración. Documento de consenso de la SEQ-AEHH-SEOM-SEMI. Rev Esp Quimioterap. 2003; 16: 343-60.

32. Strinden WD, Helgerson RB, Maki DG. Candida septic thrombosis of the great central veins associated with central catheters. Clinical features and management. Ann Surg. 1985; 202: 653-8.

33. Van Rooden CJ, Schippers EF, Barge RM, Rosendaal FR, Guiot HF, van der Meer FJ, *et al.* Infectious complications of central venous catheters increase the risk of catheter-related thrombosis in hematology patients: a prospective study. J Clin Oncol 2005; 23: 2655-60.

34. Sharma BR. Infections in patients with severe burns: causes and prevention thereof. Infect Dis Clin N Am. 2007; 21: 745-59.

35. Fowler VG Jr., Scheld WM, Bayer AS. Endocarditis and intravascular infections. En: Mandell GL, Bennett JE, Dolin R, editores. Mandell, Douglas and Bennett's. Principles and practice of infectious diseases. 7th ed. Philadelphia: Churchill Livingstone; 2010. p. 1067-112.

36. Johnson RA, Zajac RA, Evans ME. Suppurative thrombophlebitis: correlation between pathogen and underlying disease. Infect Control. 1986; 7: 582-5.

37. Arnow PM, Quimosing EM, Beach M. Consequences of intravascular catheter sepsis. Clin Infect Dis. 1993; 16: 778-84.

38. Baker CC, Petersen SR, Sheldon GF. Septic phlebitis: a neglected disease. Am J Surg. 1979; 138: 97.

39. Raad II, Narro J, Khan A, Tarrand J, Vartivarian S, Bodey GP. Serious complications of vascular catheter-related Staphylococcus aureus bacteremia in cancer patients. Eur J Clin Microbiol Infect Dis. 1992; 11: 675-82.

40. Garrison RN, Richardson JD, Fry DE. Catheter-associated septic thrombophlebitis. South Med J. 1982; 75: 917-9.

41. Constans J, Salmi LR, Sevestre-Pietri MA, Perusat S, Nguon M, Degeilh M, *et al.* A clinical prediction score for upper extremity deep venous thrombosis. Thromb Haemost. 2008; 99: 202-7.

42. Ghanem GA, Boktour M, Warneke C, Pham-Williams T, Kassis C, Bahna P, *et al.* Catheter-related Staphylococcus aureus bacteremia in cancer patients: high rate of complications with therapeutic implications. Medicine (Balt). 2007; 86: 54-60.

43. Khan EA, Correa AG, Baker CJ. Suppurative thrombophlebitis in children: a ten-year experience. Pediatr Infect Dis J. 1997; 16: 63-7.

44. Falk PS, Scuderi PE, Sherertz RJ, Motsinger SM. Infected radial artery pseudoaneurysms occurring after percutaneous cannulation. Chest. 1992; 101: 490-5.

45. Crowley AL, Peterson GE, Benjamin DK Jr, Rimmer SH, Todd C, Cabell CH, *et al.* Venous thrombosis in patients with short- and long-term central venous catheter-associated Staphylococcus aureus bacteremia. Crit Care Med. 2008; 36: 385-90.

46. Verghese A, Widrich WC, Arbeit RD. Central venous septic thrombophlebitis – the role of medical therapy. Medicine (Balt). 1985; 64: 394-400.

47. Kaufman J, Demas C, Stark K, Flancbaum L. Catheter-related septic central venous thrombosis – current therapeutic options. West J Med. 1986; 145: 200-3.

48. Verso M, Agnelli G. Venous thromboembolism associated with long-term use of central venous catheters in cancer patients. J Clin Oncol. 2003; 21: 3665-75.

49. Timsit JF, Farkas JC, Boyer JM, Martin JB, Misset B, Renaud B, *et al.* Central vein catheter-related thrombosis in intensive care patients: incidence, risks factors, and relationship with catheter-related sepsis. Chest. 1998; 114: 207-13.

50. Fowler VG Jr, Justice A, Moore C, Benjamin DK Jr, Woods CW, Campbell S, *et al.* Risk factors for hematogenous complications of intravascular catheter-associated Staphylococcus aureus bacteremia. Clin Infect Dis. 2005; 40: 695-703.

51. Munster AM. Septic thrombophlebitis. A surgical disorder. JAMA. 1974; 230: 1010-1.

52. Pruitt BA Jr, McManus WF, Kim SH, Treat RC. Diagnosis and treatment of cannula--related intravenous sepsis in burn patients. Ann Surg. 1980; 191: 546-54.

53. Torres-Rojas JR, Stratton CW, Sanders CV, Horsman TA, Hawley HB, Dascomb HE, *et al.* Candidal suppurative peripheral thrombophlebitis. Ann Intern Med. 1982; 96: 431-5.

54. Falagas ME, Vardakas KZ, Athanasiou S. Intravenous heparin in combination with antibiotics for the treatment of deep vein septic thrombophlebitis: a systematic review. Eur J Pharmacol. 2007; 557: 93-8.

55. Topiel MS, Bryan RT, Kessler CM, Simoin GL. Case report: treatment of silastic catheter-induce central vein septic thrombophlebitis. Am J Med Sci. 1986; 291: 425-8.

56. Martínez-Luengas F, Álvarez-Dardet C, León de Lope M, Suárez A, Gálvez J, Perea EJ. Bacteriemia secundaria a cánulas percutáneas intravasculares. Med Clin. 1985; 84: 734-7.

57. Maradona JA, López Alonso J, Pérez F, García G, Arribas JM. Bacteriemia por Staphylococcus aureus en adultos relacionada con el empleo de catéteres o dispositivos intravasculares. Rev Clin Esp. 1987; 180: 147-50.

58. Jensen AG, Espersen F, Skinhoj P, Rosdahl VT, Frimodt-Moller N. Increasing frequency of vertebral osteomyelitis following Staphylococcus aureus bacteraemia in Denmark 1980-1990. J Infect. 1997; 34: 113-8.

59. Jensen AG, Espersen F, Skinhoj P, Frimodt-Moller N. Bacteremic Staphylococcus aureus spondylitis. Arch Intern Med. 1998; 158: 509-17.

60. O'Grady NP, Alexander M, Burns LA, Dellinger EP, Garland J, Heard SO, *et al.;* Healthcare Infection Control Practices Advisory Committee (HICPAC). Guidelines for the prevention of intravascular catheter-related infections. Clin Infect Dis. 2011; 52: e162-93.

61. Catton JA, Dobbins BM, Kite P, Wood JM, Eastwood K, Sugden S, *et al.* In situ diagnosis of intravascular catheter-related bloodstream infection: a comparison of quantitative culture, differential time to positivity, and endoluminal brushing. Crit Care Med. 2005; 33: 787-91.

62. Estudio de prevalencia de las infecciones nosocomiales en España (EPINE) 2011. Sociedad Española de Medicina Preventiva, Salud Pública e Higiene. 22º Estudio. Informe global de España. Disponible en: http: //hws.vhebron. net/epine/Descargas/EPINE%202011%20 ESPA%C3%91A%20Resumen.pdf

63. Richet H, Hubert B, Nitemberg G, Andremont A, Buu-Hoi A, Ourbak P, *et al.* Prospective multicenter study of vascular-catheter-related complications and risk factors for positive central-catheter cultures in intensive care unit patients. J Clin Microbiol. 1990; 28: 2520-5.

64. Plit ML, Lipman J, Eidelman J, Gavaudan J. Catheter related infection. A plea for consensus with review and guidelines. Intensive Care Med. 1988; 14: 503-9.

65. Lazarus HM, Creger RJ, Bloom AD, Shenk R. Percutaneous placement of femoral central venous catheter in patients undergoing transplantation of bone marrow. Surg Gynecol Obstet. 1990; 170: 403-6.

66. Bone RC, Balk RA, Cerra FB, Dellinger RP, Fein AM, Knaus WA, *et al.* Definitions for sepsis and organ failure and guidelines for the use of innovative therapies in sepsis. The ACCP/ SCCM Consensus Conference Committee. American College of Chest Physicians/Society of Critical Care Medicine. Chest. 1992; 101: 1644-55.

67. Deshpande KS, Hatem C, Ulrich HL, Currie BP, Aldrich TK, Bryan-Brown CW, *et al.* The incidence of infectious complications of central venous catheters at the subclavian, internal jugular, and femoral sites in an intensive

care unit population. Crit Care Med. 2005; 33: 13-20.

68. Tarpatzi A, Avlamis A, Papaparaskevas J, Daikos GL, Stefanou I, Katsandri A, *et al.* Incidence and risk factors for central vascular catheter-related bloodstream infections in a tertiary care hospital. New Microbiol. 2012; 35: 429-37.

69. Chopra V, Anand S, Krein SL, Chenoweth C, Saint S. Bloodstream infection, venous thrombosis, and peripherally inserted central catheters: reappraising the evidence. Am J Med. 2012; 125: 733-41.

70. Klevens RM, Edwards JR, Richards CL Jr, Horan TC, Gaynes RP, Pollock DA, *et al.* Estimating health care-associated infections and deaths in U.S. hospitals, 2002. Public Health Rep. 2007; 122: 160-6.

71. Raad I, Hanna H, Maki D. Intravascular catheter-related infections: advances in diagnosis, prevention, and management. Lancet Infect Dis. 2007; 7: 645-57.

72. Fernández-Hidalgo N, Almirante B, Tornos P, Pigrau C, Sambola A, Igual A, *et al.* Contemporary epidemiology and prognosis of health care-associated infective endocarditis. Clin Infect Dis. 2008; 47: 1287-97.

73. Benito N, Miró JM, de Lazzari E. Cabell CH, del Río A, Altclas J, *et al.* ICE-PCS (International Collaboration on Endocarditis Prospective Cohort Study) Investigators. Health care-associated native valve endocarditis: importance of non-nosocomial acquisition. Ann Intern Med. 2009; 150: 586-94.

74. Lomas JM, Martínez-Marcos FJ, Plata A, Ivanova R, Gálvez J, Ruiz J, *et al.* Healthcare-associated infective endocarditis: an undesirable effect of healthcare universalization. Clin Microbiol Infect. 2010; 16: 1683-90.

75. Revilla A, López J, Villacorta E, et al. Isolated right-sided valvular endocarditis in non-intravenous drug users. Rev Esp Cardiol. 2008; 61: 1253-9.

76. Cartón JA, Prez F, Velasco L, Maradona JA, Vázquez F, Arribas JM. Endocarditis derecha por Staphylococcus epidermidis asociada a catéteres venosos centrales: una causa ignorada de fiebre nosocomial potencialmente curable. Enferm Infec Microbiol Clin. 1986; 4: 123-6.

77. Belzunegui J, Intxausti JJ, De Dios JR, Del Val N, Rodríguez Valverde V, González C, *et al.* Haematogenous vertebral osteomyelitis in the elderly. Clin Rheumatol. 2000; 19: 344-7.

78. Hadjipavlou AG, Mader JT, Necessary JT, Muffoletto AJ. Hematogenous pyogenic spinal infections and their surgical management. Spine (Phila Pa 1976). 2000; 25: 1668-79.

79. Jaramillo-de la Torre JJ, Bohinski RJ, Kuntz C. Vertebral osteomyelitis. Neurosurg Clin N Am. 2006; 17: 339-51.

80. D'Agostino C, Scorzolini L, Massetti AP, Carnevalini M, d'Ettorre G, Venditti M, *et al.* A seven-year prospective study on spondylodiscitis: epidemiological and microbiological features. Infection. 2010; 38: 102-7.

81. Cosgrove SE, Qi Y, Kaye KS, Harbarth S, Karchmer AW, Carmeli Y. The impact of methicillin resistance in Staphylococcus aureus bacteremia on patient outcomes: mortality, length of stay, and hospital charges. Infect Control Hosp Epidemiol. 2005; 26: 166-74.

82. Saleem MR, Mustafa S, Drew PJ, Lewis A, Shah Y, Shankar J, *et al.* Endophthalmitis, a rare metastatic bacterial complication of haemodialysis catheter-related sepsis. Nephrol Dial Transplant. 2007; 22: 939-41.

83. Okada AA, Johnson RP, Liles WC, D'Amico DJ, Baker AS. Endogenous bacterial endophthalmitis. Report of a ten-year retrospective study. Ophthalmology. 1994; 101: 832-8.

84. Bickels J, Ben-Sira L, Kessker A, Wientroub S. Primary piomiositis. J Bone Joint Surg Am. 2002; 84: 2277-86.

85. Capdevilla Morell JA, Mauri M, Delgado M. Fiebre en paciente portador de catéteres centrales. Rev Clin Esp. 2011; 211: 301-6.

86. Weber DJ, Rutala WA. Central line-associated bloodstream infections: prevention and management. Infect Dis Clin N Am. 2011; 25: 77-102.

Capítulo 7

Aportación de los modelos experimentales *in vitro* e *in vivo* a la terapéutica de las infecciones relacionadas con catéteres vasculares

N. Fernández Hidalgo, Y. Meije, J. Gavaldà

Servei de Malalties Infeccioses
Hospital Universitari Vall d'Hebron
Universitat Autònoma de Barcelona
Barcelona

Correspondencia:
joan.gavalda@vhir.org

Introducción

El sellado del catéter con un antibiótico efectivo a dosis altas en combinación con la administración sistémica de un antimicrobiano es un tratamiento aceptado en las infecciones relacionadas con catéteres venosos centrales de larga duración causadas por especies de estafilococos coagulasa negativos y por bacilos gramnegativos. Sin embargo, esta estrategia es cuestionada en el caso de las infecciones producidas por *Staphylococcus aureus* o *Candida* spp., para las cuales tanto las guías de tratamiento[1,2] como las evidencias que se encuentran en la literatura[3-5] recomiendan la retirada del catéter como opción más segura. En los pacientes sin otros accesos vasculares o con diátesis hemorrágica, el sellado del catéter puede considerarse como una alternativa terapéutica siempre que estén hemodinámicamente estables y bajo un estricto seguimiento médico.[1,6]

Ciertos antibióticos son más eficaces que otros frente a las bacterias que crecen en las biopelículas, y los diferentes grupos de investigación han fundamentado su búsqueda en moléculas y antimicrobianos capaces de penetrar, alterar o alcanzar altas concentraciones en ellas. En este capítulo, centrándonos en *Staphylococcus* spp. y en *Candida* spp., revisaremos la aportación de los modelos *in vitro* e *in vivo* a la terapéutica de las infecciones relacionadas con catéteres vasculares de larga duración.

1 Modelos *in vitro*

1.1 *Estudio* in vitro *de la biopelícula*

1.1.1 *Estudios de sensibilidad de antimicrobianos y agentes no antimicrobianos frente a microorganismos de biopelículas*

Las bacterias de las biopelículas pueden ser hasta mil veces más resistentes a los antibióticos que esas mismas bacterias en modo planctónico.[7,8] El principal problema relacionado con el estudio de la resistencia de las biopelículas a los antimicrobianos es la falta de métodos estandarizados de uso sistemático. La mayoría de los modelos de biopelículas microbianas son laboriosos y requieren un manejo experto y el uso de equipos especializados, en general no disponibles en los laboratorios de microbiología.

Los modelos utilizados incluyen el uso de discos de catéter, tubos de diferentes materiales colocados en recipientes estériles de vidrio o plástico, filtros de celulosa, microfermentadores y matrices de cultivo de tejidos, entre otros. Por otro lado, la formación de las biopelículas puede realizarse en condiciones estáticas o de flujo.

Aunque, como hemos comentado, no hay ningún método estandarizado para el estudio de la sensibilidad de las bacterias en las biopelículas a los diferentes antibióticos, el descrito por Amorena *et al.*[9] y el *Calgary Biofilm Device*[10] destacan por su facilidad para adaptarse al diagnóstico clínico. El primero se realiza sobre una placa de microtitulación con múltiples pocillos, donde la biopelícula que se ha formado en diferentes períodos de tiempo se expone a los tratamientos antimicrobianos. La viabilidad bacteriana tras 24 horas de tratamiento antibiótico se cuantifica de forma automatizada midiendo por bioluminiscencia la cantidad de trifosfato de adenosina.[9] El *Calgary Biofilm Device* utiliza una placa similar de microtitulación con una tapa que dispone de 96 púas que se introducen y ajustan en cada uno de los pocillos. Las biopelículas formadas sobre estas púas son trasladadas posteriormente a una placa con caldo sin antibiótico, donde son liberadas mediante sonicación. El número de bacterias supervivientes se cuantifica realizando recuentos en placas de agar sólido o midiendo la densidad óptica del cultivo mediante espectrofotometría.[10]

1.1.2 *Estudios de imagen: microscopía confocal y electrónica*

Las técnicas de imagen se han convertido en una herramienta indispensable para la investigación de la estructura tridimensional de la biopelícula. Durante cientos de años, las lentes de aumento y la microscopía óptica tradicional fueron los principales métodos para la observación. Sin embargo, la microscopía electrónica y la confocal han permitido un conocimiento mucho más exhaustivo de las propiedades y del comportamiento de las biopelículas, así como sobre la eficacia de los diferentes

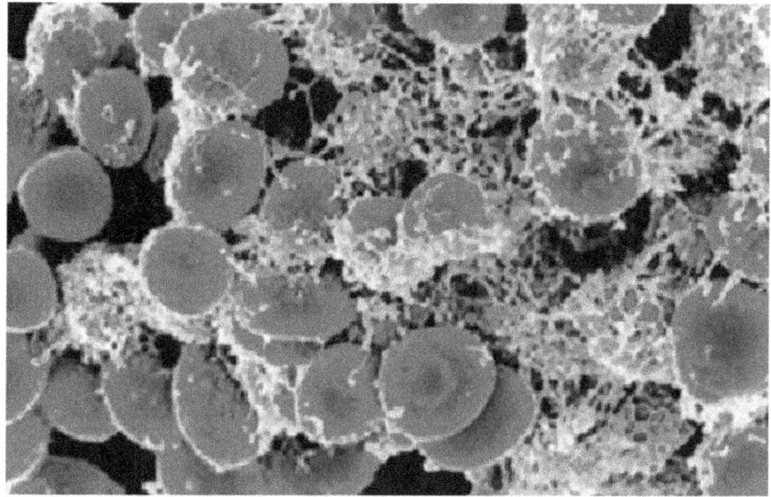

Figura 1. Biopelícula de S. epidermidis *en una matriz de exopolisacárido. Imagen tomada con microscopio electrónico de barrido. (National Institutes of Health/Science Photo Library.)*

antimicrobianos en la erradicación de los microorganismos presentes en ellas.[11] El microscopio láser confocal de barrido (CSLM, *confocal laser scanning microscopy*) permite documentar la morfología y la fisiología de la biopelícula *in situ* en cuatro dimensiones.[12] De igual forma, el microscopio electrónico de transmisión (TEM, *transmission electron microscopy*) y el microscopio electrónico de barrido (SEM, *scanning electron microscope*) son aplicaciones valiosas en el estudio de la biopelícula gracias a las propiedades ondulatorias de los electrones, que permiten generar imágenes de los objetos que no pueden verse a simple vista ni con el microscopio óptico. Las figuras 1 a 3 muestran diferentes imágenes de SEM y de CSLM de microorganismos crecidos en biopelículas.

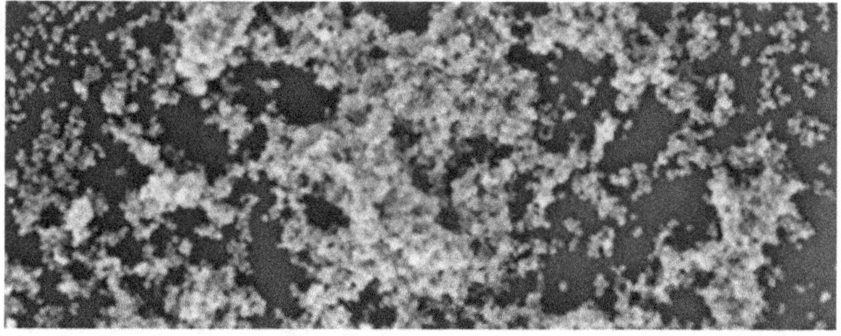

Figura 2. Biopelícula de S. aureus *resistente a la meticilina sobre una superficie de gel de agar. Imagen tomada con microscopio electrónico de barrido. (Paul Gunning/Science Photo Library.)*

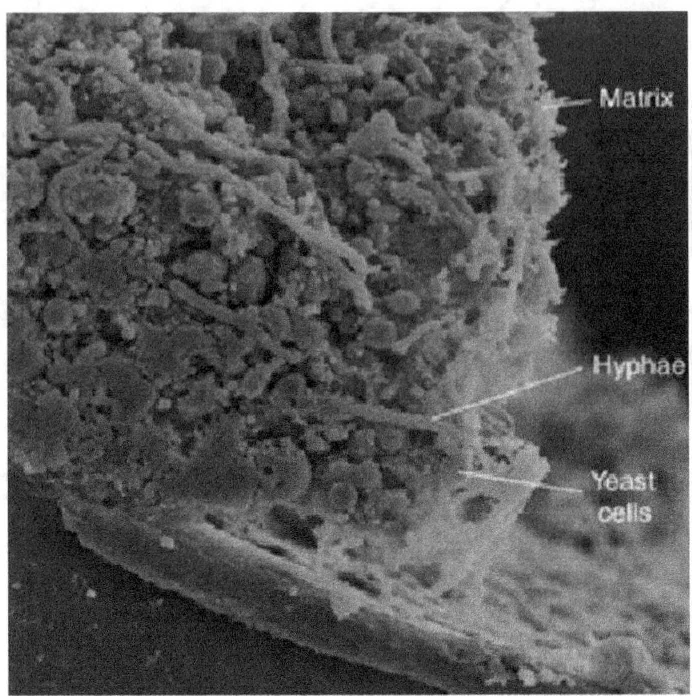

Figura 3. Biopelícula de C. albicans. *Sección transversal de un catéter vascular procedente de un modelo de infección de catéter central en rata. Imagen tomada mediante microscopio electrónico de barrido. Las levaduras y las hifas están rodeadas por la matriz de la biopelícula. (Nett J, Andes D. Candida albicans biofilm development, modeling a host-pathogen interaction. Curr Opin Microbiol. 2006; 9: 340-5.)*

1.2 *Aportación de los modelos* in vitro *a la terapéutica de las infecciones relacionadas con catéteres*

La eliminación de células planctónicas del torrente sanguíneo no implica su eliminación de la biopelícula, ya que las células dispersadas presentan una mayor sensibilidad a los antimicrobianos y las concentraciones aparentemente bactericidas pueden ser ineficaces frente a las bacterias de las biopelículas. Por tanto, las pruebas microbiológicas habituales para evaluar la sensibilidad antibiótica a los diferentes microorganismos no suelen predecir el éxito terapéutico en las infecciones relacionadas con catéteres.

La probabilidad de lograr la erradicación de las biopelículas podría mejorarse mediante el diseño de estudios dirigidos a identificar agentes, antimicrobianos y no antimicrobianos, activos frente a los microorganismos de las biopelículas. Estos estudios deben simular de manera razonable la formación de la biopelícula en el catéter para poder estudiar adecuadamente las propiedades del medio de crecimiento, el estadio de madurez o la densidad celular.

1.2.1 Antimicrobianos

1.2.1.1 *Staphylococcus* spp.

La información aportada por los estudios *in vitro* sobre la actividad de los diferentes antimicrobianos en las biopelículas frente a especies de *Staphylococcus* establece que, en general, los que penetran en la matriz, como la daptomicina,[13] la rifampicina[14] y las fluoroquinolonas,[15] tienen una gran eficacia. Sin embargo, aquellos antimicrobianos que inhiben la síntesis de la pared celular, como por ejemplo los glucopéptidos, suelen ser menos eficaces. Los glucopéptidos tienen propiedades que ensombrecen su actividad frente a la biopelícula, como es su mala penetración o la inhibición por el *slime*.[16]

Los estudios han demostrado que la daptomicina es el antibiótico más eficaz y más rápidamente bactericida.[17] Sin embargo, requiere una concentración alta de calcio en la solución, lo cual invalida su uso con un quelante del calcio como es el ácido etilendiaminotetraacético (EDTA). Por otro lado, hay una base para asumir que la combinación de fármacos con diferentes mecanismos de acción es favorable. Los macrólidos parecen reducir la sustancia extracelular polimérica de la biopelícula y permiten una mayor penetración de otros agentes antimicrobianos.[18,19] Diversos estudios con rifampicina también han demostrado su efecto sinérgico en la biopelícula.[14] Sin embargo, y en general para las infecciones relacionadas con catéteres en las cuales la formación de la biopelícula es en general reciente, las combinaciones de antimicrobianos probablemente no sean necesarias y se simplifica con el sellado del catéter.

- *Staphylococcus epidermidis*

  Varios estudios han demostrado una menor actividad de la vancomicina, en comparación con otros antimicrobianos, frente a *S. epidermidis* que crecen en biopelículas. Esto se debe en parte, como ya se ha comentado, a una pobre penetración en las biopelículas.[15,17]

  La daptomicina es uno de los antibióticos más eficaces, con una excelente actividad *in vitro* frente a *S. epidermidis* en biopelículas. Ha resultado más eficaz que el linezolid y la rifampicina utilizando concentraciones iguales a las plasmáticas frente a *S. epidermidis* en biopelículas.[14] LaPlante *et al.*[20] demostraron que la daptomicina en dosis de 5 mg/ml como sellado antibiótico erradicaba las colonias de *S. epidermidis* tras 72 horas en un modelo de catéter *in vitro*. En otro modelo *in vitro* que simulaba las condiciones *in vivo* mediante un sistema de cultivo continuo, la daptomicina fue más eficaz que la vancomicina.[17] La eficiencia de la daptomicina frente a *S. epidermidis* en las biopelículas se debe a su facilidad para penetrar en ellas. De hecho, accede a las partes más profundas en tan sólo uno o dos minutos.[21] Esto podría ser porque la daptomicina inhibe la síntesis y la maduración del *slime*, componente fundamental de la biopelícula.[13]

La rifampicina también es eficaz, sobre todo en concentraciones alrededor de la concentración mínima inhibitoria (CMI).[14] Sin embargo, la aparición de cepas resistentes durante el tratamiento ha limitado su uso en monoterapia.[22] Por último, con linezolid se han observado respuestas variables y en ocasiones dependientes del tipo de cepa.[14,23]

- *STAPHYLOCOCCUS AUREUS*

  La eficacia de la vancomicina y la daptomicina frente a *S. aureus* que crecen en las biopelículas es parecida a la comentada anteriormente frente a *S. epidermidis*. La capacidad erradicadora de la vancomicina es lenta y limitada.[20,24-26] Sin embargo, estudios con daptomicina han mostrado que este antibiótico es rápidamente bactericida frente a *S. aureus* que crece en biopelículas.[20,27]

  Lee *et al.*[25] observaron que 5 mg/ml de vancomicina, ciprofloxacino o rifampicina pueden erradicar a *S. aureus* de las biopelículas tras cinco días de tratamiento en un modelo *in vitro*.[25] Sin embargo, otro estudio observó que la vancomicina a dosis de 15 mg/l no conseguía erradicar a *S. aureus* de la biopelícula, y tan sólo su asociación con rifampicina o tigeciclina mejoraba su eficacia.[26] LaPlante *et al.*[20] observaron que aunque la vancomicina tenía actividad bactericida, la daptomicina a dosis de 5 mg/ml fue el único tratamiento capaz de erradicar las colonias de *S. aureus* de las biopelículas en los catéteres.[20] Otro estudio halló que la daptomicina fue más eficaz que la vancomicina para disminuir las colonias de *S. aureus* resistente a la meticilina (SARM) en biopelículas tras 24 horas de exposición al antibiótico.[27] La acción tan favorable de la daptomicina sobre las biopelículas de *S. aureus* parece deberse a su actividad en la inhibición de la síntesis del *slime,* con lo que se previene la formación de la biopelícula o se disgrega su estructura, tanto en la fase inicial como en la madura.[13]

  La asociación de rifampicina con vancomicina o linezolid mostró un aumento de actividad en la erradicación completa de la biopelícula, y su asociación con daptomicina, minociclina o tigeciclina presentó el mismo efecto de una forma más precoz. Sin embargo, su administración en monoterapia se asocia con aparición de resistencias.[27] El linezolid no ha mostrado una buena eficacia *in vitro* para el tratamiento de *S. aureus* en biopelículas.[24] La minociclina tiene una buena actividad frente a las colonias de SARM de la biopelícula.[27,28] Los resultados con tigeciclina han sido contradictorios.[26,27] Por último, la telavancina, un nuevo lipoglucopéptido, también ha mostrado una buena actividad frente a *S. aureus* y *S. epidermidis*.[29]

1.2.1.2 *Candida* spp.

En general, la resistencia a los antifúngicos de las especies de *Candida* que crecen en las biopelículas es multifactorial. Puede ser inducida como respuesta a la exposición concreta a un antifúngico o como resultado de un cambio genético de tipo irreversible por una exposición prolongada al fármaco. En concreto, en las biopelículas pueden producirse alteraciones en las moléculas diana de los antifúngicos, aparición de sistemas enzimáticos de bombas de expulsión, disminución de la difusión del antifúngico al interior de la biopelícula, fenómenos de tolerancia y existencia de células persistentes *(persister cells)* en el interior de la biopelícula. Las *persister cells* son una población (alrededor del 1 %) de variantes fenotípicas de la población inicial (no son una variante mutante) que sobreviven en los cultivos de biopelículas a concentraciones muy por encima de las CMI.

La resistencia a los azoles en las especies de *Candida* que crecen en biopelículas está determinada por dos mecanismos. En las fases iniciales de la formación de la biopelícula, aparecen unas bombas de expulsión determinadas genéticamente.[30,31] Por otra parte, las alteraciones en la composición del esterol, con concentraciones disminuidas de ergosterol en las etapas intermedias y finales de la formación de la biopelícula de *Candida*, son otro de los mecanismos que inducen una disminución de la eficacia de los azoles.[32]

El mecanismo de acción de las equinocandinas no se conoce en profundidad, y sorprende su eficacia teniendo en cuenta que por su gran tamaño deberían tener problemas para penetrar en el interior de la biopelícula. Es posible que, como las equinocandinas inhiben la síntesis del β-(1,3)-glucano, uno de los componentes principales de la matriz extracelular de la biopelícula de *Candida* spp., resida aquí en parte su mecanismo de acción.[33-36]

También se desconoce el mecanismo de acción de las formulaciones lipídicas de amfotericina B, y como ocurre con las equinocandinas, su gran tamaño no favorecería su difusión hacia el interior de la biopelícula. En este caso, su capacidad de dispersión en fosfolípidos facilitaría el paso a través de la matriz extracelular de la biopelícula.[32]

Los nuevos triazoles (voriconazol y posaconazol) muestran una eficacia similar a la del fluconazol frente a las especies de *Candida* crecidas en biopelículas.[37-39]

En un modelo *in vitro* de catéter para evaluar amfotericina B liposómica frente a *Candida albicans, Candida glabrata* y *Candida parapsilosis* en biopelículas se observó que, a dosis de 1 mg/m, inhibía sustancialmente, aunque no por completo, la actividad metabólica de la biopelícula.[40] Raad *et al.*[41] también observaron que la amfotericina B complejo lipídico presentaba actividad, aunque moderada, frente a las biopelículas de *C. albicans* y *C. parapsilosis*.

Las equinocandinas, sin embargo, han mostrado una excelente actividad *in vitro* frente a las biopelículas de *Candida*.[42] Katragkou *et al.*[37] hallaron que la caspofungina y la anidulafungina mantienen su actividad de forma adecuada frente a cepas de *C. albicans* y *C. parapsilosis* cuando crecen en biopelículas. Del mismo modo, Cateau *et al.*[43] objetivaron que la caspofungina y la micafungina eran claramente efectivas en la reducción y el control de las biopelículas fúngicas al usarlas como soluciones de sellado del catéter en un modelo *in vitro*.

En cuanto a la formación de la biopelícula, hay diferencias según las especies de *Candida* spp., principalmente por la cantidad de polisacárido en la matriz del componente extracelular, que pueden ser objetivables en la exploración con CSLM.[44]

A diferencia de las otras especies de *Candida*, en las cuales no se objetiva una diferencia muy significativa entre las equinocandinas y las formulaciones lipídicas de la amfotericina B frente a *C. parapsilosis,* las equinocandinas, y en concreto la anidulafungina, son más eficaces que la amfotericina B liposómica. Este hecho se ha comprobado en estudios *in vitro*[45,46] y en el modelo animal en nuestro laboratorio, como comentaremos más adelante.

1.2.2   *Agentes no antimicrobianos*

1.2.2.1   *Staphylococcus* spp.

Cationes metálicos como el calcio, el magnesio y el hierro están implicados en el mantenimiento de la matriz de la estructura en la biopelícula. Los agentes quelantes pueden desestabilizar esta estructura, y algunos, como el EDTA, tienen propiedades antimicrobianas frente a bacterias y hongos en asociación con minociclina, tigeciclina o gentamicina.[28,47,48] El citrato de sodio, otro agente quelante, también ha mostrado actividad antimicrobiana *in vitro* al inhibir la formación de biopelículas de varias cepas de *S. aureus* y de estafilococos coagulasa negativos.[49,50]

También se ha sugerido la eficacia del etanol.[51] Sin embargo, Raad *et al.*[52] hallaron que el etanol sólo era eficaz contra las biopelículas de *S. aureus* en combinación con minociclina y EDTA, por lo que serán necesarios nuevos estudios para establecer con claridad la actividad del etanol sobre la biopelícula.

La adición de N-acetilcisteína a la tigeciclina ha demostrado ser sinérgica y erradicar SARM de la biopelícula del catéter a las cuatro horas de exposición.[53]

Otras sustancias, como los biocidas oxidantes y la taurolidina, así como los bacteriófagos y los inhibidores del *quorum sensing,* que no incorporan los antimicrobianos, pueden prevenir o erradicar las biopelículas de los catéteres vasculares.[54] El *quorum sensing* es una señalización célula a célula que desempeña un papel en la unión celular y en la formación de biopelículas. Con suficientes densidades de población, estas señales alcanzan las concentraciones requeridas para la activación de los genes implicados en la diferenciación de la biopelícula.[55] Algunos estudios *in vitro* han demostrado que el péptido inhibidor de la molécula de detección de *quorum* RNA III impide que los estafilococos formen biopelículas en una variedad de superficies, y que puede ser eficaz junto con antibióticos para la erradicación de la biopelícula.[56]

La contribución de la heparina en la formación de las biopelículas es discutida. Shanks *et al.*[57] observaron que la heparina utilizada como anticoagulante en el sellado del catéter estimulaba la formación *in vitro* de biopelícula de *S. aureus*. Sin embargo, en un estudio de LaPlante *et al.*[20] se observó que, para *S. epidermidis*, la adición de heparina mejoraba la actividad de la vancomicina frente a la formación de biopelículas.

1.2.2.2   *Candida* spp.

Se han estudiado diversas moléculas por su actividad antifúngica frente a biopelículas de especies de *Candida*. Además de antibióticos como la doxiciclina y la tigeciclina a dosis altas, algunos agentes no antimicrobianos, como la heparina y los parabenos, han mostrado una actividad importante.[58-60]

Otros antibióticos con posible actividad antifúngica incluyen la combinación de rifampicina con minociclina o ciprofloxacino.[61] La asociación de EDTA con tetrasodio,[48] minociclina o amfotericina en complejo lipídico también ha demostrado un efecto antifúngico sinérgico.[41]

La DNAasa, que escinde selectivamente el DNA extracelular, parece mejorar la actividad de la amfotericina desoxicolato.[62] También se ha observado que otras sustancias, como el quitosano,[63] la taurolidina más citrato,[64] el ácido acetilsalicílico y los esteroides antiinflamatorios[65] pueden tener actividad sobre las biopelículas de *Candida* spp.

Diferentes estudios *in vitro* indican que el etanol tiene una excelente actividad frente a especies de *Candida*.[52,66,67] Recientemente se ha demostrado que una concentración de etanol del 10 % inhibe el 99 % de las colonias de *Candida* que crecen en biopelículas.[66]

1.3   Estabilidad de los antimicrobianos en el sellado

Además de la necesidad del uso de antibióticos que penetren en las biocapas y alcancen altas concentraciones *in situ*, otro factor determinante de la efectividad del tratamiento es la estabilidad de las soluciones antimicrobianas utilizadas. Varios trabajos *in vitro* han estudiado la estabilidad de diferentes antibióticos (cefazolina, ciprofloxacino, colistina, gentamicina, vancomicina, linezolid y daptomicina), solos o en combinación con heparina, tras una incubación a 25 °C o 37 °C, y han hallado una adecuada estabilidad.[20,68,69]

2   Modelos *in vivo*

Las biopelículas son ecosistemas microbianos complejos organizados sobre superficies vivas o inertes. En su formación no sólo intervienen microorganismos con capacidad para producir una matriz extracelular de exopolisacáridos a su alrededor y de cooperar entre ellos mediante *quorum-sensing*. En el caso particular de las biopelículas que se forman sobre catéteres vasculares hay una multitud de factores que interaccionan alterando su constitución, tales como la agregación de las plaquetas, la dinámica de fluidos y el sistema inmunitario, entre otros.

Aunque diversos modelos *in vitro* han intentado tener en cuenta algunos de estos factores específicos, es sumamente difícil que sus resultados sean reproducibles por completo en pacientes concretos. Por ello, los modelos animales siguen siendo imprescindibles para validar los tratamientos antibióticos sin retirar el catéter, con la técnica denominada «sellado antibiótico».

Hasta la fecha, el modelo animal más utilizado para estudiar el tratamiento conservador de las infecciones relacionadas con catéteres mediante la técnica del sellado antibiótico es el de conejo. Desde la descripción del modelo de cateterización de una vía venosa central realizado por Walsh *et al.*[70] se han realizado diversas modificaciones para adaptar la técnica a los diferentes objetivos.[71-78] El tamaño del conejo permite una cómoda inserción del catéter, y por otro lado, el diámetro del catéter utilizado es similar al de los usados en los humanos, lo que garantiza la reproducibilidad de los resultados.

Otro modelo ampliamente utilizado es el de rata, que presenta como ventajas respecto al conejo su menor coste de estabulación y su menor labilidad.[56,79-83] También se han descrito otros modelos, como el de perro,[84] pero no están justificados debido a su posición en un nivel más alto de la escala filogenética y además tienen un mayor coste de estabulación.

2.1 Modelo en conejo del tratamiento conservador de las infecciones relacionadas con catéteres

En el Laboratorio de Enfermedades Infecciosas del Hospital Universitari Vall d'Hebron (Barcelona) se utilizan conejos de la raza New Zealand con un peso aproximado de 2 kg, estabulados en cajas individuales y sin restricción en la ingesta de agua y pienso.

2.1.1 Inserción del catéter

Se anestesia al animal mediante una inyección intramuscular de ketamina (100 mg/kg) y xilacina (20 mg/kg). Se realiza una incisión laterocervical para exponer la bifurcación de la vena yugular. Se liga la vena yugular interna cranealmente y se cateteriza el extremo caudal con un catéter de silicona estéril (de 0,45 y 0,77 pulgadas de diámetro interno y externo, respectivamente). De los 18 cm de longitud del catéter, ocho quedan dentro de la luz vascular para asegurar que el extremo distal se encuentra en la vena cava superior. Se fija el catéter con puntos de seda y se comprueba su permeabilidad mediante aspiración de sangre e infusión de solución salina estéril. Se tuneliza el catéter a través del tejido celular subcutáneo hasta la región interescapular, donde la porción externa se une a una conexión extraíble unida a su vez a un reservorio desechable, que se fija con puntos de seda a la piel. Se coloca un chaleco al conejo para la protección del sistema.

2.1.2   Inoculación del catéter

Tras su inserción, el catéter se inocula con una suspensión del microorganismo objeto de estudio. En los casos de *S. aureus* y *S. epidermidis*, la cepa es subcultivada en caldo TSA durante 24 horas a 37 °C y atmósfera ambiente. Las colonias del subcultivo son suspendidas en caldo TSB con un 0,5 % de dextrosa e incubadas en un baño de agitación hasta alcanzar una turbidez equivalente al 0,5 de McFarland (10^8 unidades formadoras de colonias [UFC]/ml). Para las especies de *Candida,* la cepa es subcultivada en medio de Sabouraud con un 8 % de dextrosa durante 48 horas a 35 °C y atmósfera ambiente. Las colonias del subcultivo se suspenden en medio antibiótico 3 con un 8 % de dextrosa hasta alcanzar una concentración final de 10^7 UFC/ml. Cabe destacar que en los estudios experimentales se utilizan cepas aisladas de pacientes con bacteriemia o fungemia relacionada con un catéter demostrada.

Para la longitud y el diámetro del catéter descrito se utilizan 0,3 ml de la suspensión, que es el volumen necesario para cubrir toda la superficie interna minimizando el riesgo de metástasis sépticas a distancia.

El tiempo que permanece la suspensión en el interior del catéter depende del microorganismo estudiado: 18 horas para *S. aureus* y *S. epidermidis,* y 48 horas para las distintas especies de *Candida.*

2.1.3   Sellado antibiótico del catéter

Justo antes de iniciar el sellado antibiótico se retira cuidadosamente el inóculo mediante aspiración con jeringa. Se recambian el reservorio desechable y la conexión por otros estériles. Entonces se rellena de nuevo el sistema con 0,33 ml de la solución antibiótica en estudio o con solución salina en los controles.

El tiempo que permanece el antibiótico en la superficie interna del catéter también depende del microorganismo estudiado: 24 horas para *S. aureus* y *S. epidermidis,* y 48 horas para *Candida* spp.

2.1.4   Estudios de eficacia

Al final de periodo de tratamiento se sacrifica al animal mediante inyección intravenosa de pentotal sódico. Se retira el catéter cuidadosamente para su evaluación microbiológica mediante técnica aséptica. Se cortan los 4 cm distales para realizar un cultivo cuantitativo. Se instilan 2 ml de solución salina a través de luz del catéter y se repite la maniobra con el mismo suero. A continuación se secciona longitudinalmente este segmento y se sumerge en 4 ml de solución salina estéril para ser sonicado a 50 Hz durante 10 minutos. Se lava dos veces el producto de la instilación y el del sonicado mediante centrifugación, y el precipitado es resuspendido en solución salina. Tras el segundo lavado se resuspende el precipitado en 1 ml de solución salina y se diluye de forma seriada. Para asegurar que se recuperan y cuentan todas las células viables, se cultivan pequeñas alícuotas de las diluciones, así como del volumen restante no diluido, por duplicado, en placas de agar Columbia de sangre de cordero al 5 % durante 48 horas a 37 °C y atmósfera ambiente. Tras la incubación, se cuentan las colonias. Los resultados se expresan como $\log_{10}$ del total de UFC.

2.1.5   Análisis estadístico

Con un objetivo meramente metodológico, se asigna una UFC a aquellos catéteres que dan un resultado negativo en el cultivo. El porcentaje de cultivos negativos se compara utilizando la prueba exacta de Fisher. Los $\log_{10}$ de las UFC recuperadas de las puntas de los catéteres se comparan utilizando la prueba U de Mann-Whitney.

2.2   Aportación de los modelos animales a la terapéutica de las infecciones relacionadas con catéteres

2.2.1   Infecciones estafilocócicas

Las tablas 1 a 3 muestran la experiencia del Laboratorio de Enfermedades Infecciosas del Hospital Vall d'Hebron en el tratamiento conservador de las infecciones relacionadas con catéteres por estafilococos en el modelo experimental de conejo.

De estos trabajos puede concluirse que la vancomicina, aun siendo el antibiótico más utilizado para el tratamiento conservador de estas infecciones, tiene una efectividad moderada, similar a la del linezolid, frente a *S. aureus* (tanto sensibles como resistentes a la meticilina) y *S. epidermidis*. El ciprofloxacino presenta una efectividad ligeramente superior a la de la vancomicina en cepas de *S. aureus* sensible a la meticilina (SASM).[72,77] Estos hallazgos son comparables con los de un estudio de un grupo italiano realizado en el modelo de rata con una única cepa de SASM.[79]

La gentamicina en dosis altas (40.000 mg/l) es rápidamente bactericida y puede negativizar en 24 horas un porcentaje importante de catéteres infectados por SASM y SARM. También la daptomicina en dosis altas (50.000 mg/l) ha demostrado ser rápidamente bactericida tanto en cepas de SASM y SARM como en *S. epidermidis*. Además, en el caso de SASM y SARM, 50.000 mg/l de daptomicina son más eficaces que 5.000 mg/l, consiguiendo un mayor porcentaje de negativización de catéteres y una mayor reducción en el número de UFC en ellos. Sin embargo, dosis altas de vancomicina (10.000 mg/l) no consiguen mejores resultados que las dosis convencionales de 2.000 mg/l.

	SASM (ATCC 29213)		SASM (ATCC 6538P)	
Tratamiento	**Cultivo negativo/total cultivos (%)**	**Log$_{10}$ total de UFC Media (DE)**	**Cultivo negativo/total cultivos (%)**	**Log$_{10}$ total de UFC Media (DE)**
Control (solución salina)	0/9 (0)	5,50 (1,89)	0/8 (0)	5,64 (1,32)
Linezolid (2.000 mg/l)	1/8 (13)	3,49 (1,87)[a]	0/8 (0)	4,93 (0,59)
Vancomicina (2.000 mg/l)	1/7 (14)	4,38 (1,91)[a]	0/9 (0)	4,97 (1,13)
Gentamicina (40.000 mg/l)	7/11 (64)[a]	1,24 (1,35)[a,b]	7/8 (88)[a]	0,54 (0,66)[c,d]
Ciprofloxacino (2.000 mg/l)	0/8 (0)	2,98 (1,83)[a]	0/8 (0)	2,95 (1,50)[c]
	SARM 7		SARM 16	
Tratamiento	**Cultivo negativo/total cultivos (%)**	**Log$_{10}$ total de UFC Media (DE)**	**Cultivo negativo/total cultivos (%)**	**Log$_{10}$ total de UFC Media (DE)**
Control (solución salina)	0/15 (0)	5,90 (1,13)	0/9 (0)	5,94 (1,36)
Linezolid (2.000 mg/l)	0/10 (0)	5,13 (0,94)[a]	0/12 (0)	4,64 (1,62)
Vancomicina (2.000 mg/l)	0/13 (0)	5,11 (1,05)[a]	0/13 (0)	5,00 (1,41)
Gentamicina (40.000 mg/l)	4/10 (40)[a]	2,19 (1,78)[a,e]	2/8 (25)[a]	3,00 (2,67)

SASM: *S. aureus* sensible a la meticilina; SARM: *S. aureus* resistente a la meticilina; UFC: unidades formadoras de colonias; DE: desviación estándar.
[a] p < 0,05 frente a control; [b] p < 0,05 frente al resto de grupos de tratamiento; [c] p < 0,01 frente a control, linezolid y vancomicina; [d] p < 0,01 frente a ciprofloxacino; [e] p < 0,01 frente a linezolid y vancomicina.

Tabla 1. Tratamiento de las infecciones relacionadas con catéteres experimentales causadas por S. aureus *sensible y resistente a la meticilina con linezolid, vancomicina, gentamicina y ciprofloxacino.*[77]

	SASM (ATCC 6538P)		SARM 16	
Tratamiento	**Cultivo negativo/total cultivos (%)**	**Log$_{10}$ total de UFC Mediana (RIC)**	**Cultivo negativo/total cultivos (%)**	**Log$_{10}$ total de UFC Mediana (RIC)**
Control (solución salina)	0/12 (0)	6,08 (5,54-7,36)	0/12 (0)	6,15 (5,62-6,38)
Daptomicina (50.000 mg/l)	9/12 (75)[a]	0 (0-0,58)[b,c]	11/13 (85)[f]	0 (0-0)[f]
Daptomicina (5.000 mg/l)	1/5 (20)	1,74 (0,71-2,39)[d,e]	1/6 (17)	3,07 (1,36- 5,16)[d]
Vancomicina (2.000 mg/l)	1/11 (9)	2,64 (1,43-3,32)[d]	2/11 (18)	2,71 (2,07-3,04)[d]
Vancomicina (10.000 mg/l)	0/10 (0)	3,61 (2,56-4,43)[d]	–	–

UFC: unidades formadoras de colonias; RIC: rango intercuartílico.
[a] p < 0,05 frente al resto de los grupos de tratamiento; [b] p < 0,001 frente a control y vancomicina; [c] p < 0,05 frente a daptomicina 5.000 mg/l; [d] p < 0,01 frente a control; [e] p < 0,05 frente a vancomicina 5.000 mg/l; [f] p < 0,01 frente a control, daptomicina 5.000 mg/l y vancomicina 2.000 mg/l.

Tabla 2. Tratamiento de las infecciones relacionadas con catéteres experimentales causadas por S. aureus *sensible y resistente a la meticilina con diferentes dosis de daptomicina y vancomicina.*[86]

	S. epidermidis 14C		**S. epidermidis** 94C	
Tratamiento	**Cultivo negativo/total cultivos (%)**	**Log$_{10}$ total de UFC Mediana (RIC)**	**Cultivo negativo/total cultivos (%)**	**Log$_{10}$ total de UFC Mediana (RIC)**
Control (solución salina)	0/7 (0)	5,5 (5,1-6,4)	0/7 (0)	5,8 (5,2-6,5)
Daptomicina 50.000 mg/l	9/10 (90)[a]	0 (0-0)[a]	6/7 (86)[a]	0 (0-0)[a]
Vancomicina 10.000 mg/l	0/6 (0)	4,1 (3,2-4,7)[b]	0/6 (0)	4,7 (3,6-5,3)[b]

UFC: unidades formadoras de colonias; RIC: rango intercuartílico.
[a] p < 0,01 frente a control y vancomicina; [b] p < 0,05 frente a control.

Tabla 3. Tratamiento de las infecciones relacionadas con catéteres experimentales causadas por S. epidermidis *resistente a la cloxacilina con daptomicina, gentamicina y vancomicina.*[87]

Estudios en humanos deberán corroborar estos hallazgos, en especial en las infecciones por estafilococos coagulasa negativos, que son los microorganismos con más frecuencia involucrados en este tipo de infecciones.[4] En episodios producidos por *S. aureus,* si excepcionalmente se plantea la técnica del sellado antibiótico,[1] estaría justificado el uso de daptomicina o gentamicina en altas concentraciones.

2.2.2 Infecciones fúngicas

Las tablas 4 a 6 muestran la experiencia del Laboratorio de Enfermedades Infecciosas del Hospital Vall d'Hebron en el tratamiento conservador de las infecciones relacionadas con catéteres por especies de *Candida* en el modelo experimental de conejo.

	C. albicans CP174		**C. albicans** CP12	
Tratamiento	**Cultivo negativo/total cultivos (%)**	**Log$_{10}$ total de UFC Mediana (RIC)**	**Cultivo negativo/total cultivos (%)**	**Log$_{10}$ total de UFC Mediana (RIC)**
Control (solución salina)	0/15 (0)	5,12 (4,18-5,62)	0/10 (0)	5,34 (4,55-5,78)
Amfotericina B liposómica (5.000 mg/l)	18/19 (95)[a]	0 (0-0)[b]	8/12 (67)[a]	0 (0-0,34)[b,c]
Caspofungina (5.000 mg/l)	17/18 (94)[a]	0 (0-0)[b]	4/10 (40)	2,3 (0-3,9)[b]
Fluconazol (2.000 mg/l)	0/9 (0)	5,37 (3,08-5,74)	0/7 (0)	4,57 (3,69-4,74)

UFC: unidades formadoras de colonias; RIC: rango intercuartílico.
[a] p < 0,05 frente a control; [b] p < 0,01 frente a control y fluconazol; [c] p < 0,05 frente a caspofungina.

Tabla 4. Tratamiento de las infecciones relacionadas con catéteres experimentales causadas por C. albicans *con amfotericina B liposómica, caspofungina y fluconazol.*[88]

	C. glabrata	
Tratamiento	**Cultivo negativo/total cultivos (%)**	**Log_{10} total de UFC Mediana (RIC)**
Control (solución salina)	0/12 (0)	5,09 (4,71-5,57)
Amfotericina B liposómica (5.000 mg/l)	8/14 (54)[a]	0 (0-1,19)[a]
Caspofungina (5.000 mg/l)	6/9 (67)[a]	0 (0-3,33)[a]
Fluconazol (2.000 mg/l)	0/8 (0)	4,68 (4,13-5,71)

UFC: unidades formadoras de colonias; RIC: rango intercuartílico.
[a] p < 0,05 frente a control y fluconazol.

Tabla 5. Tratamiento de las infecciones relacionadas con catéteres experimentales causadas por una cepa de C. glabrata *con amfotericina B liposómica, caspofungina y fluconazol.*[89]

	C. parapsilosis CP12		C. parapsilosis CP54	
Tratamiento	**Cultivo negativo/total cultivos (%)**	**Log_{10} total de UFC Mediana (RIC)**	**Cultivo negativo/total cultivos (%)**	**Log_{10} total de UFC Mediana (RIC)**
Control (solución salina)	0/8 (0)	4,76 (2,4-5,4)	0/8 (0)	4,64 (3,56-6,01)
Amfotericina B liposómica (5.000 mg/l)	3/10 (30)	3,04 (0-3,86)[b]	1/6 (23)	2,07 (1,11-3,52)[b]
Anidulafungina (3.333 mg/l)	5/8 (63)[a]	0 (0-1,17)[a]	8/11 (73)[a]	0 (0-0,69)[a]

UFC: unidades formadoras de colonias; RIC: rango intercuartílico.
[a] p < 0,01 frente a control y amfotericina B; [b] p < 0,05 frente a control.

Tabla 6. Tratamiento de las infecciones relacionadas con catéteres experimentales causadas por C. parapsilosis *con amfotericina B liposómica y anidulafungina.*

En primer lugar, debemos señalar que la efectividad del tratamiento depende de la especie de *Candida* causante de la infección. Así, la amfotericina B liposómica parece ser el antifúngico más activo frente a *C. albicans*. Las equinocandinas muestran más actividad que la amfotericina B frente a *C. glabrata* y *C. parapsilosis,* y similar frente a *C. albicans* (esto último corroborado por estudios de otros autores).[74-76,85] En todos los casos, el fluconazol muestra una actividad marginal.

En segundo lugar, aunque se considera que *C. parapsilosis* es menos sensible a las equinocandinas que a otros antifúngicos, en el modelo experimental se observa un efecto paradójico. El sellado con anidulafungina consiguió más altos porcentajes de negativización de los catéteres infectados por *C. parapsilosis* que si se utilizaba amfotericina B liposómica.

En tercer lugar, teniendo en cuenta la efectividad global de los diferentes antifúngicos frente a las distintas especies de *Candida*, y que *C. parapsilosis* es la especie más asociada con las infecciones relacionadas con catéteres, en caso de que se plantee realizar tratamiento conservador el antifúngico de elección empírica sería una equinocandina.

3 Conclusiones

Los estudios *in vitro* y los modelos animales han ayudado a avanzar en el conocimiento del tratamiento conservador de las infecciones relacionadas con catéteres vasculares de larga duración causadas por estafilococos coagulasa negativos mediante la técnica de sellado antibiótico. A partir de estos estudios deberían realizarse ensayos clínicos que nos permitan llevar estos resultados a la práctica clínica.

En casos muy seleccionados de infecciones causadas por *S. aureus* y por especies de *Candida*, y ante la escasez de estudios clínicos, podría plantearse la utilización de las estrategias que han demostrado ser eficaces en los modelos animales.

Bibliografía

1. Mermel LA, Allon M, Bouza E, Craven DE, Flynn P, O'Grady NP, *et al.* Clinical practice guidelines for the diagnosis and management of intravascular catheter-related infection: 2009 update by the Infectious Diseases Society of America. Clin Infect Dis. 2009; 49: 1-45.
2. Pappas PG, Kauffman CA, Andes D, Benjamin DK, Jr., Calandra TF, Edwards JE, Jr., *et al.* Clinical practice guidelines for the management of candidiasis: 2009 update by the Infectious Diseases Society of America. Clin Infect Dis. 2009; 48: 503-35.
3. Fortun J, Grill F, Martín-Dávila P, Bláquez J, Tato M, Sánchez-Corral J, *et al.* Treatment of long-term intravascular catheter-related bacteraemia with antibiotic-lock therapy. J Antimicrob Chemother. 2006; 58: 816-21.
4. Fernández-Hidalgo N, Almirante B, Calleja R, Ruiz I, Planes AM, Rodríguez D, *et al.* Antibiotic-lock therapy for long-term intravascular catheter-related bacteraemia: results of an open, non-comparative study. J Antimicrob Chemother. 2006; 57: 1172-80.
5. Maya ID, Carlton D, Estrada E, Allon M. Treatment of dialysis catheter-related Staphylococcus aureus bacteremia with an antibiotic lock: a quality improvement report. Am J Kidney Dis. 2007; 50: 289-95.
6. Simon A, Bode U, Beutel K. Diagnosis and treatment of catheter-related infections in paediatric oncology: an update. Clin Microbiol Infect. 2006; 12: 606-20.
7. Mah TF, O'Toole GA. Mechanisms of biofilm resistance to antimicrobial agents. Trends Microbiol. 2001; 9: 34-9.
8. Stewart PS, Costerton JW. Antibiotic resistance of bacteria in biofilms. Lancet. 2001; 358: 135-8.
9. Amorena B, Gracia E, Monzón M, Leiva J, Oteiza C, Pérez M, *et al.* Antibiotic susceptibility assay for Staphylococcus aureus in biofilms developed in vitro. J Antimicrob Chemother. 1999; 44: 43-55.
10. Ceri H, Olson ME, Stremick C, Read RR, Morck D, Buret A. The Calgary Biofilm Device: new technology for rapid determination of antibiotic susceptibilities of bacterial biofilms. J Clin Microbiol. 1999; 37: 1771-6.
11. Neu TR, Manz B, Volke F, Dynes JJ, Hitchcock AP, Lawrence JR. Advanced imaging techniques for assessment of structure, compo-

sition and function in biofilm systems. FEMS Microbiol Ecol. 2010; 72: 1-21.

12. Palmer RJ, Jr., Sternberg C. Modern microscopy in biofilm research: confocal microscopy and other approaches. Curr Opin Biotechnol. 1999; 10: 263-8.

13. Roveta S, Marchese A, Schito GC. Activity of daptomycin on biofilms produced on a plastic support by Staphylococcus spp. Int J Antimicrob Agents. 2008; 31: 321-8.

14. Leite B, Gomes F, Teixeira P, Souza C, Pizzolitto E, Oliveira R. In vitro activity of daptomycin, linezolid and rifampicin on Staphylococcus epidermidis biofilms. Curr Microbiol. 2011; 63: 313-7.

15. Salem AH, Elkhatib WF, Ahmed GF, Noreddin AM. Pharmacodynamics of moxifloxacin versus vancomycin against biofilms of methicillin-resistant Staphylococcus aureus and epidermidis in an in vitro model. J Chemother. 2010; 22: 238-42.

16. Singh R, Ray P, Das A, Sharma M. Penetration of antibiotics through Staphylococcus aureus and Staphylococcus epidermidis biofilms. J Antimicrob Chemother. 2010; 65: 1955-8.

17. García I, Conejo MC, Ojeda A, Rodríguez-Baño J, Pascual A. A dynamic in vitro model for evaluating antimicrobial activity against bacterial biofilms using a new device and clinical-used catheters. J Microbiol Methods. 2010; 83: 307-11.

18. Parra-Ruiz J, Vidaillac C, Rose WE, Rybak MJ. Activities of high-dose daptomycin, vancomycin, and moxifloxacin alone or in combination with clarithromycin or rifampin in a novel in vitro model of Staphylococcus aureus biofilm. Antimicrob Agents Chemother. 2010; 54: 4329-34.

19. Sano M, Hirose T, Nishimura M, Takahashi S, Matsukawa M, Tsukamoto T. Inhibitory action of clarithromycin on glycocalyx produced by MRSA. J Infect Chemother. 1999; 5: 10-5.

20. LaPlante KL, Mermel LA. In vitro activity of daptomycin and vancomycin lock solutions on staphylococcal biofilms in a central venous catheter model. Nephrol Dial Transplant. 2007; 22: 2239-46.

21. Stewart PS, Davison WM, Steenbergen JN. Daptomycin rapidly penetrates a Staphylococcus epidermidis biofilm. Antimicrob Agents Chemother. 2009; 53: 3505-7.

22. Svensson E, Hanberger H, Nilsson M, Nilsson LE. Factors affecting development of rifampicin resistance in biofilm-producing Staphylococcus epidermidis. J Antimicrob Chemother. 1997; 39: 817-20.

23. Curtin J, Cormican M, Fleming G, Keelehan J, Colleran E. Linezolid compared with eperezolid, vancomycin, and gentamicin in an in vitro model of antimicrobial lock therapy for Staphylococcus epidermidis central venous catheter-related biofilm infections. Antimicrob Agents Chemother. 2003; 47: 3145-8.

24. Wiederhold NP, Coyle EA, Raad, II, Prince RA, Lewis RE. Antibacterial activity of linezolid and vancomycin in an in vitro pharmacodynamic model of gram-positive catheter-related bacteraemia. J Antimicrob Chemother. 2005; 55: 792-5.

25. Lee JY, Ko KS, Peck KR, Oh WS, Song JH. In vitro evaluation of the antibiotic lock technique (ALT) for the treatment of catheter-related infections caused by staphylococci. J Antimicrob Chemother. 2006; 57: 1110-5.

26. Rose WE, Poppens PT. Impact of biofilm on the in vitro activity of vancomycin alone and in combination with tigecycline and rifampicin against Staphylococcus aureus. J Antimicrob Chemother. 2009; 63: 485-8.

27. Raad I, Hanna H, Jiang Y, Dvorak T, Reitzel R, Chaiban G, et al. Comparative activities of daptomycin, linezolid, and tigecycline against catheter-related methicillin-resistant Staphylococcus bacteremic isolates embedded in biofilm. Antimicrob Agents Chemother. 2007; 51: 1656-60.

28. Raad I, Chatzinikolaou I, Chaiban G, Hanna H, Hachem R, Dvorak T, et al. In vitro and ex vivo activities of minocycline and EDTA against microorganisms embedded in biofilm on catheter surfaces. Antimicrob Agents Chemother. 2003; 47: 3580-5.

29. Gander S, Kinnaird A, Finch R. Telavancin: in vitro activity against staphylococci in a biofilm model. J Antimicrob Chemother. 2005; 56: 337-43.

30. Mukherjee PK, Chandra J, Kuhn DM, Ghannoum MA. Mechanism of fluconazole resistance in Candida albicans biofilms: phase-specific role of efflux pumps and membrane sterols. Infect Immun. 2003; 71: 4333-40.

31. Albertson GD, Niimi M, Cannon RD, Jenkinson HF. Multiple efflux mechanisms are

involved in Candida albicans fluconazole resistance. Antimicrob Agents Chemother. 1996; 40: 2835-41.

32. Tobudic S, Kratzer C, Lassnigg A, Presterl E. Antifungal susceptibility of Candida albicans in biofilms. Mycoses. 2012; 55: 199-204.

33. Al-Fattani MA, Douglas LJ. Biofilm matrix of Candida albicans and Candida tropicalis: chemical composition and role in drug resistance. J Med Microbiol. 2006; 55(Pt 8): 999-1008.

34. Nett J, Lincoln L, Marchillo K, Massey R, Holoyda K, Hoff B, *et al.* Putative role of beta-1,3 glucans in Candida albicans biofilm resistance. Antimicrob Agents Chemother. 2007; 51: 510-20.

35. Walker LA, Gow NA, Munro CA. Fungal echinocandin resistance. Fungal Genet Biol. 2010; 47: 117-26.

36. Kofla G, Ruhnke M. Pharmacology and metabolism of anidulafungin, caspofungin and micafungin in the treatment of invasive candidosis: review of the literature. Eur J Med Res. 2011; 16: 159-66.

37. Katragkou A, Chatzimoschou A, Simitsopoulou M, Dalakiouridou M, Diza-Mataftsi E, Tsantali C, *et al.* Differential activities of newer antifungal agents against Candida albicans and Candida parapsilosis biofilms. Antimicrob Agents Chemother. 2008; 52: 357-60.

38. Tobudic S, Lassnigg A, Kratzer C, Graninger W, Presterl E. Antifungal activity of amphotericin B, caspofungin and posaconazole on Candida albicans biofilms in intermediate and mature development phases. Mycoses. 2010; 53: 208-14.

39. Kuhn DM, George T, Chandra J, Mukherjee PK, Ghannoum MA. Antifungal susceptibility of Candida biofilms: unique efficacy of amphotericin B lipid formulations and echinocandins. Antimicrob Agents Chemother. 2002; 46: 1773-80.

40. Toulet D, Debarre C, Imbert C. Could liposomal amphotericin B (L-AMB) lock solutions be useful to inhibit Candida spp. biofilms on silicone biomaterials? J Antimicrob Chemother. 2012; 67: 430-2.

41. Raad, II, Hachem RY, Hanna HA, Fang X, Jiang Y, Dvorak T, *et al.* Role of ethylene diamine tetra-acetic acid (EDTA) in catheter lock solutions: EDTA enhances the antifungal activity of amphotericin B lipid complex against Candida embedded in biofilm. Int J Antimicrob Agents. 2008; 32: 515-8.

42. Ku TS, Bernardo SM, Lee SA. In vitro assessment of the antifungal and paradoxical activity of different echinocandins against Candida tropicalis biofilms. J Med Microbiol. 2011; 60(Pt 11): 1708-10.

43. Cateau E, Rodier MH, Imbert C. In vitro efficacies of caspofungin or micafungin catheter lock solutions on Candida albicans biofilm growth. J Antimicrob Chemother. 2008; 62: 153-5.

44. Ramage G, Mowat E, Jones B, Williams C, López-Ribot J. Our current understanding of fungal biofilms. Crit Rev Microbiol. 2009; 35: 340-55.

45. Fiori B, Posteraro B, Torelli R, Tumbarello M, Perlin DS, Fadda G, *et al.* In vitro activities of anidulafungin and other antifungal agents against biofilms formed by clinical isolates of different Candida and Aspergillus species. Antimicrob Agents Chemother. 2011; 55: 3031-5.

46. Melo AS, Bizerra FC, Freymuller E, Arthington-Skaggs BA, Colombo AL. Biofilm production and evaluation of antifungal susceptibility amongst clinical Candida spp. isolates, including strains of the Candida parapsilosis complex. Med Mycol. 2011; 49: 253-62.

47. Root JL, McIntyre OR, Jacobs NJ, Daghlian CP. Inhibitory effect of disodium EDTA upon the growth of Staphylococcus epidermidis in vitro: relation to infection prophylaxis of Hickman catheters. Antimicrob Agents Chemother. 1988; 32: 1627-31.

48. Percival SL, Kite P, Eastwood K, Murga R, Carr J, Arduino MJ, *et al.* Tetrasodium EDTA as a novel central venous catheter lock solution against biofilm. Infect Control Hosp Epidemiol. 2005; 26: 515-9.

49. Shanks RM, Sargent JL, Martínez RM, Graber ML, O'Toole GA. Catheter lock solutions influence staphylococcal biofilm formation on abiotic surfaces. Nephrol Dial Transplant. 2006; 21: 2247-55.

50. Takla TA, Zelenitsky SA, Vercaigne LM. Effectiveness of a 30% ethanol/4% trisodium citrate locking solution in preventing biofilm formation by organisms causing haemodialysis catheter-related infections. J Antimicrob Chemother. 2008; 62: 1024-6.

51. Qu Y, Istivan TS, Daley AJ, Rouch DA, Deighton MA. Comparison of various antimicrobial agents as catheter lock solutions: preference for ethanol in eradication of coagulase-negative staphylococcal biofilms. J Med Microbiol. 2009; 58(Pt 4): 442-50.

52. Raad I, Hanna H, Dvorak T, Chaiban G, Hachem R. Optimal antimicrobial catheter lock solution, using different combinations of minocycline, EDTA, and 25-percent ethanol, rapidly eradicates organisms embedded in biofilm. Antimicrob Agents Chemother. 2007; 51: 78-83.

53. Aslam S, Trautner BW, Ramanathan V, Darouiche RO. Combination of tigecycline and N-acetylcysteine reduces biofilm-embedded bacteria on vascular catheters. Antimicrob Agents Chemother. 2007; 51: 1556-8.

54. Donlan RM. Biofilm elimination on intravascular catheters: important considerations for the infectious disease practitioner. Clin Infect Dis. 2011; 52: 1038-45.

55. Donlan RM. Biofilms: microbial life on surfaces. Emerg Infect Dis. 2002; 8: 881-90.

56. Cirioni O, Giacometti A, Ghiselli R, Dell'Acqua G, Orlando F, Mocchegiani F, *et al.* RNAIII-inhibiting peptide significantly reduces bacterial load and enhances the effect of antibiotics in the treatment of central venous catheter-associated Staphylococcus aureus infections. J Infect Dis. 2006; 193: 180-6.

57. Shanks RM, Donegan NP, Graber ML, Buckingham SE, Zegans ME, Cheung AL, *et al.* Heparin stimulates Staphylococcus aureus biofilm formation. Infect Immun. 2005; 73: 4596-606.

58. Miceli MH, Bernardo SM, Ku TS, Walraven C, Lee SA. In vitro analyses of the effects of heparin and parabens on Candida albicans biofilms and planktonic cells. Antimicrob Agents Chemother. 2012; 56: 148-53.

59. Miceli MH, Bernardo SM, Lee SA. In vitro analyses of the combination of high-dose doxycycline and antifungal agents against Candida albicans biofilms. Int J Antimicrob Agents. 2009; 34: 326-32.

60. Ku TS, Palanisamy SK, Lee SA. Susceptibility of Candida albicans biofilms to azithromycin, tigecycline and vancomycin and the interaction between tigecycline and antifungals. Int J Antimicrob Agents. 2010; 36: 441-6.

61. Sherertz RJ, Boger MS, Collins CA, Mason L, Raad II. Comparative in vitro efficacies of various catheter lock solutions. Antimicrob Agents Chemother. 2006; 50: 1865-8.

62. Martins M, Henriques M, López-Ribot JL, Oliveira R. Addition of DNase improves the in vitro activity of antifungal drugs against Candida albicans biofilms. Mycoses. 2012; 55: 80-5.

63. Martínez LR, Mihu MR, Tar M, Cordero RJ, Han G, Friedman AJ, *et al.* Demonstration of antibiofilm and antifungal efficacy of chitosan against candidal biofilms, using an in vivo central venous catheter model. J Infect Dis. 2010; 201: 1436-40.

64. Shah CB, Mittelman MW, Costerton JW, Parenteau S, Pelak M, Arsenault R, *et al.* Antimicrobial activity of a novel catheter lock solution. Antimicrob Agents Chemother. 2002; 46: 1674-9.

65. Alem MA, Douglas LJ. Prostaglandin production during growth of Candida albicans biofilms. J Med Microbiol. 2005; 54(Pt 11): 1001-5.

66. Rane HS, Bernardo SM, Walraven CJ, Lee SA. In vitro analyses of ethanol activity against Candida albicans biofilms. Antimicrob Agents Chemother. 2012; 56: 4487-9.

67. Balestrino D, Souweine B, Charbonnel N, Lautrette A, Aumeran C, Traore O, *et al.* Eradication of microorganisms embedded in biofilm by an ethanol-based catheter lock solution. Nephrol Dial Transplant. 2009; 24: 3204-9.

68. Anthony TU, Rubin LG. Stability of antibiotics used for antibiotic-lock treatment of infections of implantable venous devices (ports). Antimicrob Agents Chemother. 1999; 43: 2074-6.

69. Morales-Molina JA, Mateu-de Antonio J, Grau S, Segura M, Acosta P. La estabilidad como factor para considerar en las soluciones de sellado antibiótico. Enferm Infecc Microbiol Clin. 2010; 28: 104-9.

70. Walsh TJ, Bacher J, Pizzo PA. Chronic silastic central venous catheterization for induction, maintenance and support of persistent granulocytopenia in rabbits. Lab Anim Sci. 1988; 38: 467-71.

71. Segura M, Alia C, Valverde J, Franch G, Torres Rodríguez JM, Sitges-Serra A. Assessment of a new hub design and the semiquantitative

catheter culture method using an in vivo experimental model of catheter sepsis. J Clin Microbiol. 1990; 28: 2551-4.

72. Capdevila JA, Gavaldà J, Fortea J, López P, Martín MT, Gomis X, et al. Lack of antimicrobial activity of sodium heparin for treating experimental catheter-related infection due to Staphylococcus aureus using the antibiotic-lock technique. Clin Microbiol Infect. 2001; 7: 206-12.

73. Raad I, Hachem R, Tcholakian RK, Sherertz R. Efficacy of minocycline and EDTA lock solution in preventing catheter-related bacteremia, septic phlebitis, and endocarditis in rabbits. Antimicrob Agents Chemother. 2002; 46: 327-32.

74. Schinabeck MK, Long LA, Hossain MA, Chandra J, Mukherjee PK, Mohamed S, et al. Rabbit model of Candida albicans biofilm infection: liposomal amphotericin B antifungal lock therapy. Antimicrob Agents Chemother. 2004; 48: 1727-32.

75. Shuford JA, Rouse MS, Piper KE, Steckelberg JM, Patel R. Evaluation of caspofungin and amphotericin B deoxycholate against Candida albicans biofilms in an experimental intravascular catheter infection model. J Infect Dis. 2006; 194: 710-3.

76. Mukherjee PK, Long L, Kim HG, Ghannoum MA. Amphotericin B lipid complex is efficacious in the treatment of Candida albicans biofilms using a model of catheter-associated Candida biofilms. Int J Antimicrob Agents. 2009; 33: 149-53.

77. Fernández-Hidalgo N, Gavaldà J, Almirante B, Martín MT, Onrubia PL, Gomis X, et al. Evaluation of linezolid, vancomycin, gentamicin and ciprofloxacin in a rabbit model of antibiotic-lock technique for Staphylococcus aureus catheter-related infection. J Antimicrob Chemother. 2010; 65: 525-30.

78. Chandra J, Long L, Ghannoum MA, Mukherjee PK. A rabbit model for evaluation of catheter-associated fungal biofilms. Virulence. 2011; 2: 466-74.

79. Giacometti A, Cirioni O, Ghiselli R, Orlando F, Mocchegiani F, Silvestri C, et al. Comparative efficacies of quinupristin-dalfopristin, linezolid, vancomycin, and ciprofloxacin in treatment, using the antibiotic-lock technique, of experimental catheter-related infection due

to Staphylococcus aureus. Antimicrob Agents Chemother. 2005; 49: 4042-5.

80. Ghiselli R, Giacometti A, Cirioni O, Mocchegiani F, Silvestri C, Orlando F, et al. Pretreatment with the protegrin IB-367 affects Gram-positive biofilm and enhances the therapeutic efficacy of linezolid in animal models of central venous catheter infection. J Parenter Enteral Nutr. 2007; 31: 463-8.

81. Van Praagh AD, Li T, Zhang S, Arya A, Chen L, Zhang XX, et al. Daptomycin antibiotic lock therapy in a rat model of staphylococcal central venous catheter biofilm infections. Antimicrob Agents Chemother. 2011; 55: 4081-9.

82. Chauhan A, Lebeaux D, Ghigo JM, Beloin C. Full and broad-spectrum in vivo eradication of catheter-associated biofilms using gentamicin-EDTA antibiotic lock therapy. Antimicrob Agents Chemother. 2012; 56: 6310-8.

83. Chauhan A, Lebeaux D, Decante B, Kriegel I, Escande MC, Ghigo JM, et al. A rat model of central venous catheter to study establishment of long-term bacterial biofilm and related acute and chronic infections. PLoS One. 2012; 7: e37281.

84. Bach A, Just A, Berthold H, Ehmke H, Kirchheim H, Borneff-Lipp M, et al. Catheter-related infections in long-term catheterized dogs. Observations on pathogenesis, diagnostic methods, and antibiotic lock technique. Zentralbl Bakteriol. 1998; 288: 541-52.

85. Lazzell AL, Chaturvedi AK, Pierce CG, Prasad D, Uppuluri P, López-Ribot JL. Treatment and prevention of Candida albicans biofilms with caspofungin in a novel central venous catheter murine model of candidiasis. J Antimicrob Chemother. 2009; 64: 567-70.

86. Gavaldà J, Martín MT, Fernández N, Gomis X, Sordé R, Cabral E, et al. Assessment of antibiotic lock technique (ALT) with daptomycin (DAP), vancomycin (VAN), or gentamicin (GEN) for the treatment of S. aureus (SA) experimental catheter infection (CI). 50th Interscience Conference on Antimicrobial Agents and Chemotherapy. Boston, MA; 2010. Poster No. B-065.

87. Gavaldà J, Orbegozo C, Fernández-Hidalgo N, Gomis X, Almirante B, Pahissa A. Assessment of antibiotic lock technique with daptomycin, vancomycin for the treatment of coagulase-negative staphylococci experimental

catheter infection. 22nd European Congress of Clinical Microbiology and Infectious Diseases. London, UK; 2012. Poster No. 2060.

88. Gavaldà J, López PM, Martín MT, Fernández-Hidalgo N, Gomis X, Pahissa A. Efficacy of amphotericin B liposomal (AmB) or caspofungin (CS) in the treatment of experimental Candida catheter infection (CI) using the antifungal-lock technique (ALT). 48th Interscience Conference on Antimicrobial Agents and Chemotherapy. Washington, DC; 2008. Poster No. M-1560.

Capítulo 8

Tratamiento sistémico de la bacteriemia por catéter

J. Parra Ruiz,[1] A. Bravo Molina,[2] F. Anguita Santos,[1] J. Hernández Quero[1]

[1] **Servicio de Enfermedades Infecciosas**
Hospital Universitario San Cecilio
Granada

[2] **Servicio de Angiología y Cirugía Vascular**
Hospital Universitario San Cecilio
Granada

Correspondencia:
Dr. Jorge Parra Ruiz
jordi@ugr.es

Sinopsis

El tratamiento de la bacteriemia relacionada con un catéter requiere una toma de decisiones rápida y eficaz para disminuir la enorme morbimortalidad que llevan aparejadas. El tratamiento empírico, que ha de iniciarse ante la sospecha de la bacteriemia y tras obtener muestras para cultivo, tiene que incluir antibióticos activos frente a cocos grampositivos resistentes a la meticilina y la ampicilina, y frente a bacilos gramnegativos resistentes, así como la retirada del catéter cuando sea posible. Una vez conocidos los resultados microbiológicos, el tratamiento tiene que ajustarse al informe de sensibilidad antimicrobiana de los patógenos detectados. Como norma general, la duración del tratamiento antibiótico ha de ser de 7 a 14 días en aquellas situaciones en que no haya complicaciones (como metástasis sépticas, inestabilidad hemodinámica o endocarditis infecciosa); en el caso de haber alguna, deberá prolongarse durante 4 a 6 semanas.

1 Medidas generales

Si bien las medidas generales del tratamiento de las infecciones relacionadas con catéteres se comentan en otros capítulos, cabe señalar de nuevo que hay determinadas circunstancias en que es necesario retirar el catéter, ya que, con independencia del tratamiento antibiótico sistémico empleado, no retirarlo se asociará con una menor probabilidad de curación del cuadro infeccioso. Así, la presencia de sepsis grave, inestabilidad hemodinámica, endocarditis o embolia séptica a distancia, supuración por el orificio de punción y persistencia de hemocultivos positivos tras 72 horas de haber iniciado el tratamiento antibiótico, son motivos que obligan a reconsiderar la decisión de mantener el catéter.[1]

Si se opta por no retirar el catéter, el tratamiento antibiótico se administra por vía sistémica y con sellado del catéter con una solución antibiótica, antiséptica o ambas. El tratamiento con sellado antimicrobiano se comenta en otro capítulo, por lo que aquí nos centraremos en el tratamiento sistémico. Éste puede administrarse a través de la luz del catéter infectado o, preferiblemente, mediante otro acceso venoso con el fin de preservar la luz o luces del catéter origen de la infección para efectuar su sellado antimicrobiano de manera óptima.

Una vez comenzado el tratamiento hay que extraer dos muestras para hemocultivo y valorar la esterilización de la bacteriemia. La persistencia de cultivos positivos es un criterio absoluto de retirada del catéter.[1,2]

2 Tratamiento antibiótico sistémico

Como norma general, dada la potencial gravedad de estas infecciones y el aumento de la supervivencia de los pacientes con instauración precoz de un tratamiento antibiótico activo en situaciones de sepsis, la antibioticoterapia ha de iniciarse antes de tener los resultados de los cultivos y de los estudios de sensibilidad.[3] Con posterioridad, el espectro del antibiótico tiene que ajustarse al informe microbiológico.

2.1 *Tratamiento antibiótico empírico*

El tratamiento antibiótico empírico se basa en el estado clínico del paciente (gravedad clínica, comorbilidad, etc.), en los factores de riesgo asociados a la infección (duración de la cateterización y localización del catéter), en la utilización previa de antibióticos y en los microorganismos más frecuentemente implicados en las infecciones relacionadas con catéteres. Los patógenos que con más frecuencia causan bacteriemia relacionada con un catéter son los estafilococos coagulasa negativos y *Staphylococcus aureus*, y en un alto porcentaje de los casos son resistentes a la meticilina, por lo que el tratamiento empírico deberá incluir fármacos activos frente a estas especies resistentes. Los antimicrobianos que poseen actividad frente a estas especies resistentes y que, en principio, podrían ser utilizados en el tratamiento empírico de infecciones por especies resistentes serían la vancomicina, la teicoplanina, la daptomicina, el linezolid y la tigeciclina.

Debido a la creciente evidencia sobre el aumento progresivo de la concentración mínima inhibitoria (CMI) de la vancomicina frente a ciertas cepas de *S. aureus*, junto a la mayor tasa de fracaso en estos casos,[4,5] probablemente este antibiótico no deba ser de elección empírica cuando se sospecha una infección por *S. aureus* resistente a la meticilina (SARM). Por otro lado, Kim *et al.*[6] demostraron que el tratamiento con vancomicina en las bacteriemias por *S. aureus* sensible a la meticilina (SASM) se asociaba con un aumento de la mortalidad en comparación con el tratamiento con betalactámicos (37 % frente a 18 %, p = 0,02) con una *odds ratio* (OR) asociada al aumento de mortalidad en los tratamientos con vancomicina, en comparación con los betalactámicos, de 3,3 (intervalo de confianza del 95 % [IC95 %]: 1,2-3,95). Con posterioridad, Schweizer *et al.*[7] compararon nuevamente de manera retrospectiva la mortalidad de los pacientes con bacteriemia por SASM tratados con vancomicina y la de los tratados con nafcilina o cefazolina, y detectaron un aumento de la mortalidad asociada al tratamiento con vancomicina (20 % con vancomicina frente a 3 % con cefazolina y 7 % con nafcilina, p < 0,01). La probabilidad de supervivencia de los sujetos tratados con vancomicina fue casi un 80 % inferior a la de los que no la recibieron en ningún momento, con una *hazard ratio* (HR) ajustada de 0,21 (IC95 %: 0,09-0,47). Al evaluar el efecto del cambio de tratamiento a nafcilina o cefazolina, en comparación con seguir con vancomicina, tras conocerse que los microorganismos eran sensibles a la meticilina, se observó un aumento de la mortalidad asociado al mantenimiento del tratamiento con vancomicina, de manera que los sujetos que no fueron cambiados al betalactámico tuvieron menor probabilidad de sobrevivir que los que sí se cambiaron (HR: 0,31; IC95 %: 0,10-0,95).

Respecto a la tigeciclina, si bien su amplio espectro la haría ideal para el tratamiento en monoterapia de estas infecciones, sus propias características farmacocinéticas y farmacodinámicas (gran volumen de distribución y, por tanto, bajas concentraciones séricas), desaconsejan su empleo en el tratamiento de las infecciones relacionadas con catéteres.[8]

En el caso del linezolid, según los resultados de un ensayo clínico de fase III[9] podría ser una alternativa, pero algunas dudas sobre su eficacia como tratamiento empírico sin documentar una infección por cocos grampositivos[10] hacen prudente reservar su empleo como alternativa a otras opciones.

Estos datos, tomados en conjunto, llevan a que el tratamiento empírico más adecuado en la actualidad sea la daptomicina. Sus características farmacocinéticas y farmacodinámicas, que le confieren una mayor eficacia a dosis más altas, y la escasa incidencia de efectos secundarios cuando se utiliza en dosis elevadas,[11-13] sugieren que la dosis de daptomicina debería ser de 8-10 mg/kg de peso al día. Por otro lado, si bien es cierto que no se han comparado las eficacias de la daptomicina y de la cloxacilina, se sabe que, al menos en el tratamiento de la bacteriemia complicada y de la endocarditis derecha por SASM, la monoterapia con daptomicina, en dosis de 6 mg/kg de peso al día, no es inferior al tratamiento con cloxacilina más gentamicina (44,6 % para daptomicina frente a 48,6 % con cloxacilina más gentamicina, p = 0,74),[14] por lo que es razonable asumir que la monoterapia con daptomicina es una opción tan aconsejable como el tratamiento con cloxacilina, máxime si se tiene en cuenta la optimización del tratamiento en la actualidad de acuerdo con el conocimiento más adecuado de sus parámetros farmacocinéticos y farmacodinámicos.

Tradicionalmente, la cobertura de otros patógenos variaba en función de las características individuales del paciente; así, en aquellos con neutropenia o con sepsis grave la cobertura de bacilos gramnegativos, incluyendo los no fermentadores (*Pseudomonas* spp. y *Acinetobacter* spp.), se consideraba apropiada. En la actualidad, los bacilos gramnegativos se han convertido en una causa frecuente de infecciones relacionadas con catéteres; en algunas series[15] han sido los causantes de hasta el 40 % de las bacteriemias relacionadas con catéteres, por lo que su cobertura tendría que ser una práctica habitual. El espectro antibiótico para esta cobertura ampliada dependerá de la prevalencia de las resistencias en cada hospital, y por ello es fundamental un estrecho contacto con los laboratorios de microbiología para conocer el mapa de resistencias del centro, y resulta complicado establecer recomendaciones exactas acerca del tratamiento antibiótico empírico más adecuado para cubrir a los bacilos gramnegativos.

Finalmente hay que señalar que *Candida* spp. está implicada con cierta frecuencia en las infecciones relacionadas con catéteres,[16] por lo que cabe considerarla en el tratamiento empírico de los pacientes con sepsis grave que además cumplan alguno de los siguientes criterios: nutrición parenteral total, uso prolongado de antibioticoterapia de amplio espectro, neoplasia hematológica, trasplante de precursores hematopoyéticos o de órgano sólido, localización femoral del catéter o colonización múltiple por *Candida* spp. En estos casos, además de la cobertura antibiótica es recomendable incluir un antifúngico, que puede ser una equinocandina o un azol. Se prefieren las equinocandinas en caso de exposición reciente a los azoles (tres meses previos) y en zonas donde la prevalencia de infecciones por *Candida krusei* o *Candida glabrata* sea alta.[1,17]

En la tabla 1 se resumen las indicaciones del tratamiento antibiótico empírico para las infecciones relacionadas con catéteres. Una vez conocidos el o los microorganismos

Situación clínica	Pauta recomendada	Pauta alternativa
Estabilidad hemodinámica	DAP (8-10 mg/kg al día)[12,13] + CEF o PIPE-TAZO	VAN (15-20 mg/kg cada 8-12 h) + CEF o PIPE-TAZO
Sepsis grave, *shock* séptico	DAP (8-10 mg/kg al día) + CEF o PIPE-TAZO o MER + ANID o CAS o MIC	VAN (dosis de carga 25-30 mg/kg seguida de dosis de 15-20 mg/kg cada 8-12 h)[5,30] + CEF o PIPE-TAZO o MER + ANID o CAS o MIC

DAP: daptomicina; VAN: vancomicina; CEF: cefepima; PIPE-TAZO: piperacilina-tazobactam; MER: meropenem; ANID: anidulafungina; CAS: caspofungina; MIC: micafungina.

Tabla 1. Recomendaciones para el tratamiento empírico de las infecciones relacionadas con catéteres.

implicados, si es necesario se procede al ajuste del tratamiento de acuerdo con los resultados microbiológicos.

2.2 Tratamiento antibiótico dirigido

El tratamiento antibiótico dirigido variará según la identificación del microorganismo causante de la infección y su patrón de sensibilidad antimicrobiana. Con el objeto de estructurar de un modo más docente este apartado, los tratamientos se detallarán de acuerdo con el microorganismo implicado, sin realizar una revisión de todos los antimicrobianos a utilizar. En la tabla 2 se recogen las recomendaciones para el tratamiento dirigido en función de los diferentes microorganismos. Debido a que las infecciones relacionadas por catéteres producidas por levaduras se tratarán en otro lugar, en este capítulo se abordarán de manera exclusiva los aspectos terapéuticos de las infecciones bacterianas.

2.2.1 Estafilococos coagulasa negativos

Como ya hemos señalado, los estafilococos coagulasa negativos son los microorganismos que con más frecuencia están implicados en las bacteriemias relacionadas con catéteres, y presentan una serie de características que los hacen particularmente difíciles de tratar. En primer lugar, la interpretación de los cultivos positivos para estafilococos coagulasa negativos puede ser complicada, porque además de ser la causa más habitual de las bacteriemias relacionadas con catéteres también son la primera causa de contaminación de los hemocultivos, por lo que es necesario discriminar de manera adecuada entre una verdadera bacteriemia y una contaminación.[18] Elzi *et al.*[19] han descrito un algoritmo predictivo basado en una serie de factores de riesgo fácilmente identificables en la cabecera del paciente. La presencia de criterios de síndrome de respuesta inflamatoria sistémica, como fiebre o hipotermia (OR: 2,93; IC95 %: 1,91-4,5), taquicardia (OR: 2,29; IC95 %: 1,50-3,50), taquipnea (OR: 2,4; IC95 %: 1,30-4,43) y leucocitosis o leucocitopenia (OR: 4,15; IC95 %: 2,17-6,36), junto a ser portador de un catéter venoso central (OR: 5,38; IC95 %: 3,25-8,88), se asociaron de manera significativa con una bacteriemia verdadera. La probabilidad de bacteriemia verdadera por estafilococos coagulasa negativos aumentaba en función del número de criterios presentes, y los autores establecieron que la presencia de tres de los criterios de síndrome de respuesta inflamatoria sistémica o dos de ellos junto a ser portador de un catéter venoso central suponía una probabilidad de bacteriemia verdadera superior al 70 %. Datos similares han comunicado Leth *et al.*[20] en un estudio prospectivo realizado durante 30 días en un hospital danés. Por ello, ante un paciente con sospecha de bacteriemia relacionada con catéter y la existencia de al menos dos criterios de síndrome de respuesta inflamatoria sistémica, podemos considerar que se trata de una bacteriemia verdadera por estafilococos coagulasa negativos.

Microorganismo	Pauta recomendada	Pauta alternativa
SASM	CLO 2 g/4 h i.v. ± GENT 5,1 mg/kg cada 24 h i.v. o DAP (8-10 mg/kg al día)[12,13]	VAN (15-20 mg/kg cada 8-12 h) o LNZ 600 mg cada 12 h i.v.
SARM	DAP (8-10 mg/kg al día)	VAN (dosis de carga 25-30 mg/kg seguida de dosis de 15-20 mg/kg cada 8-12 h)[5,30] o LNZ 600 mg cada 12 h i.v.
Enterococos sensibles a la ampicilina	AMP 2 g cada 4 h i.v. ± CRO 2 g cada 24 h i.v. o GENT 5,1 mg/kg cada 24 h i.v.	LNZ 600 mg cada 12 h i.v. o DAP 8-10 mg/kg cada 24 h o VAN (15-20 mg/kg cada 8-12 h)
Enterococos resistentes a la ampicilina	VAN (15-20 mg/kg cada 8-12 h) ± GENT 5,1 mg/kg cada 24 h i.v.	LNZ 600 mg cada 12 h i.v. o DAP 8-10 mg/kg cada 24 h
Enterobacterias	CTX 2 g cada 8 h i.v. o CRO 2 g cada 24 h i.v.	CIP 400 mg cada 12 h i.v. o ERT 1 g cada 24 h i.v.*
P. aeruginosa	MER 1 g cada 8 h i.v. o PIPE-TAZO 4/0,5 g cada 6 h i.v. ± TOBR 5,1 mg/kg cada 24 h i.v. o AMK 15 mg/kg cada 24 h i.v.	IMP 0,5-1 g cada 6-8 h i.v. o CEF 2 g cada 12 h i.v. o CIP 400 mg cada 8 h i.v. ± TOBR 5,1 mg/kg cada 24 h i.v. o AMK 15 mg/kg cada 24 h i.v.

*En caso de cepas productoras de betalactamasas de espectro extendido o enterobacterias ampC.
SASM: *S. aureus* sensible a la meticilina; SARM: *S. aureus* resistente a la meticilina; AMK: amikacina; AMP: ampicilina; CIP: ciprofloxacino; CRO: ceftriaxona; CTX: cefotaxima; DAP: daptomicina; ERT: ertapenem; CEF: cefepima; GENT: gentamicina; IMP: imipenem; MER: meropenem; TOBR: tobramicina; CLO: cloxacilina; PIPE-TAZO: piperacilina-tazobactam; VAN: vancomicina.

Tabla 2. Recomendaciones para el tratamiento dirigido de las bacteriemias relacionadas con catéteres.

No hay estudios aleatorizados que evalúen el tratamiento de las bacteriemias relacionadas con catéteres producidas por estafilococos coagulasa negativos, pero hay consenso general sobre que habitualmente tienen un curso benigno, sobre todo cuando se retira el catéter de forma precoz, y que no suelen asociarse con sepsis grave ni con el desarrollo de metástasis sépticas. La mayoría de los expertos aconsejan tratamiento antibiótico durante cinco a siete días tras la retirada del catéter. No obstante, puesto que muchas de estas bacteriemias se resuelven de manera espontánea después de retirar el catéter que las origina, si no hay otros dispositivos protésicos de riesgo (como marcapasos, implantes ortopédicos o válvulas cardíacas, fundamentalmente), ni evidencia de infección profunda metastásica, puede suspenderse el tratamiento antibiótico, en caso de haberse iniciado, si el paciente queda afebril. En los portadores de otros dispositivos protésicos de riesgo se aconseja retirar el catéter y administrar tratamiento sistémico, y si los hemocultivos persisten positivos a pesar del tratamiento antibiótico deberá descartarse una colonización de dichos dispositivos. Una vez descartada, probablemente 10 a 14 días de tratamiento sistémico serán suficientes.[21]

2.2.2　Staphylococcus aureus

Como norma general, el tratamiento de la bacteriemia relacionada con catéter producida por *S. aureus* consiste en la retirada del catéter y antibioticoterapia sistémica.[1] Tras retirar el catéter, si los hemocultivos posteriores son negativos a las 72 horas del inicio del tratamiento, podría colocarse un nuevo catéter venoso central en un lugar diferente.

Como ya se ha señalado en el apartado del tratamiento empírico, después de conocer el resultado microbiológico de infección por *S. aureus* ha de iniciarse tratamiento con daptomicina en dosis de 8-10 mg/kg de peso cada 24 horas, a la espera del antibiograma. Una vez obtenido el antibiograma, si se trata de SASM puede modificarse el tratamiento y comenzar con cloxacilina, o bien podría plantearse mantener el tratamiento con daptomicina hasta el final, pues recientes datos publicados[22] indican que la eficacia de la daptomicina fue idéntica para SASM y SARM en el tratamiento de la endocarditis infecciosa, con tasas de respuesta por encima del 90 % (91 % para endocarditis derecha y 89 % para endocarditis izquierda), con dosis de daptomicina superiores a 8 mg/kg.

Ya hemos mencionado que no se dispone de estudios directos que hayan comparado la cloxacilina y la daptomicina, pero extrapolando los del registro de la daptomicina[14] parece que ésta, a dosis bajas, no es inferior a la cloxacilina más gentamicina, por lo que consideramos que la recomendación de mantener el tratamiento con dosis altas de daptomicina en caso de SASM es adecuada.

Recientemente se ha observado un aumento del efecto bactericida de la daptomicina, a dosis altas, asociada con fosfomicina, frente a SASM y SARM.[23] Los autores comunicaron el tratamiento de tres pacientes con endocarditis infecciosa izquierda con la asociación de daptomicina (10 mg/kg de peso al día) y fosfomicina (2 g/6 h). Con posterioridad evaluaron *in vitro* la eficacia de la asociación sobre siete cepas de SASM y cinco de SARM, y hallaron sinergia frente a once de ellas (79 %). Así mismo, la asociación de daptomicina y cloxacilina o nafcilina se ha mostrado eficaz en el tratamiento de las bacteriemias persistentes por SARM.[24]

Por todo ello, si bien en las bacteriemias relacionadas con catéteres por SASM, de acuerdo con las guías actuales, puede modificarse el tratamiento y comenzar con un betalactácmico antiestafilocócico (cloxacilina o cefazolina, esta última de elección en caso de hemodiálisis), consideramos igualmente recomendable el tratamiento con daptomicina a dosis altas. Esta recomendación se sustenta en la numerosa evidencia obtenida *in vitro*, así como en las experiencias publicadas sobre tratamiento en pacientes. Finalmente, por sus características farmacocinéticas y farmacodinámicas, su utilización en régimen de administración única diaria y su escasa venotoxicidad, la daptomicina permite que estos pacientes, en general con accesos venosos difíciles, se beneficien de poder tener el catéter sellado la mayor parte del tiempo o de la durabilidad de una vía venosa alternativa, en caso de no poder utilizar el reservorio. Esto supone una enorme ventaja con respecto a la cloxacilina, que por sus propiedades farmacocinéticas y farmacodinámicas debe administrarse cada 4 horas y a dosis altas, o preferiblemente en infusión continua,[25,26] y precisa un acceso venoso ocupado continuamente por un antibiótico con una venotoxicidad de moderada a alta,[27] en especial tras dos días de tratamiento,[28] lo que podría hacernos decantar por el empleo de daptomicina para el tratamiento de las bacteriemias relacionadas con catéteres causadas por SASM.

En las infecciones por SARM, con independencia de la CMI de la vancomicina, la opinión de los autores de este capítulo es que el tratamiento de elección ha de ser la daptomicina, y que la vancomicina, por la dificultad para alcanzar concentraciones terapéuticas,[29] la posible nefrotoxicidad con las dosis necesarias para el tratamiento de las infecciones por SARM (con CMI de 1 mg/l y valores valle de 15-20 mg/l)[5,30,31] que persiste incluso tras ajustar por otras covariables potencialmente nefrotóxicas,[32] la necesidad de monitorizar sus concentraciones, la posibilidad de que se trate de cepas con un fenotipo de heterorresistencia a la vancomicina[33] (hasta un 8 % en algunas series[34]), y la menor eficacia en las infecciones por SARM,[4] tiene que considerarse una estrategia alternativa, reservada para aquellos pacientes en que no puedan utilizarse otras opciones terapéuticas.

En caso de fracaso terapéutico con betalactámicos antiestafilocócicos (SASM) o con daptomicina (SASM o SARM), la asociación de fosfomicina o cloxacilina con daptomicina se ha mostrado sinérgica tanto en estudios *in vitro* como en series de casos.[18,22-24]

No hay estudios aleatorizados que permitan establecer la duración óptima del tratamiento antibiótico. En la actualidad, se basa en la existencia o no de factores predictivos de complicaciones. Diversos estudios han demostrado que determinados factores, como dispositivos intravasculares, comorbilidad potencialmente inmunodepresora (diabetes mellitus, infección por el virus de la inmunodeficiencia humana o toma de inmunosupresores), patología valvular cardíaca predisponente a endocarditis infecciosa, tromboflebitis supurada, hemodiálisis o no retirada del catéter, se asocian con una mayor incidencia de complicaciones hematológicas asociadas a la bacteriemia por *S. aureus*.[2,35]

En los pacientes con factores de riesgo de aparición de complicaciones, o que ya las presenten (abscesos sépticos a distancia), el tratamiento se prolongará por espacio de 4-6 semanas.[35-37] Si no hay factores de mal pronóstico, la fiebre ha desaparecido en las primeras 72 horas y se ha retirado el catéter, probablemente 10 a 14 días de tratamiento serán suficientes.[1]

Es importante señalar que los pacientes con bacteriemia por *S. aureus* tienen un alto riesgo de desarrollar una endocarditis infecciosa (25 % a 30 %),[38,39] por lo que es recomendable realizar una ecocardiografía en la mayoría de estos casos. Posiblemente serían excepciones aquellos pacientes en quienes haya desaparecido la fiebre en las primeras 72 horas tras la retirada del catéter y no tengan una valvulopatía ni una cardiopatía predisponente, o no sean portadores de dispositivos protésicos intracardíacos. Debido a la baja sensibilidad de la ecocardiografía transtorácica, muchos autores recomiendan la ecocadiografía transesofágica.[40] Sin embargo, como en la primera semana esta última también tiene poca sensibilidad para el diagnóstico de endocarditis en dicha situación clínica, es recomendable demorar su realización hasta 5 a 7 días después del inicio de la clínica.[40] En aquellos pacientes con patología valvular predisponente en quienes no pueda realizarse una ecocadiografía transesofágica, sería recomendable mantener el tratamiento durante 4 a 6 semanas.

2.2.3　Enterococcus *spp.*

En las bacteriemias relacionadas con catéteres producidas por *Enterococcus* spp. sensibles a la ampicilina hay un amplio consenso en cuanto a que este antimicrobiano constituye el tratamiento de elección, y a que debe reservarse el empleo de otros para aquellas situaciones en que no pueda utilizarse la ampicilina.

Si bien las guías actuales recomiendan utilizar vancomicina frente a los enterococos resistentes a la ampicilina,[1] es posible que por varios de los motivos antes expuestos para *S. aureus* y por las cada vez más numerosas publicaciones con resultados favorables del tratamiento con linezolid y daptomicina en las bacteriemias por enterococos, haya argumentos para defender que estas otras opciones son más eficaces que la vancomicina.

En la actualidad se dispone de datos *in vitro* e *in vivo* sobre la eficacia del linezolid en el tratamiento de las bacteriemias por enterococos resistentes y sensibles a la vancomicina. Miyazaki *et al.*[41] compararon la eficacia *in vitro* y en un modelo animal de bacteriemia del linezolid y la vancomicina, y no encontraron diferencias entre los dos fármacos frente a *Enterococcus faecalis* sensible a la vancomicina.

Respecto al tratamiento en humanos, recientemente se ha publicado un estudio retrospectivo que evaluó el resultado clínico y microbiológico de bacteriemias por enterococos tratadas con linezolid (138 pacientes) o con daptomicina (63 pacientes).[42]

Al final del periodo de tratamiento, los resultados fueron muy similares tanto en la tasa de curación clínica (74 % para linezolid y 75 % para daptomicina) como en la de erradicación microbiológica (94 % con ambos tratamientos). Tan sólo hubo diferencias (p = 0,0321) en las recurrencias, que fueron más con daptomicina (12 %) que con linezolid (3 %), aunque el mayor número de pacientes con neoplasias o con hepatopatías en el grupo de daptomicina podría explicar estas diferencias. El linezolid también se ha comparado con quinupristina-dalfopristina en el tratamiento de bacteriemias por *Enterococcus faecium*, y los resultados han sido similares en cuanto a mortalidad (48 % con linezolid y 41 % con quinupristina-dalfopristina) y respuesta microbiológica (60 % para linezolid y 66 % para quinupristina-dalfopristina). Sin embargo, sí se observaron diferencias significativas en cuanto a la persistencia de la bacteriemia, que fue del 18 % con quinupristina-dalfopristina y del 5 % con linezolid, con una mortalidad del 48 % y del 41 %, respectivamente (p = 0,04). Así mismo, el desarrollo de resistencias fue del 11 % con quinupristina-dalfopristina y del 0 % con linezolid (p = 0,02),[43] lo que sugiere un mayor beneficio del tratamiento con linezolid. También se conocen datos de otro estudio retrospectivo que comparó la eficacia de la daptomicina y el linezolid en el tratamiento de bacteriemias por enterococos en 98 pacientes (68 tratados con linezolid y 30 con daptomicina).[44] En ambos grupos, la eficacia microbiológica fue muy alta (90 % para daptomicina y 88,2 % para linezolid; p = 0,92), y aunque la mortalidad, el tiempo hasta la desaparición de la bacteriemia y el número de recidivas fueron mayores en el grupo tratado con daptomicina, las diferencias no fueron estadísticamente significativas, por lo que se considera que ambos fármacos pueden utilizarse para el tratamiento de las bacteriemias por *Enterococcus* spp.

En el caso de la daptomicina, dentro del registro de su uso postautorización (denominado Registro CORE *[Cubicin Outcomes Registry and Experience])* se han evaluado los resultados en el tratamiento de bacteriemias por cocos grampostivos, incluyendo los enterococos.[45] En este registro se consideraron los enterococos tanto resistentes como sensibles a la vancomicina (el 74 % de *E. faecalis* eran sensibles a ella) y los resultados globales fueron satisfactorios, ya que 139 de los 159 pacientes evaluables (87 %) presentaron éxito clínico, definido como curación o mejoría, con una curación del 58 % y del 41 % para *E. faecium* y *E. faecalis*, respectivamente. Si bien no se evaluaron por separado los resultados para enterococos sensibles y resistentes a la vancomicina, la ausencia de diferencias estadísticamente significativas entre el resultado del tratamiento de *E. faecium* (mayoritariamente resistentes a la vancomicina) y *E. faecalis* (mayoritariamente sensibles a la vancomicina) permiten inferir que tampoco hubo diferencias en cuanto a la respuesta en función de la sensibilidad o la resistencia a la vancomicina. No obstante, al igual que con los estafilococos, el tratamiento con daptomicina tiene que realizarse con dosis altas (8-12 mg/kg al día).

Finalmente, hay que señalar la controversia existente acerca del empleo de monoterapia (ampicilina) o biterapia (ampicilina mas gentamicina o ceftriaxona) en las bacteriemias relacionadas con catéteres producidas por enterococos sensibles a la ampicilina. Si bien parece no haber un claro beneficio con el tratamiento combinado en las bacteriemias no complicadas, los datos más recientes derivados de un estudio sobre 61 episodios de bacteriemia relacionada con catéteres producidas por enterococos apoyan el empleo del tratamiento en asociación cuando se decide mantener el catéter, ya que en esos casos la tasa de curación con la terapia combinada fue estadísticamente superior que con un agente activo en monoterapia (4/4 frente a 1/5; $p < 0{,}05$).[46]

En cuanto a la duración del tratamiento, hay cierto consenso en que será de 10 a 14 días, con independencia del mantenimiento o no del catéter, siempre y cuando no haya embolias sépticas a distancia ni endocarditis infecciosa.[1]

2.2.4 *Bacilos gramnegativos*

Como ya se ha mencionado, el tratamiento empírico de las bacteriemias relacionadas con catéteres tiene que incluir un antibiótico activo frente a bacilos gramnegativos resistentes que, dependiendo de la ecología local, podría ser piperacilina-tazobactam, cefepima o un carbapenémico con actividad frente a *Pseudomonas* spp.

Si el informe microbiológico inicial indica bacteriemia relacionada con un catéter producida por un bacilo gramnegativo, en el momento actual se aconseja utilizar biterapia[47] y considerar pasar a monoterapia tras valorar los resultados del estudio de sensibilidad antimicrobiana del patógeno detectado, hasta completar los 10 a 14 días de tratamiento recomendados.[1] En caso de infección por *Pseudomonas aeruginosa*, a partir de los datos existentes, que muestran que sí parece haber un beneficio en cuanto a disminución de la mortalidad con el tratamiento combinado,[48] no debe reducirse el número de antibióticos activos y se completarán con biterapia los 10 a 14 días de tratamiento.

Bibliografía

1. Mermel LA, Allon M, Bouza E, Craven DE, Flynn P, O'Grady NP, *et al.* Clinical practice guidelines for the diagnosis and management of intravascular catheter-related infection: 2009 update by the Infectious Diseases Society of America. Clin Infect Dis. 2009; 49: 1-45.

2. Fowler VG, Jr., Justice A, Moore C, Benjamin DK Jr, Woods CW, Campbell S, *et al.* Risk factors for hematogenous complications of intravascular catheter-associated Staphylococcus aureus bacteremia. Clin Infect Dis. 2005; 40: 695-703.

3. Kumar A, Roberts D, Wood KE, Light B, Parrillo JE, Sharma S, *et al.* Duration of hypotension before initiation of effective antimicrobial therapy is the critical determinant of survival in human septic shock. Crit Care Med. 2006; 34: 1589-96.

4. Soriano A, Marco F, Martínez JA, Pisos E, Almela M, Dimova VP, *et al.* Influence of vancomycin minimum inhibitory concentration on the treatment of methicillin-resistant Staphylococcus aureus bacteremia. Clin Infect Dis. 2008; 46: 193-200.

5. Rybak MJ, Lomaestro BM, Rotschafer JC, Moellering RC, Craig WA, Billeter M, *et al.* Vancomycin therapeutic guidelines: a summary of consensus recommendations from the Infectious Diseases Society of America, the American Society of Health-System Pharmacists, and the Society of Infectious Dis-

eases Pharmacists. Clin Infect Dis. 2009; 49: 325-7.

6. Kim SH, Kim KH, Kim HB, Kim NJ, Kim EC, Oh MD, *et al.* Outcome of vancomycin treatment in patients with methicillin-susceptible Staphylococcus aureus bacteremia. Antimicrob Agents Chemother. 2008; 52: 192-7.

7. Schweizer ML, Furuno JP, Harris AD, Johnson JK, Shardell MD, McGregor JC, *et al.* Comparative effectiveness of nafcillin or cefazolin versus vancomycin in methicillin-susceptible Staphylococcus aureus bacteremia. BMC Infect Dis. 2011; 11: 279.

8. Giamarellou H, Poulakou G. Pharmacokinetic and pharmacodynamic evaluation of tigecycline. Expert Opin Drug Metab Toxicol. 2011; 7: 1459-70.

9. Wilcox MH, Tack KJ, Bouza E, Herr DL, Ruf BR, Ijzerman MM, *et al.* Complicated skin and skin-structure infections and catheter-related bloodstream infections: noninferiority of linezolid in a phase 3 study. Clin Infect Dis. 2009; 48: 203-12.

10. Lustberg ME, Schlesinger LS, Mangino JE. Concerns about "Complicated skin and skin-structure infections and catheter-related bloodstream infections: noninferiority of linezolid in a phase 3 study". Clin Infect Dis. 2009; 49: 313; author reply 4-5.

11. Benvenuto M, Benziger DP, Yankelev S, Vigliani G. Pharmacokinetics and tolerability of daptomycin at doses up to 12 milligrams per kilogram of body weight once daily in healthy volunteers. Antimicrob Agents Chemother. 2006; 50: 3245-9.

12. Safdar N, Andes D, Craig WA. In vivo pharmacodynamic activity of daptomycin. Antimicrob Agents Chemother. 2004; 48: 63-8.

13. Parra-Ruiz J, Peña-Monje A, Tomas-Jiménez C, Pomares-Mora J, Hernandez-Quero J. Eficacia y seguridad de daptomicina en dosis elevadas (>/= 8 mg/kg/dia). Enferm Infecc Microbiol Clin. 2011; 29: 425-7.

14. Fowler VG, Jr., Boucher HW, Corey GR, Abrutyn E, Karchmer AW, Rupp ME, *et al.* Daptomycin versus standard therapy for bacteremia and endocarditis caused by Staphylococcus aureus. N Engl J Med. 2006; 355: 653-65.

15. Marcos M, Soriano A, Inurrieta A, Martínez JA, Romero A, Cobos N, *et al.* Changing epidemiology of central venous catheter-related bloodstream infections: increasing prevalence of Gram-negative pathogens. J Antimicrob Chemother. 2011; 66: 2119-25.

16. Pfaller MA, Diekema DJ. Epidemiology of invasive candidiasis: a persistent public health problem. Clin Microbiol Rev. 2007; 20: 133-63.

17. Almirante B, Rodríguez D, Park BJ, Cuenca-Estrella M, Planes AM, Almela M, *et al.* Epidemiology and predictors of mortality in cases of Candida bloodstream infection: results from population-based surveillance, Barcelona, Spain, from 2002 to 2003. J Clin Microbiol. 2005; 43: 1829-35.

18. Rahkonen M, Luttinen S, Koskela M, Hautala T. True bacteremias caused by coagulase negative Staphylococcus are difficult to distinguish from blood culture contaminants. Eur J Clin Microbiol Infect Dis. 2012; 31: 2639-44.

19. Elzi L, Babouee B, Vogeli N, Laffer R, Dangel M, Frei R, *et al.* How to discriminate contamination from bloodstream infection due to coagulase-negative staphylococci: a prospective study with 654 patients. Clin Microbiol Infect. 2012; 18: E355-61.

20. Leth RA, Forman BE, Kristensen B. Predicting bloodstream infection via systemic inflammatory response syndrome or biochemistry. J Emerg Med. 2012 Sep 19. doi: 10.1016/j.jemermed.2012.07.059. (Epub ahead of print.)

21. Weber DJ, Rutala WA. Central line-associated bloodstream infections: prevention and management. Infect Dis Clin North Am. 2011; 25: 77-102.

22. Dohmen PM, Guleri A, Capone A, Utili R, Seaton RA, González-Ramallo VJ, *et al.* Daptomycin for the treatment of infective endocarditis: results from a European registry. J Antimicrob Chemother. 2012 Nov 28. (Epub ahead of print.)

23. Miró JM, Entenza JM, Del Río A, Velasco M, Castañeda X, García de la Mària C, *et al.* High-dose daptomycin plus fosfomycin is safe and effective in treating methicillin-susceptible and methicillin-resistant Staphylococcus aureus endocarditis. Antimicrob Agents Chemother. 2012; 56: 4511-5.

24. Dhand A, Bayer AS, Pogliano J, Yang SJ, Bolaris M, Nizet V, *et al.* Use of antistaphylococcal beta-lactams to increase daptomycin activity in eradicating persistent bacteremia due to methicillin-resistant Staphylococcus aureus:

role of enhanced daptomycin binding. Clin Infect Dis. 2011; 53: 158-63.

25. López E, Soy D, Miana MT, Codina C, Ribas J. Algunas reflexiones acerca de la administración de antibióticos betalactámicos en infusión continua. Enferm Infecc Microbiol Clin. 2006; 24: 445-52.

26. Mouton JW, Vinks AA. Continuous infusion of beta-lactams. Curr Opin Crit Care. 2007; 13: 598-606.

27. Lanbeck P, Odenholt I, Paulsen O. Dicloxacillin: a higher risk than cloxacillin for infusion phlebitis. Scand J Infect Dis. 2003; 35: 397-400.

28. Svedhem A, Alestig K, Jertborn M. Phlebitis induced by parenteral treatment with flucloxacillin and cloxacillin: a double-blind study. Antimicrob Agents Chemother. 1980; 18: 349-52.

29. Thomson AH, Staatz CE, Tobin CM, Gall M, Lovering AM. Development and evaluation of vancomycin dosage guidelines designed to achieve new target concentrations. J Antimicrob Chemother. 2009; 63: 1050-7.

30. Rybak M, Lomaestro B, Rotschafer JC, Moellering R Jr, Craig W, Billeter M, *et al.* Therapeutic monitoring of vancomycin in adult patients: a consensus review of the American Society of Health-System Pharmacists, the Infectious Diseases Society of America, and the Society of Infectious Diseases Pharmacists. Am J Health Syst Pharm. 2009; 66: 82-98.

31. Lodise TP, Patel N, Lomaestro BM, Rodvold KA, Drusano GL. Relationship between initial vancomycin concentration-time profile and nephrotoxicity among hospitalized patients. Clin Infect Dis. 2009; 49: 507-14.

32. van Hal SJ, Paterson DL, Lodise TP. Systematic review and meta-analysis of vancomycin-induced nephrotoxicity associated with dosing schedules that maintain troughs between 15 and 20 milligrams per liter. Antimicrob Agents Chemother. 2013; 57: 734-44.

33. Pitz AM, Yu F, Hermsen ED, Rupp ME, Fey PD, Olsen KM. Vancomycin susceptibility trends and prevalence of heterogeneous vancomycin-intermediate Staphylococcus aureus in clinical methicillin-resistant S. aureus isolates. J Clin Microbiol. 2011; 49: 269-74.

34. Khatib R, Jose J, Musta A, Sharma M, Fakih MG, Johnson LB, *et al.* Relevance of vancomycin-intermediate susceptibility and heteroresistance in methicillin-resistant Staphylococcus aureus bacteraemia. J Antimicrob Chemother. 2011; 66: 1594-9.

35. Fowler VG, Jr., Olsen MK, Corey GR, Woods CW, Cabell CH, Reller LB, *et al.* Clinical identifiers of complicated Staphylococcus aureus bacteremia. Arch Intern Med. 2003; 163: 2066-72.

36. Chang FY, Peacock JE, Jr., Musher DM, Triplett P, MacDonald BB, Mylotte JM, *et al.* Staphylococcus aureus bacteremia: recurrence and the impact of antibiotic treatment in a prospective multicenter study. Medicine (Baltimore). 2003; 82: 333-9.

37. Chang FY, MacDonald BB, Peacock JE, Jr., Musher DM, Triplett P, Mylotte JM, *et al.* A prospective multicenter study of Staphylococcus aureus bacteremia: incidence of endocarditis, risk factors for mortality, and clinical impact of methicillin resistance. Medicine (Baltimore). 2003; 82: 322-32.

38. Abraham J, Mansour C, Veledar E, Khan B, Lerakis S. Staphylococcus aureus bacteremia and endocarditis: the Grady Memorial Hospital experience with methicillin-sensitive S. aureus and methicillin-resistant S. aureus bacteremia. Am Heart J. 2004; 147: 536-9.

39. Sullenberger AL, Avedissian LS, Kent SM. Importance of transesophageal echocardiography in the evaluation of Staphylococcus aureus bacteremia. J Heart Valve Dis. 2005; 14: 23-8.

40. Naber CK, Baddour LM, Giamarellos-Bourboulis EJ, Gould IM, Herrmann M, Hoen B, *et al.* Clinical consensus conference: survey on Gram-positive bloodstream infections with a focus on Staphylococcus aureus. Clin Infect Dis. 2009; 48(Suppl 4): S260-70.

41. Miyazaki S, Fujikawa T, Kobayashi I, Matsumoto T, Tateda K, Yamaguchi K. The in vitro and in vivo antibacterial characterization of vancomycin and linezolid against vancomycin-susceptible and -resistant enterococci. J Antimicrob Chemother. 2002; 50: 971-4.

42. Twilla JD, Finch CK, Usery JB, Gelfand MS, Hudson JQ, Broyles JE. Vancomycin-resistant Enterococcus bacteremia: an evaluation of treatment with linezolid or daptomycin. J Hosp Med. 2012; 7: 243-8.

43. Chong YP, Lee SO, Song EH, Lee EJ, Jang EY, Kim SH, *et al.* Quinupristin-dalfopristin versus linezolid for the treatment of vancomycin-

resistant Enterococcus faecium bacteraemia: efficacy and development of resistance. Scand J Infect Dis. 2010; 42: 491-9.

44. Mave V, García-Díaz J, Islam T, Hasbun R. Vancomycin-resistant enterococcal bacteraemia: is daptomycin as effective as linezolid? J Antimicrob Chemother. 2009; 64: 175-80.

45. Mohr JF, Friedrich LV, Yankelev S, Lamp KC. Daptomycin for the treatment of enterococcal bacteraemia: results from the Cubicin Outcomes Registry and Experience (CORE). Int J Antimicrob Agents. 2009; 33: 543-8.

46. Sandoe JA, Witherden IR, Au-Yeung HK, Kite P, Kerr KG, Wilcox MH. Enterococcal intravascular catheter-related bloodstream infection: management and outcome of 61 consecutive cases. J Antimicrob Chemother. 2002; 50: 577-82.

47. Micek ST, Welch EC, Khan J, Pervez M, Doherty JA, Reichley RM, *et al.* Empiric combination antibiotic therapy is associated with improved outcome against sepsis due to Gram-negative bacteria: a retrospective analysis. Antimicrob Agents Chemother. 2010; 54: 1742-8.

48. Safdar N, Handelsman J, Maki DG. Does combination antimicrobial therapy reduce mortality in Gram-negative bacteraemia? A meta-analysis. Lancet Infect Dis. 2004; 4: 519-27.

Capítulo 9

Candidemia y catéter vascular

D. Rodríguez-Pardo, B. Almirante

**Servicio de Enfermedades Infecciosas
Hospital Universitari Vall d'Hebron
Universitat Autònoma de Barcelona
Barcelona**

Correspondencia:
Dra. Dolors Rodríguez-Pardo
dolorodriguez@vhebron.net

1 Epidemiología general de la candidemia

1.1 Incidencia

En los últimos años se ha detectado un aumento de la incidencia de las infecciones invasivas por *Candida*, en especial de las candidemias, debido fundamentalmente al mayor número de pacientes en situación de riesgo para su adquisición. En estudios recientes se ha comprobado que este patógeno es el cuarto agente causal de bacteriemias y fungemias adquiridas en las instituciones sanitarias, en EE.UU. y en otros países.[1-4] En conjunto, las diferentes especies de *Candida* representan casi el 80 % de todos los hongos patógenos causantes de infecciones hospitalarias. Más de un 5 % de los pacientes hospitalizados desarrollan una infección nosocomial, y alrededor de un 5 % pueden estar ocasionadas por especies de *Candida*.[3]

La incidencia de las infecciones invasivas por *Candida* spp. se estima, de manera fundamental, mediante estudios prospectivos de tipo poblacional. En las últimas décadas se han publicado diversos trabajos que han reportado una incidencia anual que oscila entre valores inferiores a 2 y superiores a 20 por cada 100.000 habitantes (véase la tabla 1). Las tasas varían mucho según los países, con las cifras más altas en determinados estados de EE.UU. y en Dinamarca. En Europa, la incidencia de candidemia varía de dos a cinco episodios por cada 100.000 habitantes en la mayoría de los países.[5-20] Los factores relacionados con esta incidencia tan variable son de tipo demográfico, por la comorbilidad asociada y por diferencias en la práctica médica, en especial en cuanto al uso de catéteres vasculares durante tiempo prolongado (en muchas ocasiones en régimen ambulatorio), así como por los patrones de utilización de los antimicrobianos. También podría influir la frecuencia de realización de pruebas diagnósticas a los pacientes, sobre todo hemocultivos y el tipo de sistema utilizado, ya que los estudios poblacionales se basan en un registro de casos con cultivos positivos para *Candida* spp. de muestras sanguíneas. A pesar de estas variaciones en la incidencia en los diferentes países, la frecuencia de candidiasis invasiva es superior a la de cualquier otra infección fúngica y comparable a la de muchas de las infecciones bacterianas invasivas.[17,21,22]

En los estudios poblacionales destaca que la candidemia afecta de manera fundamental a pacientes en edades extremas de la vida (neonatos y mayores de 65 años), como queda reflejado en la tabla 1, aunque también se ha observado una gran variabilidad en la incidencia en estas poblaciones en las diferentes áreas geográficas. En EE.UU., por causas no bien identificadas, se ha detectado una mayor incidencia de candidemia en sujetos de raza negra en comparación con los de raza caucásica.[21]

Desde el punto de vista de la ubicación de los pacientes, se ha comprobado que entre un 10 % y un 30 % de los episodios de candidemia se diagnostican en pacientes

| | | | Nº casos/100.000 habitantes y año | | |
Región	Años	Lugar	Total	Pacientes <1 año	Pacientes >65 años
Europa	91-03	Noruega	2,4	10,3	7
	95-99	Islandia	4,9	11,3	19
	95-99	Finlandia	1,9	9,4	5,2
	02-03	Barcelona	4,9	38,8	12
	03-04	Dinamarca	11		
	05-06	Escocia	4,8		
	06	Dinamarca	11,9	25,1	
	10-11	España	8,1	96,4	
América del Norte	92-93	San Francisco y Atlanta	8	75	26
	98-00	Connecticut y Baltimore	7,1-24,0		
	98-01	Iowa	6		
	08-11	Atlanta y Baltimore	13,3-26,2	34,3-46,2	59,1-72,4
	99-04	Calgary	2,8	19	15
Australia	01-04	Todo el país	1,8	24,8	13,7
América del Sur	03-04	Brasil	2,5		

Tabla 1. Incidencia de candidemia en estudios de vigilancia poblacionales.[5-20]

no ingresados en hospitales, aunque la aparición de la infección está claramente relacionada con los cuidados sanitarios que los enfermos reciben en régimen ambulatorio (fundamentalmente uso de catéteres vasculares, quimioterapia, nutrición parenteral o hemodiálisis).[8,10,11] En las unidades de cuidados intensivos (UCI), la incidencia de candidemia es alrededor de 10 veces superior a la observada en las áreas de hospitalización convencional para pacientes médicos o quirúrgicos, aunque globalmente sólo un tercio de los pacientes están ingresados en dichas unidades en el momento del diagnóstico de la infección.[23,24]

La incidencia de candidemia también es mucho mayor en los pacientes con cáncer y en los diabéticos. La mayoría de los enfermos afectados son portadores de catéteres venosos centrales, temporales o permanentes, en el momento de la detección de la infección fúngica invasiva.[21,25]

Los avances experimentados en el cuidado de los niños prematuros han condicionado un aumento de la incidencia de candidiasis neonatal. Por ello, *Candida* spp. se ha convertido en un importante agente causal de infecciones neonatales, con unas cifras relevantes de morbilidad y mortalidad asociadas, en especial en aquellos con un peso al nacer inferior a 1.000 o 1.500 g.[26,27] En estudios poblacionales realizados en EE.UU., la incidencia anual de candidemia fue de 1,53 por 1.000 días de hospitalización en los neonatos ingresados en la UCI, y claramente superior en relación con el bajo peso al nacer (2,68 por 1.000 días de hospitalización para aquellos con un peso inferior a 1.000 g).[26] *C. albicans* es la especie más detectada, y en esta población también es muy frecuente *C. parapsilosis;* las restantes especies de *Candida* son muy infrecuentes.[28]

En la población pediátrica, la candidemia se observa fundamentalmente en los neonatos ingresados en la UCI, en pacientes graves y en aquellos en situaciones clínicas de inmunodepresión. La mortalidad en este grupo de pacientes es menor del 20 %, bastante inferior a la observada en la población adulta.[29,30] En los últimos años se ha descrito un cambio importante en la distribución de las especies de *Candida* causantes de infección invasiva, con un aumento sustancial de las especies diferentes a *C. albicans* y con una mayor frecuencia de resistencia al fluconazol.[30,31]

1.2 *Distribución por especies de* Candida

Aunque se han descrito más de 17 especies como agentes causales de candidiasis invasiva, más del 90 % están producidas por cinco especies: *C. albicans, C. glabrata, C. parapsilosis, C. tropicalis* y *C. krusei.*[32]

En las últimas dos décadas, la proporción de infecciones causadas por especies de *Candida* no *albicans* ha aumentado exponencialmente,[33] y en la actualidad, del 50 % al 80 % de los casos de candidemia se deben a dichas especies.[34] La utilización de fluconazol se ha considerado uno de los factores principales en el cambio epidemiológico de la candidiasis invasiva, en particular en el aumento de *C. glabrata* y *C. krusei,*[35] aunque en un reciente estudio no se ha demostrado la relación entre el uso previo de fluconazol y la detección de estas especies.[36] Los pacientes con trasplante hematológico, los que han recibido previamente azoles y los neonatos se consideran con mayor riesgo de desarrollar una candidemia por una especie diferente a *C. albicans*.[37]

En el mayor estudio multicéntrico europeo realizado hasta la fecha sobre candidemia (2.089 episodios), el 46% de los casos estaban producidos por especies no *albicans*, se detectaron con más frecuencia en pacientes con neoplasias hematológicas (65%) y se apreció un aumento en la incidencia de *C. glabrata* con el incremento de la edad de los enfermos.[38] Sin embargo, en el subanálisis de la contribución española al estudio europeo (290 episodios), en el cual se observó una incidencia anual media de 3,5 por 100.000 habitantes, *C. albicans* constituyó el 43% de los aislados y la suma de *C. glabrata* y *C. krusei* alcanzó el 11%.[39]

En estudios de vigilancia epidemiológica como el ARTEMIS, que recaba datos sobre candidiasis invasiva en 127 centros hospitalarios de 39 países desde hace 11 años, también se ha apreciado un descenso gradual de los aislados de *C. albicans* (del 73,3% al 62,3%), junto con un incremento progresivo de *C. parapsilosis* (del 4,2% al 7,3%) y de *C. tropicalis* (del 4,6% al 7,5%), entre los años 1997 y 2003.[21] En este macroestudio también se observa la paulatina emergencia de especies más infrecuentes (como *C. guilliermondii, C. kefyr, C. rugosa* y *C. famata)*, que llegan a multiplicar por diez sus aislados durante el período estudiado, aunque su repercusión global sigue siendo muy baja si se compara con las especies mayoritarias.

En la tabla 2 puede apreciarse la variabilidad temporal y geográfica de las distintas especies de *Candida* aisladas en hemocultivo en 24 estudios multicéntricos realizados en los últimos años.[40] En todos ellos, *C. albicans* continúa siendo la especie predominante, aunque su frecuencia varía según el área geográfica estudiada, desde un 37% en Latinoamérica hasta un 70% en Noruega. En los estudios españoles, su frecuencia varía entre el 43% y el 51% de todos los aislados.[8,39,41]

Aunque *C. glabrata* se ha convertido en un patógeno cuya incidencia sigue en aumento en EE.UU. (24% en 2004), y constituye la segunda causa de candidemia en Norteamérica, su tasa de detección en hemocultivos en otras regiones es muy inferior (13% en Lombardía y Noruega, 10% en Asia-Pacífico y Europa, 7% en Latinoamérica). En España su incidencia también es baja (8-12%), siempre por detrás de *C. parapsilosis* (véase la tabla 2).[8,39,41-44] La explicación que justifique esta variabilidad geográfica en los aislados de *C. glabrata* se desconoce, pero podría ser fruto de diversos factores: longevidad de los pacientes, enfermedad de base (especialmente neoplasias) o exposición previa a los azoles. Durante mucho tiempo se ha relacionado el uso previo de fluconazol con la emergencia de especies menos sensibles a este antifúngico *(C. glabrata, C. krusei)*, pero en los estudios publicados en los últimos años no ha podido demostrarse esta relación,[36,45] y parece que la edad del paciente, la gravedad de la enfermedad de base y la exposición a determinados antibacterianos (piperacilina-tazobactam, vancomicina) son más determinantes en el desarrollo de una candidemia por *C. glabrata*.

Lugar del estudio	Años	Nº de aislados	Especie (%)						
			C. albicans	*C. glabrata*	*C. parapsilosis*	*C. tropicalis*	*C. krusei*	*C. guilliermondii*	*C. lusitaniae*
EE.UU.	92-93	837	52	12	21	10	4		
	93-95	79	56	15	15	10			
	95-97	1.593	46	20	14	12	2	<1	1
	95-98	934	53	20	10	12	3		
	98-00	935	45	24	13	12	2		
	08-11	2675	38	29	17	10	2		2
Canadá	92-94	415	69	8	10	7	1	<1	1
Norteamérica	01-04	2.773	51	22	14	7	2	<1	<1
Latinoamérica	95-96	145	37	4	25	24	1	2	
	01-04	1.565	50	7	16	20	2	4	<1
Asia	01-04	1.344	56	10	16	14	2	<1	<1
Taiwan	94-00	1.095	50	12	14	21	<1		
Europa	92-94	249	49	10	11	11	9		
	97-99	2.089	56	14	13	7	2	1	1
	01-04	2.515	60	10	12	9	5	1	<1
Noruega	91-03	1.415	70	13	6	7	2	<1	<1
Dinamarca	03-04	307	63	20	4	4	3	<1	<1
	06	316	53	21	5	4	6	<1	<1
Lombardía	97-99	569	58	13	15	6	1	2	<1
España	97-99	293	43	8	29	10	3	2	
	01-06	1.997	47	12	19	10	5	3	1
	02-03	351	51	9	23	10	4		
	09	1357	45	11	29	8	2	<1	1
	10-11	752	45	13	25	8	2	2	1

Tabla 2. Variaciones geográficas en la distribución de especies de Candida *aisladas en hemocultivo en diferentes estudios multicéntricos.*[40]

A diferencia de otras especies, *C. parapsilosis* es exógena, habitualmente comensal de la piel y las mucosas, y tiene una gran facilidad para formar biopelículas en catéteres o biomateriales, sobrevivir en el ambiente hospitalario, transmitirse a través de las manos e infectar a niños y neonatos. Su frecuencia como agente causal de candidemias ha aumentado en los últimos años, sobre todo en Latinoamérica, Lombardía y España, donde es la segunda especie más detectada en hemocultivo después de *C. albicans* (véase la tabla 2).[8,19,20,39,42,43] Afortunadamente, las infecciones invasivas por *C. parapsilosis* se asocian a una baja tasa de letalidad; además, debido a su origen exógeno, la correcta higiene de las manos y el manejo adecuado de los catéteres son medidas más recomendables que la profilaxis antifúngica para la prevención de estas infecciones.[46]

La neutropenia y la mucositis, situaciones muy frecuentes en los pacientes con neoplasias hematológicas, son los factores de riesgo más habituales para el desarrollo de una infección invasiva por *C. tropicalis*. Aunque la frecuencia de esta especie ha disminuido en EE.UU., probablemente por el uso profiláctico de fluconazol, su incidencia va en aumento en otras latitudes y es la segunda especie más común como causa de candidemia en Latinoamérica (20 %) y Taiwan (21 %). En España, su incidencia (10 %) no ha variado en los distintos estudios (véase la tabla 2).

C. krusei, especie intrínsecamente resistente al fluconazol, también se detecta en mayor medida en enfermos con neoplasias hematológicas y en receptores de trasplante de progenitores hematopoyéticos. Suele ser la causa del 1 % al 9 % de todas las candidemias (véase la tabla 2), y su incidencia, en algunos centros, es mayor en los pacientes que han recibido profilaxis con fluconazol.[33] Sin embargo, en otras instituciones la asociación entre el uso previo de fluconazol y la candidemia por *C. krusei* no ha sido confirmada, y se ha relacionado a esta especie, al igual que a *C. glabrata*, con la exposición previa a piperacilina-tazobactam o vancomicina.[45]

C. guilliermondii y *C. rugosa* son dos especies emergentes con sensibilidad reducida al fluconazol y causantes de brotes infecciosos nosocomiales. Son especialmente comunes en Latinoamérica, donde pueden ser más frecuentes que *C. krusei* y llegan a representar un 3 % a un 5 % de todas las candidemias (véase la tabla 2). Además, *C. rugosa* presenta una sensibilidad reducida a la amfotericina B y es causa de candidemias relacionadas con catéteres.[24]

Por su parte, *C. inconspicua* y *C. norvegensis* son especies fenotípicamente similares a *C. krusei*, y comparten también su resistencia intrínseca al fluconazol. *C. inconspicua* ha sido causa de candidemia en pacientes con infección por el virus de la inmunodeficiencia humana o con neoplasias hematológicas, y *C. norvegensis* se aísla ocasionalmente en el norte de Europa y en Japón.[44]

2　Epidemiología de la candidemia asociada a catéteres vasculares

Los catéteres venosos centrales están considerados como el factor de riesgo más relevante para el desarrollo de una candidemia en los pacientes sin neutropenia profunda ni inmunodeficiencia grave. Alrededor de un 5 % de estos catéteres pueden ser el foco de origen de una infección bacteriémica, que estará causada por alguna especie de *Candida* hasta en un 10 % de los episodios.[47,48]

En general, la aparición de una candidemia relacionada con el catéter depende del tipo de éste, de la unidad de hospitalización, del lugar de inserción y de la duración de la cateterización. En el programa de vigilancia de las infecciones nosocomiales en Cataluña (denominado Programa VINCat) se ha comprobado, para el período 2007-2011, que la frecuencia de candidemia de catéter demostrada por hemocultivos es de un 6,5 % sobre el total de los episodios de bacteriemias originadas en este tipo de dispositivos. El 80 % de los casos se originó en un catéter venoso central, el 15 % en un catéter venoso central de inserción periférica y el 5 % restante en un catéter venoso periférico. A pesar de que en la mayoría de los hospitales el acceso por vía subclavia es el más habitual, en un 40 % de los episodios el foco de origen de las candidemias de catéter fue un catéter venoso central colocado en las venas yugular o femoral. La candidemia de catéter, globalmente, se detectó en pacientes ingresados en el área quirúrgica en 415 de los casos, en el área de críticos en el 33 % y en el área médica en el 26 % restante.[49]

Los factores relacionados con la candidemia de catéter son la neutropenia de una duración superior a ocho días, la existencia de procesos hematológicos graves, el uso del catéter para nutrición parenteral total (NPT), la duración de la cateterización en el mismo lugar de inserción, las frecuentes manipulaciones del catéter y la gravedad basal de los pacientes ingresados en la UCI (evaluada según la escala APACHE II).[47]

En las series generales de candidemia se observa que alrededor de un 30 % de los episodios se diagnostica con certeza, según los criterios actualmente validados, y que el foco de origen es un catéter vascular. La frecuencia de las diferentes especies de *Candida* es variable: el 54 % de las candidemias por *C. parapsilosis* se originan en catéteres vasculares, el 31 % de las causadas por *C. albicans*, y el 22 %, el 17 % y el 10 % de las debidas a *C. tropicalis*, *C. krusei* y *C. glabrata*, respectivamente.[8]

Debe sospecharse que el origen de una candidemia es un catéter vascular en presencia de los siguientes hallazgos: hemocultivos cualitativos positivos para *C. albicans* o *C. parapsilosis*, hemocultivos cuantitativos o un tiempo diferencial entre ellos con valores considerados significativos, uso del catéter o de alguna de sus luces para NPT, ausencia de otro posible foco de origen, y presencia de candidemia persistente a pesar de la administración de un tratamiento antifúngico adecuado.[47]

La mortalidad de la candidemia supera el 30 % al 40 % en el momento actual; sin embargo, en la mayoría de las series publicadas, la evolución de la infección está claramente influenciada por la retirada precoz de los catéteres vasculares, en especial si son su foco de origen sospechado o demostrado.[8] La candidemia por *C. parapsilosis*, que en un alto porcentaje de los casos se origina en catéteres vasculares y es muy frecuente en la población neonatal, tiene una mortalidad inferior al 10 % si los catéteres vasculares se retiran de forma precoz.[50]

3   Patogenia de la candidemia originada en un catéter vascular

La patogenia de la candidemia asociada a los catéteres vasculares está en relación con la formación de biocapas microbianas, tanto en la superficie interna como en la externa de este tipo de dispositivos.

C. albicans es la especie fúngica patógena más común productora de infecciones relacionadas con biocapas.[51] En los pacientes con candidemia, las cepas de *Candida* spp. productoras de biocapas se correlacionan con un mayor riesgo de morbilidad y mortalidad que aquellas que no las desarrollan.[52]

Las biocapas mantienen las formas sésiles de *Candida* formando unas estructuras altamente organizadas y comunicadas entre sí por diferentes mecanismos. En estas biocapas adheridas a las superficies de los catéteres se produce el crecimiento del patógeno y, a partir de ellas, la diseminación hematógena de la forma planctónica de *Candida* spp., con la consiguiente aparición de las manifestaciones clínicas de la candidemia o de la candidiasis invasiva. En las biocapas, *Candida* spp. está plenamente protegida del ambiente hostil del huésped.[53,54]

La formación de biocapas en los catéteres vasculares depende de la llegada previa de *Candida* spp. por contaminación en cualquier momento de la permanencia del dispositivo en el paciente. Las vía más frecuente de colonización de los catéteres es la exoluminal, a través de la piel *(Candida* puede ser un comensal de la piel en los pacientes hospitalizados o ser transmitida de forma exógena por el personal sanitario), por diseminación hematógena desde un foco distante de infección o por traslocación microbiana desde el tracto digestivo en los pacientes con mucositis. En los enfermos con candidemia asociada a NPT, la vía de colonización más frecuente es la endoluminal, a través de la conexión y la luz de los catéteres.[55]

Desde una perspectiva clínica, la importancia de las biocapas de *Candida* radica en su alta resistencia a la acción de los antifúngicos habituales. Los mecanismos implicados en esta resistencia intrínseca son: *1)* la dificultad de penetración del fármaco a través de la matriz de la biocapa; *2)* la disminución del metabolismo fúngico y la limitación de los nutrientes; *3)* la expresión de genes de resistencia, en especial aquellos que codifican bombas de flujo, y *4)* la presencia de las denominadas células persistentes *(persister cells).* Este mecanismo multifactorial puede incrementar hasta 4.000 veces la resistencia al fluconazol de las cepas sésiles de *Candida* en comparación con las cepas en estado planctónico.[53]

4   Manifestaciones clínicas y complicaciones de la candidemia de catéter

Las infecciones invasivas por *Candida* spp. pueden ocasionar diferentes formas clínicas de enfermedad, desde la manifestación más habitual en forma de candidemia, asociada o no con signos y síntomas de candidiasis diseminada, la candidiasis hepatoesplénica o candidiasis crónica diseminada, y las diferentes infecciones focales invasivas (ocular, cardíaca, del sistema nervioso central [SNC], del riñón y el sistema urinario, peritoneal o intraabdominal, osteoarticular o de otras localizaciones menos frecuentes).[1]

La presentación más común de la candidiasis neonatal es la afectación sanguínea, en forma de candidemia, asociada con extensión al SNC y la consiguiente meningoencefalitis, que puede condicionar la aparición de secuelas neurológicas permanentes. Otras localizaciones pueden producir endocarditis, abscesos renales, esplénicos o hepáticos, endoftalmitis, infecciones cutáneas o del tracto urinario, y osteomielitis.[56]

Las infecciones graves por *Candida* spp. en los niños pueden ocasionar procesos invasivos locales, como infecciones del tracto urinario, peritonitis, endoftalmitis, endocarditis, infecciones osteoarticulares, meningitis o candidiasis diseminada crónica o hepatoesplénica. De igual manera, pueden observarse formas de candidemia o de candidiasis diseminada aguda con afectación multivisceral por diseminación hematógena. Las formas más graves de la enfermedad se observan en niños graves ingresados en la UCI y en pacientes con procesos hematológicos y neutropenia profunda y prolongada.[29,57] En estas situaciones clínicas es frecuente la aparición de lesiones cutáneas diseminadas, en ocasiones pustulosas con base eritematosa, que son muy características de la infección diseminada por *Candida*.

4.1 *Candidemia y candidiasis diseminada*

Las manifestaciones clínicas de la candidemia son muy variables y oscilan desde cuadros febriles sin foco aparente hasta un síndrome séptico indistinguible de cualquier infección sistémica bacteriana grave. Si hay diseminación hematógena de la enfermedad pueden afectarse múltiples órganos o vísceras (ojos, riñones, válvulas cardíacas o cerebro), y producir síntomas asociados con dichas localizaciones. En la exploración clínica es fundamental valorar el estado hemodinámico para evaluar la gravedad de la sepsis, y comprobar si hay lesiones cutáneas características u oculares compatibles con endoftalmitis (mediante una exploración oftalmológica practicada por un especialista).[1,58]

La frecuencia de la afectación ocular en los pacientes con candidemia es variable, entre un 2 % y un 25 % según los estudios. El tratamiento antifúngico adecuado ha condicionado un descenso de esta localización de la infección diseminada y ha hecho que se limite su extensión, desde sólo una coriorretinitis hasta cuadros más graves de vitritis o panoftalmitis.[59]

Las lesiones cutáneas características de la candidemia (véase la figura 1) pueden aparecer tanto en sujetos neutropénicos como en aquellos sin neutropenia asociada. Estas lesiones suelen aparecer de manera súbita y en general son agrupaciones de pústulas no dolorosas sobre una base eritematosa, con una distribución difusa o localizada en una o varias regiones del cuerpo (véase la figura 2). El tamaño de las

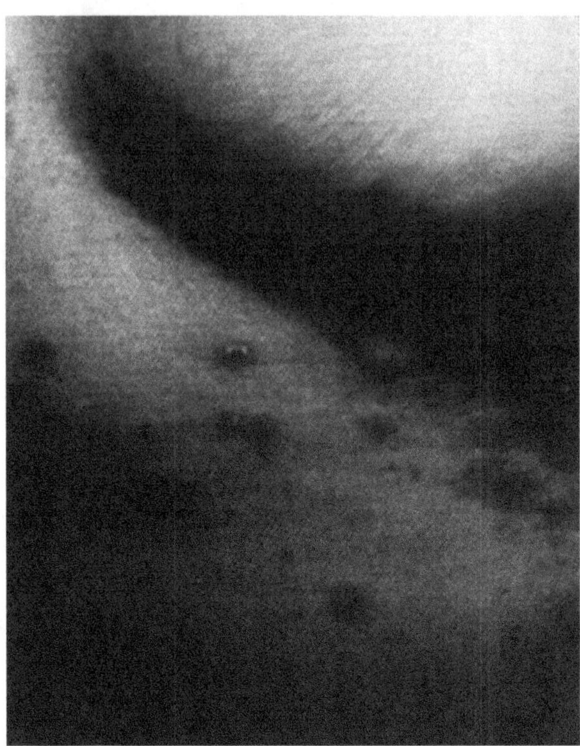

Figura 1.Lesiones cutáneas en un paciente con leucocitosis y candidemia originada en un catéter vascular permanente tipo Porth-a-Cath®.

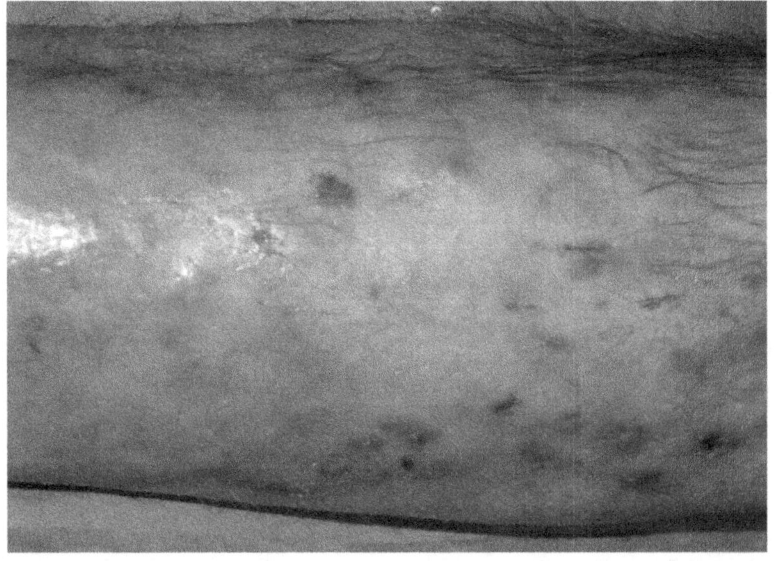

Figura 2. Lesiones cutáneas en un paciente receptor de un trasplante hepático con candidiasis diseminada.

lesiones puede ser desde puntiformes, y pasar desapercibidas a la exploración física, hasta nodulares de varios centímetros de diámetro con necrosis central. En los pacientes con neutropenia profunda, las lesiones tienden a ser maculares en lugar de pustulosas. El reconocimiento de las lesiones cutáneas compatibles con candidiasis diseminada es importante para llegar al diagnóstico, mediante examen histológico y cultivo del material obtenido por punción o rascado, en los pacientes con hemocultivos negativos.[1]

Aunque es infrecuente, algunos enfermos pueden presentar dolor en algún grupo muscular como consecuencia de la formación de microabscesos producidos por *Candida*. En la exploración física se observan signos inflamatorios moderados en la zona afectada. En los pacientes con profunda inmunodepresión, los abscesos musculares pueden ser de mayor tamaño, con respuesta lenta al tratamiento antifúngico y, en ocasiones, recidivantes.[1]

Además de estas manifestaciones periféricas características de la candidemia, los enfermos pueden tener signos de insuficiencia de diversos órganos. En las autopsias de fallecidos por candidiasis suele observarse una diseminación de la infección, que ha ocasionado microabscesos en numerosas vísceras, en especial los riñones, el corazón, el hígado, el bazo, los pulmones, los ojos y el SNC.

La presentación más común de la candidiasis neonatal es la afectación sanguínea, en forma de candidemia, asociada con extensión al SNC que da lugar a una meningoencefalitis, que puede condicionar la aparición de secuelas neurológicas permanentes. Otras localizaciones resultarán en endocarditis, abscesos renales, esplénicos o hepáticos, coriorretinitis endoftalmitis (véase la figura 3), infecciones cutáneas o del tracto urinario, y osteomielitis.[56]

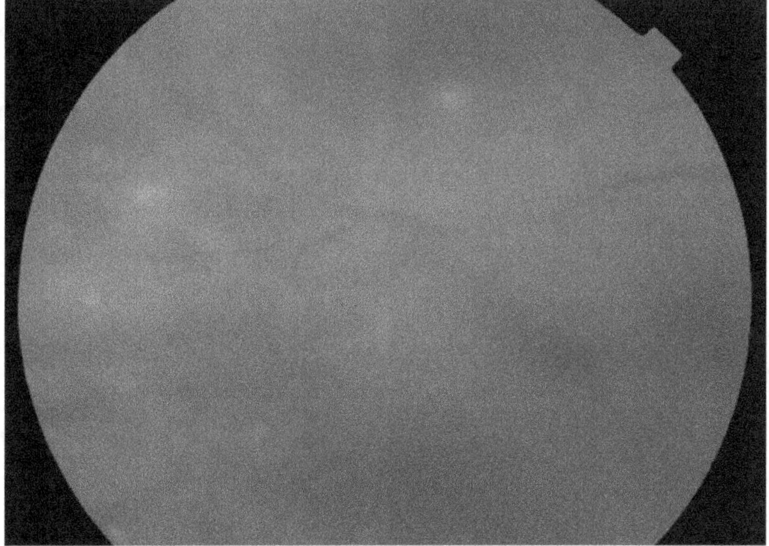

Figura 3. Lesiones coriorretinianas compatibles con afectación ocular en el curso de una candidemia.

5   Bases para el tratamiento antifúngico

5.1   *Sensibilidad antifúngica*

Se dispone de diferentes opciones terapéuticas para la candidemia, que incluyen fluconazol, formulaciones lipídicas de amfotericina B, voriconazol o una equinocandina, por lo que un aspecto básico es conocer la sensibilidad de *Candida* spp. a estos fármacos (véase la tabla 3).

La amfotericina B sigue siendo el patrón de referencia y es activa frente a todas las especies de *Candida* a excepción de *C. lusitaniae,* que es una especie con muy baja presencia en todas las series. *C. albicans, C. parapsilosis* y *C. tropicalis,* que constituyen aproximadamente el 78 % de los aislados, suelen ser muy sensibles al fluconazol, con unas tasas de resistencia inferiores al 3 %. El fluconazol no es activo frente *C. krusei,* y puede no serlo o requerir dosis altas frente *C. glabrata,* lo que se conoce como «sensibilidad dependiente de la dosis». En este sentido, estudios poblacionales realizados en Barcelona y Andalucía[8,60,61] indican que la resistencia *in vitro* al fluconazol es baja en nuestro entorno, con cifras que la sitúan alrededor del 4 %, mientras que el 7 % de las cepas (la mayor parte *C. glabrata* y *C. krusei*) requieren una concentración mínima inhibitoria (CMI) de fluconazol de 16-32 mg/l, por lo que se consideran con sensibilidad dependiente de la dosis.

	Fluconazol	Itraconazol	Voriconazol	Posaconazol	Flucitosina	Amfotericina B	Equinocandinas
C. albicans	S	S	S	S	S	S	S
C. tropicalis	S	S	S	S	S	S	S
C. parapsilosis	S	S	S	S	S	S	S a I*
C. glabrata	SDD a R	SDD a R	S-I-R	S-I-R	S	S	S
C. krusei	R	SDD a R	S a I	S a I	I a R	S	S
C. guillermondi	I a R	I a R	S-I-R	S-I-R	S	S	S a I
C. lusitaniae	S	S	S	S	S	S-I-R	S

* La resistencia a las equinocandinas en las cepas aisladas de *C. parapsilosis* es poco frecuente.
S: sensible; I: sensibilidad intermedia; R: resistente; SDD: sensibilidad dependiente de la dosis.

Tabla 3. Actividad in vitro *de los antifúngicos frente a las cinco especies más frecuentes de* Candida.

Sin embargo, la clasificación entre especies sensibles y resistentes al fluconazol varía según si se utilizan los puntos de corte propuestos por el Clinical Laboratory Standards Institute (CLSI),[62] que hasta ahora los establecía en ≤ 8 mg/l para las cepas sensibles, 16-32 mg/l para las sensibles dependiendo de la dosis y ≥ 64 mg/l para las resistentes, o los establecidos por el European Committee for Antimicrobial Susceptibility Testing (EUCAST),[63] que considera estos puntos de corte demasiado altos y ha propuesto otros basándose en análisis poblacionales y de respuesta antifúngica: ≤ 2 mg/l para las cepas sensibles, 4 mg/l para las cepas con sensibilidad intermedia y > 4 mg/l para las resistentes. Recientemente el CLSI también ha modificado sus puntos de corte para el fluconazol y ha establecido unos valores similares a los del EUCAST frente a *C. albicans, C. tropicalis* y *C. parapsilosis*.[64] Además, se considera que *C. glabrata* no tendría que tratarse con fluconazol, con independencia de la CMI para la cepa, porque desarrolla resistencia con facilidad.[65]

Teniendo en cuenta estas consideraciones, con los nuevos puntos de corte y clasificando *C. glabrata* como resistente al fluconazol, el porcentaje de resistencias a este fármaco aumenta y se sitúa alrededor del 15 %.[66] En cuanto al voriconazol, el 7,8 % de los aislados de muestras clínicas en España son resistentes a este azol, y destaca el 20 % de resistencia en *C. glabrata*.[66] Las equinocandinas son fármacos fungicidas para todas las especies de *Candida,* y aunque las CMI son más altas frente a *C. parapsilosis* que para el resto de las especies, este hecho parece no tener trascendencia clínica.[67]

Un aspecto a considerar es la capacidad de algunas especies de *Candida* de formar biopelículas sobre los materiales protésicos y los dispositivos endovasculares, como los catéteres venosos, lo cual se ha asociado a una mayor mortalidad relacionada. Estas biopelículas de *Candida* spp. se caracterizan por mostrar una resistencia variable a la amfotericina B desoxicolato y al fluconazol, mientras que las equinocandinas y las preparaciones lipídicas de amfotericina B han demostrado tener la mayor actividad antifúngica *in vitro*.[68,69]

5.2 *Modelos experimentales*

Para valorar la utilidad del tratamiento antifúngico local sobre las biopelículas de *Candida* spp. se han realizado diferentes estudios *in vitro*. Gracias a ellos se sabe que la amfotericina B desoxicolato tiene una escasa actividad,[70] mientras que en sus formulaciones lipídicas es superior.[69] La actividad de la amfotericina B complejo lipídico se potencia *in vitro* cuando se combina con ácido etilendiaminotetraacético (EDTA).[71] La actividad de los azoles es escasa, sobre todo en *C. albicans*, especie para la que se han descrito unas CMI muy altas.[72] Las equinocandinas han demostrado tener una excelente actividad frente a las biopelículas de *C. albicans*[73] y *C. tropicalis*[74] en un modelo estático de crecimiento en microplaca. En el trabajo de Oncu,[75] que comparó la actividad de la amfotericina B desoxicolato, la caspofungina, el fluconazol, el voriconazol y el itraconazol frente a biopeliculas de *C. albicans* y *C. parapsilosis* en un modelo de catéter de silicona, se demuestra que ninguno de los azoles utilizados consigue la esterilización de los segmentos del catéter, mientras que la amfotericina B y la caspofungina lo logran en el quinto día del estudio. Las limitaciones de estos modelos experimentales *in vitro* incluyen: *1)* su naturaleza estática, *2)* el uso de un inóculo inicial fúngico muy elevado y *3)* la falta de reproducibilidad del papel de la respuesta inmunitaria del huésped frente a la infección.[68] Además, puesto que en estos estudios se utiliza un número limitado de aislados de *Candida*, la generalización de los resultados puede ser cuestionable.

En cuanto a los estudios *in vivo,* es destacable el trabajo de Schinabeck *et al.,*[76] que utilizaron un modelo de catéter de silicona colonizado por *C. albicans* en ratón y observaron su esterilización en los seis animales tratados con amfotericina B liposómica y sólo en dos de los seis que recibieron fluconazol. También es relevante el estudio de Shuford *et al.*[77] en un modelo de catéter colonizado por *C. albicans* en conejos tratados durante siete días, de forma local y sistémica, con caspofungina o amfotericina B desoxicolato, en el cual se consiguió la esterilización de todos los catéteres tratados con caspofungina, de 13 de 16 tratados con amfotericina B desoxicolato y de ninguno de los del grupo control.

5.3 Estudios clínicos

La amfotericina B desoxicolato se ha considerado durante años el tratamiento de elección para las infecciones fúngicas invasivas, aunque actualmente las formulaciones lipídicas la han sustituido debido a su mejor perfil de seguridad. La amfotericina B liposómica a dosis de 3 mg/kg al día ha demostrado, en un estudio clínico prospectivo, su eficacia para el tratamiento de la candidemia.[78]

Diversos estudios clínicos avalan la utilización de fluconazol en pacientes seleccionados no neutropénicos que presentan candidemia.[79-83] El voriconazol se ha mostrado tan efectivo como la amfotericina B en el tratamiento de inducción (4-7 días), seguido de fluconazol, para el tratamiento de la candidemia en el paciente no neutropénico, y además tiene actividad antifúngica frente a la mayoría de *Candida* spp., incluyendo *C. krusei*.[81] En aquellos pacientes en quienes no se ha iniciado el tratamiento de la candidemia con fluconazol, diferentes estudios clínicos demuestran la seguridad de completar el tratamiento con este fármaco, una vez estabilizado el paciente, si la especie de *Candida* es sensible.[78,81,83-85] Aunque el posaconazol tiene una excelente actividad *in vitro* frente a la mayoría de *Candida* spp., no hay estudios clínicos que avalen su uso en los pacientes con candidemia, lo cual, unido a la ausencia de una formulación para uso intravenoso, hace que no sea una alternativa de tratamiento de la candidemia.[67]

Las equinocandinas han demostrado una buena actividad fungicida frente a todas las especies de *Candida,* según los resultados de un estudio aleatorizado.[82] A partir de estos resultados, en las guías de expertos se aconseja iniciar el tratamiento con estos fármacos cuando el paciente presenta criterios de gravedad, neutropenia o antecedente de consumo de azoles.

En el caso de los pacientes con neutropenia, no hay estudios clínicos aleatorizados con suficiente poder estadístico que valoren el tratamiento de la candidemia, aunque se han publicado estudios de tratamiento que demuestran la eficacia de las equinocandinas para esta indicación, con porcentajes de éxito del 50 % al 70 %.[78,84-86]

6 Tratamiento

Las guías clínicas de las diferentes sociedades científicas recomiendan que el tratamiento de la candidemia incluya antifúngicos por vía intravenosa, valorar la retirada de los catéteres vasculares, en especial si pueden ser el foco de la infección, y realizar una exploración del fondo del ojo para descartar una endoftalmitis o una coriorretinitis asociadas.[67,87-89]

6.1 Tratamiento antifúngico

En los pacientes con candidemia, el tratamiento antifúngico precoz es un elemento clave para que el pronóstico sea favorable. Las recomendaciones terapéuticas se encuentran recogidas en documentos de consenso e incluyen la necesidad de administrar tratamiento antifúngico a todos los pacientes con candidemia.[67,87-89]

Hasta hace unos años se consideraba que la amfotericina B era el tratamiento de elección para las infecciones fúngicas invasivas. La introducción, primero, de los azoles (en especial del fluconazol), y luego de las equinocandinas, de los nuevos azoles (como el voriconazol) y de las formulaciones lipídicas de la amfotericina B, han modificado de manera sustancial el tratamiento de las candidemias. La elección del antifúngico para el tratamiento empírico inicial dependerá de la distribución de las diferentes especies de *Candida* en esa área geográfica, de la prevalencia de la resistencia a los azoles, del estado clínico del paciente, de sus características y de si ha recibido tratamientos previos con azoles.[67,87-89]

Respecto a la distribución de las diferentes especies de *Candida* y de los porcentajes de resistencia a los antifúngicos, en nuestro medio alrededor del 50 % de las candidemias están causadas por especies de *Candida* no *albicans*, cuya resistencia a los azoles puede ser globalmente superior al 10 %.[8,19,60]

En cuanto al estado del paciente, deben considerarse características como la edad, la presencia de neutropenia y de otras condiciones asociadas (NPT, cirugía abdominal previa o exposición anterior a antimicrobianos o antifúngicos), y la situación de estabilidad hemodinámica del paciente.[67,87,89,90] Probablemente la característica de mayor relevancia es la neutropenia asociada a la candidemia, sobre todo si hay antecedentes de tratamientos o profilaxis con azoles.[67,87,89] El tratamiento empírico con fluconazol ha demostrado ser eficaz en los pacientes con candidemia que están hemodinámicamente estables, sin neutropenia asociada ni exposición previa a azoles.[79,80] No se plantea el uso de itraconazol en estas circunstancias porque tiene un espectro de actividad antifúngica similar al del fluconazol, y este último ofrece mejores características farmacocinéticas, mayor facilidad de administración y más tolerabilidad.[67] Para el tratamiento de la candidemia, el voriconazol sólo está recomendado en el paciente neutropénico, cuando además se desea una cobertura adicional para hongos filamentosos.[91]

En presencia de signos de sepsis grave, es decir, disfunción de al menos un órgano o afectación hemodinámica, así como en caso de exposición previa a los azoles (pacientes con neoplasias hematológicas que han seguido profilaxis de la infección fúngica invasiva con azoles, receptores de trasplantes, etc.) o de neutropenia, la primera opción es una equinocandina, y la amfotericina B liposómica es un tratamiento alternativo.[67,87-90]

La duración del tratamiento antifúngico no se ha valorado específicamente en ensayos clínicos controlados, pero en los pacientes sin complicaciones metastásicas se aceptan 14 días tras los primeros hemocultivos negativos y la mejoría del cuadro clínico. En los pacientes neutropénicos se suspenderá el tratamiento cuando se cumplan los criterios anteriores y además se haya resuelto la neutropenia. Una vez que el paciente se encuentra estable, y si se trata de *Candida* sensible al fluconazol, puede completarse el tratamiento con este fármaco. El diagnóstico de infección secundaria metastásica (endoftalmitis) condiciona la prolongación del tratamiento antifúngico al menos hasta completar 4 semanas.[67,87-90]

6.2   *Retirada del catéter*

Aunque las guías clínicas de diferentes sociedades científicas recomiendan que ante un paciente con candidemia se proceda a la retirada precoz de todos los catéteres,[67,87-90] éste sigue siendo un tema de debate por la falta de estudios aleatorizados bien diseñados que hayan valorado los riesgos y los beneficios de esta medida.

El catéter venoso central no siempre es el origen de la infección, pero su mantenimiento podría representar un reservorio que prolongaría la candidemia y podría incrementar el riesgo de desarrollar focos metastásicos de la infección.[89] Esto se explicaría por la gran adherencia de las especies de *Candida* a las biopelículas que se forman en los catéteres, donde, como ya se ha mencionado, se ha demostrado una significativa resistencia a la acción de algunos antifúngicos.[68] Por ello, las guías clínicas actuales recomiendan retirar los catéteres de corta permanencia en todos los casos de candidemia.[8,87-89] En la tabla 4 se recoge una selección de estudios clínicos que han analizado el efecto de la actuación sobre los catéteres en los pacientes con candidemia. Algunos, no aleatorizados, demuestran que los pacientes con candidemia a quienes se retiran los catéteres presentan una menor mortalidad o duración de la fungemia respecto a aquellos en que se mantienen.[92-106] En otras series no ha podido demostrarse el efecto protector de la retirada precoz del catéter vascular sobre la supervivencia, excepto en

Autores	Diseño del estudio	Nº pacientes	Efecto de mantener frente a retirar los catéteres
Eppes *et al.*[94]	Retrospectivo	21	Murieron 2/8 (25 %) pacientes con el catéter venoso central frente a ninguno de 13 (0 %) en los que se retiró (p = 0,13)
Dato y Dajani[93]	Retrospectivo	31	Murieron 3/5 (60 %) pacientes con el catéter venoso central frente a 2/26 (7,7 %) en los que se retiró (p = 0,02)
Goodrich *et al.*[96]	Retrospectivo	102	No se demostraron diferencias en la mortalidad, pero mantener el catéter venoso central se asoció a una mayor duración de la fungemia (p < 0,001)
Lecciones *et al.*[99]	Retrospectivo	155	Murieron 4/4 (100 %) pacientes con el catéter venoso central frente a 72/151 (48 %) en los que se retiró (p = 0,06)
Rex *et al.*[103]	Cohorte prospectiva	237	No se analizó la mortalidad. Mantener el catéter venoso central se asoció a una mayor duración de la fungemia (p < 0,001)
Stamos[104]	Retrospectivo	61	Murieron 9/19 (47 %) pacientes con el catéter venoso central frente a 4/42 (9,6 %) en los que se retiró (p = 0,002)
Nguyen *et al.*[101]	Cohorte prospectiva	360	En el análisis multivariado, mantener el catéter venoso central se asoció a una mayor mortalidad (p < 0,001)
Girmenia *et al.*[95]	Retrospectivo	35	Murieron 7/13 (54 %) pacientes con el catéter venoso central frente a 5/22 (23 %) en los que se retiró (p = 0,08)
Hung *et al.*[97]	Cohorte prospectiva	118	En el análisis multivariado, mantener el catéter venoso central se asoció a una mayor mortalidad (p < 0,001)
Anaissie *et al.*[92]	Retrospectivo	476	En el análisis multivariado, mantener el catéter venoso central se asoció a una mayor mortalidad (OR: 2,2; IC95 %: 1,6-3,2)
Nucci[102]	Cohorte prospectiva	145	En el análisis multivariado, mantener el catéter venoso central se asoció a una mayor mortalidad (OR: 4,8; IC95 %: 2,0-11,6)
Luzzati *et al.*[100]	Retrospectivo	189	En el análisis multivariado, retirar el catéter venoso central se asoció a una menor mortalidad (OR: 0,62; IC95 %: 0,38-0,99)
Karlowicz[98]	Cohorte prospectiva	104	Murieron 10/23 (43,5 %) pacientes con el catéter venoso central frente a 1/50 (2 %) en los que se retiró (p < 0,001)

Continúa

Continuación

Autores	Diseño del estudio	Nº pacientes	Efecto de mantener frente a retirar los catéteres
Garnacho-Montero *et al.*[105]	Cohorte prospectiva	188	En el análisis multivariado, la retirada del catéter venoso central en las primeras 48 h se asoció a un mejor pronóstico (HR: 0,34; IC95%: 0,16-0,70)
Slavin *et al.*[106]	Cohorte prospectiva	138	La retirada del catéter venoso central en los primeros 5 días tras la candidemia se asoció a un mejor pronóstico
Nucci *et al.*[107]	Cohorte propectiva	842	En el análisis multivariado no se demostró mejoría del pronóstico con la retirada precoz (<48 h) del catéter venoso central
Rodríguez *et al.*[108]	Cohorte prospectiva	265	En el análisis multivariado no se demostró mejoría del pronóstico con la retirada precoz (<48 h) del catéter venoso central
Rodríguez-Hernández *et al.*[60]	Cohorte prospectiva	220	En el análisis multivariado, la retirada del catéter venoso central no se asoció a una menor mortalidad

OR: *odds ratio;* IC95%: intervalo de confianza del 95%; HR: *hazard ratio.*

Tabla 4. Estudios clínicos que han analizado el efecto de mantener o de retirar los catéteres en pacientes con candidemia.

los pacientes cuyo foco de origen es el propio dispositivo.[60,107,108] En este sentido, una revisión sistemática de la literatura realizada por Nucci y Anaissie[109] concluye que, aunque la retirada del catéter posiblemente reduzca la tasa de complicaciones asociadas a la fungemia, incluyendo la mortalidad, no hay evidencia suficiente que apoye esta recomendación de forma generalizada.

No sólo es importante saber cuál es el impacto de la retirada del catéter sobre la supervivencia, sino también qué momento es el más apropiado para hacerlo y en qué subgrupo de pacientes es más efectiva esta medida (pacientes con candidemia originada en un catéter venoso central frente a pacientes con candidemia de otro origen). En un trabajo publicado por Raad[110] se concluye que cuanto más precoz es la retirada del catéter mejor es la respuesta al tratamiento antifúngico, cuando el origen de la fungemia es el propio catéter, pero si hay un foco secundario la retirada del catéter no tiene ningún impacto sobre la respuesta al tratamiento antifúngico. Coincidimos con este autor en considerar que es probable que la retirada de los catéteres venosos en aquellos pacientes en quienes éste sea el origen de la candidemia sea una actuación beneficiosa, ya que reduce el tiempo de duración de la infección y el riesgo de complicaciones secundarias, pero hay dudas sobre el beneficio de aplicar esta medida de forma sistemática, en especial en los pacientes neutropénicos y en los ingresados en la UCI. En éstos, el origen de la candidemia puede ser endógeno (por traslocación intestinal)[111] e intervienen una serie de factores que facilitan la colonización del catéter, como el traumatismo local y el uso de NPT o de antibióticos de amplio espectro. Otros argumentos en contra de la retirada sistemática de los catéteres en los pacientes con candidemia son las posibles complicaciones asociadas a la inserción de nuevos dispositivos, los problemas para su canalización en algunos casos y el alto porcentaje de catéteres retirados sospechosos de ser origen de la candidemia pero con cultivo de la punta negativo (hasta el 90 %).[98]

Pese a todas estas consideraciones, y aunque no haya estudios concluyentes que lo avalen,[109] las diferentes guías de práctica clínica para los pacientes con candidemia recomiendan la retirada de todos los catéteres, si es posible, sobre todo en los pacientes no neutropénicos (nivel de evidencia B-II).[88] La recomendación es más clara si se trata de una fungemia por *C. parapsilosis* (A-II),[87-89] porque su origen es casi siempre un catéter venoso, en el caso de sepsis grave o con signos de infección local, y si la candidemia es persistente o no se observa respuesta clínica al cabo de 72 horas del inicio del tratamiento con una pauta antifúngica correcta.[88] En los pacientes con neutropenia esta recomendación es más controvertida, ya que con frecuencia presentan trastornos de la coagulación asociados a una trombocitopenia grave y además se ha documentado un mayor papel del intestino como origen de la candidiasis diseminada.[87,111] Finalmente, las guías de práctica clínica recomiendan la retirada del catéter (incluso los tunelizados) siempre que la candidemia sea persistente.[67,87,89]

6.3 Tratamiento local (sellado antibiótico)

En los pacientes con accesos vasculares difíciles, y en aquellos casos en que su retirada puede implicar un riesgo vital, los antifúngicos como las equinocandinas, con demostrada actividad sobre la biocapa, abren una nueva ruta de investigación y la posibilidad de que en casos seleccionados (pacientes hemodinámicamente estables, portadores de catéteres de larga duración y sin otras posibilidades de acceso vascular) pueda intentarse un tratamiento conservador para la candidemia de catéter mediante técnicas de sellado con antifúngicos, junto al tratamiento sistémico.[68]

Las primeras pautas de instilación local de antifúngicos a través del catéter origen de la infección utilizaban amfotericina B desoxicolato a una concentración de 2,5 mg/ml, disuelta en solución salina o en heparina, pero diferentes estudios han demostrado que su actividad frente a las biopelículas de *Candida* spp. es reducida.[68,70] Para el fluconazol también se ha demostrado, tanto *in vitro* como en el modelo animal *in vivo*, que tiene una reducida actividad frente a las biopelículas.[72,112] Por el contrario, las formulaciones lipídicas de amfotericina B, y en especial las equinocandinas, tienen una excelente actividad frente a las biopelículas de *Candida* spp. y, por tanto, son los fármacos de elección para esta modalidad de tratamiento.[68,69] Debido a su potencial actividad antifúngica sobre las biopelículas de *Candida* spp., una posible alternativa en estudio es la utilización de antibióticos como la doxiciclina, la tigeciclina o combinaciones de minociclina o ciprofloxacino con rifampicina. También han demostrado su actividad *in vitro* frente a las biopelículas de *Candida* sustancias como el quitosano, la taurolidina, el EDTA y el etanol.[68]

Hay dudas sobre la duración del tratamiento y el intervalo de administración óptimo, pero en general se recomienda una duración de 14 días del tratamiento antifúngico local, junto al tratamiento sistémico, a partir de la negativización de los hemocultivos.[68]

6.4 Seguimiento

Las guías clínicas de diferentes sociedades científicas recomiendan que, ante un paciente con candidemia, se practiquen de forma sistemática hemocultivos de control y examen del fondo de ojo durante la primera semana de tratamiento antifúngico efectivo, con el fin de comprobar la erradicación de la fungemia y de descartar una infección secundaria metastásica.[67,87-89] La persistencia de *Candida* spp. en los segundos hemocultivos practicados a las 48 a 72 horas de la instauración de un tratamiento antifúngico efectivo se ha relacionado con una mayor mortalidad,[60] probablemente como reflejo de un tratamiento inapropiado o de la no erradicación del foco de la infección.

7   Evolución y pronóstico

La infección invasiva por *Candida* spp. presenta una alta mortalidad, entre un 10 % y un 50 %, según la especie causante de la infección.[8,17,20,22,47,60]

Diversos trabajos han intentado identificar factores pronósticos asociados a la mortalidad por candidemia, entre ellos la edad superior a 65 años, la sepsis bacteriana concomitante, la enfermedad rápidamente fatal o un índice APACHE elevado, la presencia de inestabilidad hemodinámica, la neoplasia como enfermedad de base, la cirugía abdominal previa, la presencia de un catéter venoso central, la candidemia por una especie de *Candida* resistente al fluconazol, el tratamiento sistémico con esteroides, y la ausencia o el retraso de un tratamiento antifúngico adecuado.[8,47,60,106,107] Los factores significativamente asociados con una mayor mortalidad en los pacientes con candidemia, relacionados con la enfermedad de base y su gravedad, son difícilmente modificables. Sin embargo, los factores relacionados con la atención del paciente sí son modificables. En este sentido, el impacto de un tratamiento inadecuado sobre la mortalidad atribuible a la candidemia es muy relevante y es el único factor pronóstico mejorable.

Ante la sospecha de una candidemia debe tenerse en cuenta no sólo el fármaco antifúngico a emplear sino también otras medidas que pueden influir en el pronóstico del paciente, como son la precocidad del inicio del tratamiento antifúngico y la retirada de los catéteres vasculares. Se ha comprobado que un retraso de más de 12 horas tras la extracción de la sangre del primer hemocultivo positivo en la administración de un tratamiento antifúngico adecuado es un factor predictor independiente de mortalidad hospitalaria.[113] El posible efecto beneficioso de la retirada del catéter vascular en el paciente con candidemia ya se ha comentado. En un estudio reciente, publicado por Garnacho-Montero *et al.,*[105] se demuestra el efecto protector respecto a la mortalidad de la retirada de los catéteres vasculares y del inicio de un tratamiento antifúngico adecuado en las primeras 48 horas tras la candidemia.

Como ya se ha mencionado, en casos seleccionados de pacientes con accesos vasculares difíciles, o en aquellos cuya retirada implique un riesgo vital, puede intentarse un tratamiento conservador del catéter mediante técnicas de sellado junto con el tratamiento sistémico. Con esta estrategia terapéutica se han comunicado tasas de éxito globales en el tratamiento de la candidemia de hasta el 77 %.[68]

Bibliografía

1. Pappas PG. Invasive candidiasis. Infect Dis Clin North Am. 2006; 20: 485-506.
2. Garbino J, Kolarova L, Rohner P, Lew D, Pichna P, Pittet D. Secular trends of candidemia over 12 years in adult patients at a tertiary care hospital. Medicine (Baltimore). 2002; 81: 425-33.
3. Jarvis WR. Epidemiology of nosocomial fungal infections, with emphasis on Candida species. Clin Infect Dis. 1995; 20: 1526-30.
4. Marchetti O, Bille J, Fluckiger U, Eggimann P, Ruef C, Garbino J, *et al.* Epidemiology of candidemia in Swiss tertiary care hospitals: secular trends, 1991-2000. Clin Infect Dis. 2004; 38: 311-20.
5. Sandven P, Bevanger L, Digranes A, Haukland HH, Mannsaker T, Gaustad P. Candidemia in Norway (1991 to 2003): results from a nationwide study. J Clin Microbiol. 2006; 44: 1977-81.
6. Asmundsdottir LR, Erlendsdottir H, Gottfredsson M. Increasing incidence of candidemia: results from a 20-year nationwide study in Iceland. J Clin Microbiol. 2002; 40: 3489-92.
7. Prentice HG, Kibbler CC, Prentice AG. Towards a targeted, risk-based, antifungal strategy in neutropenic patients. Br J Haematol. 2000; 110: 273-84.
8. Almirante B, Rodríguez D, Park BJ, Cuenca-Estrella M, Planes AM, Almela M, *et al.* Epidemiology and predictors of mortality in cases of Candida bloodstream infection: results from population-based surveillance, Barcelona, Spain, from 2002 to 2003. J Clin Microbiol. 2005; 43: 1829-35.
9. Arendrup MC, Fuursted K, Gahrn-Hansen B, Jensen IM, Knudsen JD, Lundgren B, *et al.* Seminational surveillance of fungemia in Denmark: notably high rates of fungemia and numbers of isolates with reduced azole susceptibility. J Clin Microbiol. 2005; 43: 4434-40.
10. Kao AS, Brandt ME, Pruitt WR, Conn LA, Perkins BA, Stephens DS, *et al.* The epidemiology of candidemia in two United States cities: results of a population-based active surveillance. Clin Infect Dis. 1999; 29: 1164-70.
11. Hajjeh RA, Sofair AN, Harrison LH, Lyon GM, Arthington-Skaggs BA, Mirza SA, *et al.* Incidence of bloodstream infections due to Candida species and in vitro susceptibilities of isolates collected from 1998 to 2000 in a population-based active surveillance program. J Clin Microbiol. 2004; 42: 1519-27.
12. Laupland KB, Gregson DB, Church DL, Ross T, Elsayed S. Invasive Candida species infections: a 5 year population-based assessment. J Antimicrob Chemother. 2005; 56: 532-7.
13. Odds FC, Hanson MF, Davidson AD, Jacobsen MD, Wright P, Whyte JA, *et al.* One year prospective survey of Candida bloodstream infections in Scotland. J Med Microbiol. 2007; 56(Pt 8): 1066-75.

14. Diekema DJ, Messer SA, Brueggemann AB, Coffman SL, Doern GV, Herwaldt LA, *et al.* Epidemiology of candidemia: 3-year results from the emerging infections and the epidemiology of Iowa organisms study. J Clin Microbiol. 2002; 40: 1298-302.

15. Colombo AL, Nucci M, Park BJ, Nouér SA, Arthington-Skaggs B, da Matta DA, *et al.* Epidemiology of candidemia in Brazil: a nationwide sentinel surveillance of candidemia in eleven medical centers. J Clin Microbiol. 2006; 44: 2816-23.

16. Chen S, Slavin M, Nguyen Q, Marriott D, Playford EG, Ellis D, *et al.* Active surveillance for candidemia, Australia. Emerg Infect Dis. 2006; 12: 1508-16.

17. Cleveland AA, Farley MM, Harrison LH, Stein B, Hollick R, Lockhart SR, *et al.* Changes in incidence and antifungal drug resistance in candidemia: results from population-based laboratory surveillance in Atlanta and Baltimore, 2008-2011. Clin Infect Dis. 2012; 55: 1352-61.

18. Arendrup MC, Bruun B, Christensen JJ, Fuursted K, Johansen HK, Kjaeldgaard P, *et al.* National surveillance of fungemia in Denmark (2004 to 2009). J Clin Microbiol. 2011; 49: 325-34.

19. Pemán J, Cantón E, Quindós G, Eraso E, Alcoba J, Guinea J, *et al.* Epidemiology, species distribution and in vitro antifungal susceptibility of fungaemia in a Spanish multicentre prospective survey. J Antimicrob Chemother. 2012; 67: 1181-7.

20. Puig M, Garnacho J, Padilla B, Zaragoza R, Aguado JM, Montejo M, *et al.* Epidemiology, risk factors for mortality and fluconazol susceptibility in a population-based surveillance for candidaemia in Spain. 22nd European Congress of Clinical Microbiology and Infectious Diseases. London, 2012. Oral communication O110.

21. Pfaller MA, Diekema DJ. Epidemiology of invasive candidiasis: a persistent public health problem. Clin Microbiol Rev. 2007; 20: 133-63.

22. Horn DL, Neofytos D, Anaissie EJ, Fishman JA, Steinbach WJ, Olyaei AJ, *et al.* Epidemiology and outcomes of candidemia in 2019 patients: data from the prospective antifungal therapy alliance registry. Clin Infect Dis. 2009; 48: 1695-703.

23. Rangel-Frausto MS, Wiblin T, Blumberg HM, Saiman L, Patterson J, Rinaldi M, *et al.* National epidemiology of mycoses survey (NEMIS): variations in rates of bloodstream infections due to Candida species in seven surgical intensive care units and six neonatal intensive care units. Clin Infect Dis. 1999; 29: 253-8.

24. Leroy O, Gangneux JP, Montravers P, Mira JP, Gouin F, Sollet JP, *et al.* Epidemiology, management, and risk factors for death of invasive Candida infections in critical care: a multicenter, prospective, observational study in France (2005-2006). Crit Care Med. 2009; 37: 1612-8.

25. Hachem RY, Boktour MR, Hanna HA, Husni RN, Torres HA, Afif C, *et al.* Amphotericin B lipid complex versus liposomal amphotericin B monotherapy for invasive aspergillosis in patients with hematologic malignancy. Cancer. 2008; 112: 1282-7.

26. Fridkin SK, Kaufman D, Edwards JR, Shetty S, Horan T. Changing incidence of Candida bloodstream infections among NICU patients in the United States: 1995-2004. Pediatrics. 2006; 117: 1680-7.

27. Stoll BJ, Hansen N, Fanaroff AA, Wright LL, Carlo WA, Ehrenkranz RA, *et al.* Late-onset sepsis in very low birth weight neonates: the experience of the NICHD Neonatal Research Network. Pediatrics. 2002; 110(2 Pt 1): 285-91.

28. Rodríguez D, Almirante B, Park BJ, Cuenca-Estrella M, Planes AM, Sanchez F, *et al.* Candidemia in neonatal intensive care units: Barcelona, Spain. Pediatr Infect Dis J. 2006; 25: 224-9.

29. Stamos JK, Rowley AH. Candidemia in a pediatric population. Clin Infect Dis.1995; 20: 571-5.

30. Blyth CC, Chen SC, Slavin MA, Serena C, Nguyen Q, Marriott D, *et al.* Not just little adults: candidemia epidemiology, molecular characterization, and antifungal susceptibility in neonatal and pediatric patients. Pediatrics. 2009; 123: 1360-8.

31. Celebi S, Hacimustafaoglu M, Ozdemir O, Ozkaya G. Nosocomial candidaemia in children: results of a 9-year study. Mycoses. 2008; 51: 248-57.

32. Pfaller MA, Diekema DJ. Rare and emerging opportunistic fungal pathogens: concern for

resistance beyond Candida albicans and Aspergillus fumigatus. J Clin Microbiol. 2004; 42: 4419-31.

33. Abi-Said D, Anaissie E, Uzun O, Raad I, Pinzcowski H, Vartivarian S. The epidemiology of hematogenous candidiasis caused by different Candida species. Clin Infect Dis. 1997; 24: 1122-8.

34. Krcmery V, Barnes AJ. Non-albicans Candida spp. causing fungaemia: pathogenicity and antifungal resistance. J Hosp Infect. 2002; 50: 243-60.

35. Girmenia C, Martino P. Fluconazole and the changing epidemiology of candidemia. Clin Infect Dis. 1998; 27: 232-4.

36. Shorr AF, Lazarus DR, Sherner JH, Jackson WL, Morrel M, Fraser VJ, *et al.* Do clinical features allow for accurate prediction of fungal pathogenesis in bloodstream infections? Potential implications of the increasing prevalence of non-albicans candidemia. Crit Care Med. 2007; 35: 1077-83.

37. Rodríguez D, Almirante B, Cuenca-Estrella M, Rodríguez-Tudela JL, Mensa J, Ayats J, *et al.* Predictors of candidaemia caused by non-albicans Candida species: results of a population-based surveillance in Barcelona, Spain. Clin Microbiol Infect. 2010; 16: 1676-82.

38. Tortorano AM, Pemán J, Bernhardt H, Klingspor L, Kibbler CC, Faure O, *et al.* Epidemiology of candidaemia in Europe: results of 28-month European Confederation of Medical Mycology (ECMM) hospital-based surveillance study. Eur J Clin Microbiol Infect Dis. 2004; 23: 317-22.

39. Pemán J, Cantón E, Gobernado M. Epidemiology and antifungal susceptibility of Candida species isolated from blood: results of a 2-year multicentre study in Spain. Eur J Clin Microbiol Infect Dis. 2005; 24: 23-30.

40. Almirante B, Pemán J. Tratamiento actual de la candidemia. Papel de anidulafungina. Enferm Infecc Microbiol Clin. 2008; 26(Supl 14): 21-8.

41. Cuenca-Estrella M, Gómez-Lopez A, Mellado E, Buitrago MJ, Monzón A, Rodríguez-Tudela JL. Head-to-head comparison of the activities of currently available antifungal agents against 3,378 Spanish clinical isolates of yeasts and filamentous fungi. Antimicrob Agents Chemother. 2006; 50: 917-21.

42. Pfaller MA, Boyken L, Hollis RJ, Messer SA, Tendolkar S, Diekema DJ. In vitro susceptibilities of Candida spp. to caspofungin: four years of global surveillance. J Clin Microbiol. 2006; 44: 760-3.

43. Tortorano AM, Biraghi E, Astolfi A, Ossi C, Tejada M, Farina C, *et al.* European Confederation of Medical Mycology (ECMM) prospective survey of candidaemia: report from one Italian region. J Hosp Infect. 2002; 51: 297-304.

44. Sandven P, Bevanger L, Digranes A, Haukland HH, Mannsaker T, Gaustad P. Candidemia in Norway (1991 to 2003): results from a nationwide study. J Clin Microbiol. 2006; 44: 1977-81.

45. Lin MY, Carmeli Y, Zumsteg J, Flores EL, Tolentino J, Sreeramoju P, *et al.* Prior antimicrobial therapy and risk for hospital-acquired Candida glabrata and Candida krusei fungemia: a case-case-control study. Antimicrob Agents Chemother. 2005; 49: 4555-60.

46. Sarvikivi E, Lyytikainen O, Soll DR, Pujol C, Pfaller MA, Richardson M, *et al.* Emergence of fluconazole resistance in a Candida parapsilosis strain that caused infections in a neonatal intensive care unit. J Clin Microbiol. 2005; 43: 2729-35.

47. Kojic EM, Darouiche RO. Candida infections of medical devices. Clin Microbiol Rev. 2004; 17: 255-67.

48. Cauda R. Candidaemia in patients with an inserted medical device. Drugs. 2009; 69(Suppl 1): 33-8.

49. Almirante B, Limón E, Freixas N, Gudiol F; VINCat Program. Laboratory-based surveillance of hospital-acquired catheter-related bloodstream infections in Catalonia. Results of the VINCat Program (2007-2010). Enferm Infecc Microbiol Clin. 2012; 30(Suppl 3): 13-9.

50. Almirante B, Rodríguez D, Cuenca-Estrella M, Almela M, Sánchez F, Ayats J, *et al.* Epidemiology, risk factors, and prognosis of Candida parapsilosis bloodstream infections: case-control population-based surveillance study of patients in Barcelona, Spain, from 2002 to 2003. J Clin Microbiol. 2006; 44: 1681-5.

51. Ramage G, Mowat E, Jones B, Williams C, López-Ribot J. Our current understanding of

fungal biofilms. Crit Rev Microbiol. 2009; 35: 340-55.

52. Tumbarello M, Posteraro B, Trecarichi EM, Fiori B, Rossi M, Porta R, *et al.* Biofilm production by Candida species and inadequate antifungal therapy as predictors of mortality for patients with candidemia. J Clin Microbiol. 2007; 45: 1843-50.

53. Ramage G, Martínez JP, López-Ribot JL. Candida biofilms on implanted biomaterials: a clinically significant problem. FEMS Yeast Res. 2006; 6: 979-86.

54. Francolini I, Donelli G. Prevention and control of biofilm-based medical-device-related infections. FEMS Immunol Med Microbiol. 2010; 59: 227-38.

55. Raad I. Intravascular-catheter-related infections. Lancet. 1998; 351: 893-8.

56. López Sastre JB, Coto Cotallo GD, Fernández Colomer B; Grupo de Hospitales Castrillo. Neonatal invasive candidiasis: a prospective multicenter study of 118 cases. Am J Perinatol. 2003; 20: 153-63.

57. Zaoutis TE, Greves HM, Lautenbach E, Bilker WB, Coffin SE. Risk factors for disseminated candidiasis in children with candidemia. Pediatr Infect Dis J. 2004; 23: 635-41.

58. Fridkin SK. The changing face of fungal infections in health care settings. Clin Infect Dis. 2005; 41: 1455-60.

59. Kannangara S, Shindler D, Kunimoto DY, Sell B, DeSimone JA. Candidemia complicated by endophthalmitis: a prospective analysis. Eur J Clin Microbiol Infect Dis. 2007; 26: 839-41.

60. Rodríguez-Hernández MJ, Ruiz-Pérez de PM, Márquez-Solero M, Martín-Rico P, Castón-Osorio JJ, Guerrero-Sánchez FM, *et al.* Candidemias: análisis multicéntrico en 16 hospitales andaluces. Enferm Infecc Microbiol Clin. 2011; 29: 328-33.

61. Cuenca-Estrella M, Rodríguez D, Almirante B, Morgan J, Planes AM, Almela M, *et al.* In vitro susceptibilities of bloodstream isolates of Candida species to six antifungal agents: results from a population-based active surveillance programme, Barcelona, Spain, 2002-2003. J Antimicrob Chemother. 2005; 55: 194-9.

62. Clinical Laboratory Standards Institute. Reference method for broth dilution antifungal susceptibility testing of yeast: approved standard. 3rd ed. CLSI document M27-A3. Wayne: Clinical Laboratory Standards Institute; 2008.

63. EUCAST technical note on fluconazole. Clin Microbiol Infect 2008; 14: 193-5.

64. Pfaller MA, Andes D, Diekema DJ, Espinel-Ingroff A, Sheehan D. Wild-type MIC distributions, epidemiological cutoff values and species-specific clinical breakpoints for fluconazole and Candida: time for harmonization of CLSI and EUCAST broth microdilution methods. Drug Resist Updat. 2010; 13: 180-95.

65. Almirante B, Cuenca-Estrella M. Candidemia: impacto de los estudios epidemiológicos en la terapéutica y en el pronóstico de una infeccion grave. Enferm Infecc Microbiol Clin. 2011; 29: 325-7.

66. Cuenca-Estrella M, Gómez-López A, Mellado E, Monzón A, Buitrago MJ, Rodríguez-Tudela JL, *et al.* Activity profile in vitro of micafungin against Spanish clinical isolates of common and emerging species of yeasts and molds. Antimicrob Agents Chemother. 2009; 53: 2192-5.

67. Pappas PG, Kauffman CA, Andes D, Benjamin DK Jr, Calandra TF, Edwards JE Jr, *et al.* Clinical practice guidelines for the management of candidiasis: 2009 update by the Infectious Diseases Society of America. Clin Infect Dis. 2009; 48: 503-35.

68. Walraven CJ, Lee SA. Antifungal lock therapy. Antimicrob Agents Chemother. 2013; 57: 1-8.

69. Kuhn DM, George T, Chandra J, Mukherjee PK, Ghannoum MA. Antifungal susceptibility of Candida biofilms: unique efficacy of amphotericin B lipid formulations and echinocandins. Antimicrob Agents Chemother. 2002; 46: 1773-80.

70. Lewis RE, Kontoyiannis DP, Darouiche RO, Raad II, Prince RA. Antifungal activity of amphotericin B, fluconazole, and voriconazole in an in vitro model of Candida catheter-related bloodstream infection. Antimicrob Agents Chemother. 2002; 46: 3499-505.

71. Raad II, Hachem RY, Hanna HA, Fang X, Jiang Y, Dvorak T, *et al.* Role of ethylene diamine tetra-acetic acid (EDTA) in catheter lock solutions: EDTA enhances the antifungal activity of amphotericin B lipid complex against Candida embedded in biofilm. Int J Antimicrob Agents. 2008; 32: 515-8.

72. Ramage G, Vande WK, Wickes BL, López-Ribot JL. Standardized method for in vitro antifungal susceptibility testing of Candida albicans biofilms. Antimicrob Agents Chemother. 2001; 45: 2475-9.

73. Miceli MH, Bernardo SM, Lee SA. In vitro analysis of the occurrence of a paradoxical effect with different echinocandins and Candida albicans biofilms. Int J Antimicrob Agents. 2009; 34: 500-2.

74. Ku TS, Bernardo SM, Lee SA. In vitro assessment of the antifungal and paradoxical activity of different echinocandins against Candida tropicalis biofilms. J Med Microbiol. 2011; 60: 1708-10.

75. Oncu S. In vitro effectiveness of antifungal lock solutions on catheters infected with Candida species. J Infect Chemother. 2011; 17: 634-9.

76. Schinabeck MK, Long LA, Hossain MA, Chandra J, Mukherjee PK, Mohamed S, et al. Rabbit model of Candida albicans biofilm infection: liposomal amphotericin B antifungal lock therapy. Antimicrob Agents Chemother. 2004; 48: 1727-32.

77. Shuford JA, Rouse MS, Piper KE, Steckelberg JM, Patel R. Evaluation of caspofungin and amphotericin B deoxycholate against Candida albicans biofilms in an experimental intravascular catheter infection model. J Infect Dis. 2006; 194: 710-3.

78. Kuse ER, Chetchotisakd P, Da Cunha CA, Ruhnke M, Barrios C, Raghunadharao D, et al. Micafungin versus liposomal amphotericin B for candidaemia and invasive candidosis: a phase III randomised double-blind trial. Lancet. 2007; 369: 1519-27.

79. Phillips P, Shafran S, Garber G, Rotstein C, Smaill F, Fong I, et al. Multicenter randomized trial of fluconazole versus amphotericin B for treatment of candidemia in non-neutropenic patients. Canadian Candidemia Study Group. Eur J Clin Microbiol Infect Dis. 1997; 16: 337-45.

80. Rex JH, Bennett JE, Sugar AM, Pappas PG, van der Horst CM, Edwards JE, et al. A randomized trial comparing fluconazole with amphotericin B for the treatment of candidemia in patients without neutropenia. Candidemia Study Group and the National Institute. N Engl J Med. 1994; 331: 1325-30.

81. Kullberg BJ, Sobel JD, Ruhnke M, Pappas PG, Viscoli C, Rex JH, et al. Voriconazole versus a regimen of amphotericin B followed by fluconazole for candidaemia in non-neutropenic patients: a randomised non-inferiority trial. Lancet. 2005; 366: 1435-42.

82. Reboli AC, Rotstein C, Pappas PG, Chapman SW, Kett DH, Kumar D, et al. Anidulafungin versus fluconazole for invasive candidiasis. N Engl J Med. 2007; 356: 2472-82.

83. Rex JH, Pappas PG, Karchmer AW, Sobel J, Edwards JE, Hadley S, et al. A randomized and blinded multicenter trial of high-dose fluconazole plus placebo versus fluconazole plus amphotericin B as therapy for candidemia and its consequences in nonneutropenic subjects. Clin Infect Dis. 2003; 36: 1221-8.

84. Mora-Duarte J, Betts R, Rotstein C, Colombo AL, Thompson-Moya L, Smietana J, et al. Comparison of caspofungin and amphotericin B for invasive candidiasis. N Engl J Med. 2002; 347: 2020-9.

85. Pappas PG, Rotstein CM, Betts RF, Nucci M, Talwar D, De Waele JJ, et al. Micafungin versus caspofungin for treatment of candidemia and other forms of invasive candidiasis. Clin Infect Dis. 2007; 45: 883-93.

86. Betts R, Glasmacher A, Maertens J, Nucci M, Talwar D, De Waele JJ, et al. Efficacy of caspofungin against invasive Candida or invasive Aspergillus infections in neutropenic patients. Cancer. 2006; 106: 466-73.

87. Aguado JM, Ruiz-Camps I, Muñoz P, Mensa J, Almirante B, Vázquez L, et al. Recomendaciones sobre el tratamiento de la candidiasis invasiva y otras infecciones por levaduras de la Sociedad Española de Enfermedades Infecciosas y Microbiología Clínica (SEIMC). Actualización 2011. Enferm Infecc Microbiol Clin. 2011; 29: 345-61.

88. Mermel LA, Allon M, Bouza E, Craven DE, Flynn P, O'Grady NP, et al. Clinical practice guidelines for the diagnosis and management of intravascular catheter-related infection: 2009 update by the Infectious Diseases Society of America. Clin Infect Dis. 2009; 49: 1-45.

89. Ullmann AJ, Akova M, Herbrecht R, Viscoli C, Arendrup MC, Arikan-Akdagli S, et al. ESCMID guideline for the diagnosis and management of Candida diseases 2012:

adults with haematological malignancies and after haematopoietic stem cell transplantation (HCT). Clin Microbiol Infect. 2012; 18(Suppl 7): 53-67.

90. Spellberg BJ, Filler SG, Edwards JE, Jr. Current treatment strategies for disseminated candidiasis. Clin Infect Dis. 2006; 42: 244-51.

91. Walsh TJ, Pappas P, Winston DJ, Lazarus HM, Petersen F, Raffalli J, et al. Voriconazole compared with liposomal amphotericin B for empirical antifungal therapy in patients with neutropenia and persistent fever. N Engl J Med. 2002; 346: 225-34.

92. Anaissie EJ, Rex JH, Uzun O, Vartivarian S. Predictors of adverse outcome in cancer patients with candidemia. Am J Med. 1998; 104: 238-45.

93. Dato VM, Dajani AS. Candidemia in children with central venous catheters: role of catheter removal and amphotericin B therapy. Pediatr Infect Dis J. 1990; 9: 309-14.

94. Eppes SC, Troutman JL, Gutman LT. Outcome of treatment of candidemia in children whose central catheters were removed or retained. Pediatr Infect Dis J. 1989; 8: 99-104.

95. Girmenia C, Martino P, De BF, Gentile G, Boccanera M, Monaco M, et al. Rising incidence of Candida parapsilosis fungemia in patients with hematologic malignancies: clinical aspects, predisposing factors, and differential pathogenicity of the causative strains. Clin Infect Dis. 1996; 23: 506-14.

96. Goodrich JM, Reed EC, Mori M, Fisher LD, Skerrett S, Dandliker PS, et al. Clinical features and analysis of risk factors for invasive candidal infection after marrow transplantation. J Infect Dis. 1991; 164: 731-40.

97. Hung CC, Chen YC, Chang SC, Luh KT, Hsieh WC. Nosocomial candidemia in a university hospital in Taiwan. J Formos Med Assoc. 1996; 95: 19-28.

98. Karlowicz MG. Should central venous catheters be removed as soon as candidemia is detected in neonates? Pediatrics. 2000; 106; e63.

99. Lecciones JA, Lee JW, Navarro EE, Witebsky FG, Marshall D, Steinberg SM, et al. Vascular catheter-associated fungemia in patients with cancer: analysis of 155 episodes. Clin Infect Dis. 1992; 14: 875-83.

100. Luzzati R, Amalfitano G, Lazzarini L, Soldani F, Bellino S, Solbiati M. et al. Nosocomial candidemia in non-neutropenic patients at an Italian tertiary care hospital. Eur J Clin Microbiol Infect Dis. 2000; 19: 602-7.

101. Nguyen MH, Peacock JE, Jr., Tanner DC, Morris AJ, Nguyen ML, Snydman DR, et al. Therapeutic approaches in patients with candidemia. Evaluation in a multicenter, prospective, observational study. Arch Intern Med. 1995; 155: 2429-35.

102. Nucci M. Risk factors for death in patients with candidemia. Infect Control Hosp Epidemiol. 1998; 19: 846-50.

103. Rex JH, Bennett JE, Sugar AM, Pappas PG, Serody J, Edwards JE, et al. Intravascular catheter exchange and duration of candidemia. NIAID Mycoses Study Group and the Candidemia Study Group. Clin Infect Dis. 1995; 21: 994-6.

104. Stamos JK. Candidemia in a pediatric population. Clin Infect Dis. 1995; 20: 571-5.

105. Garnacho-Montero J, Díaz-Martín A, García-Cabrera E, Ruiz Pérez de Pipaon M, Hernández-Caballero C, Lepe-Jiménez JA. Impact on hospital mortality of catheter removal and adequate antifungal therapy in Candida spp. bloodstream infections. J Antimicrob Chemother. 2013; 68: 206-13.

106. Slavin MA, Sorrell TC, Marriott D, Thursky KA, Nguyen Q, Ellis DH, et al. Candidaemia in adult cancer patients: risks for fluconazole-resistant isolates and death. J Antimicrob Chemother. 2010; 65: 1042-51.

107. Nucci M, Anaissie E, Betts RF, Dupont BF, Wu C, Buell DN, et al. Early removal of central venous catheter in patients with candidemia does not improve outcome: analysis of 842 patients from 2 randomized clinical trials. Clin Infect Dis. 2010; 51: 295-303.

108. Rodríguez D, Park BJ, Almirante B, Cuenca-Estrella M, Planes AM, Mensa J, et al. Impact of early central venous catheter removal on outcome in patients with candidaemia. Clin Microbiol Infect. 2007; 13: 788-93.

109. Nucci M, Anaissie E. Should vascular catheters be removed from all patients with candidemia? An evidence-based review. Clin Infect Dis. 2002; 34: 591-9.

110. Raad I. Management of central venous catheters in patients with cancer and candidemia. Clin Infect Dis. 2004; 38: 119-27.
111. Telenti A, Steckelberg JM, Stockman L, Edson RS, Roberts GD, *et al.* Quantitative blood cultures in candidemia. Mayo Clin Proc. 1991; 66: 1120-3.
112. Andes D, Nett J, Oschel P, Albrecht R, Marchillo K, Pitula A. Development and characterization of an in vivo central venous catheter Candida albicans biofilm model. Infect Immun. 2004; 72: 6023-31.
113. Morrell M, Fraser VJ, Kollef MH. Delaying the empiric treatment of candida bloodstream infection until positive blood culture results are obtained: a potential risk factor for hospital mortality. Antimicrob Agents Chemother. 2005; 49: 3640-5.

Capítulo 10

Tratamiento conservador de la bacteriemia relacionada con catéteres

N. Fernández-Hidalgo, B. Almirante

**Servicio de Enfermedades Infecciosas
Hospital Universitari Vall d'Hebron
Universitat Autònoma de Barcelona
Barcelona**

Correspondencia:
Dra. N. Fernández-Hidalgo
nufernan@gmail.com

Introducción

Las bacteriemias relacionadas con catéteres vasculares son una causa importante de morbilidad y mortalidad en los pacientes portadores de dispositivos, temporales o permanentes, para tratamientos como la hemodiálisis, la nutrición parenteral total o la administración de quimioterapia u otras afines. La frecuencia de esta complicación es variable, pero puede alcanzar cifras de uno a dos episodios por cada 1.000 días de uso del catéteres, y ser el motivo de su retirada precoz hasta en un 25 % de los pacientes.[1,2]

Los catéteres venosos centrales se clasifican en tres categorías: *a)* no tunelizados, colocados generalmente durante períodos de tiempo que no superan las cuatro a seis semanas; *b)* tunelizados (tipos Broviac, Hickman, Groshom y Quinton), y *c)* reservorios implantables subcutáneos permanentes (tipo *Port-a-Cath*®). El tipo de catéter implicado en la bacteriemia influye de manera importante en el tratamiento de ésta. En las infecciones relacionadas con catéteres colocados con técnica quirúrgica (los tunelizados y los reservorios) siempre es aconsejable valorar un tratamiento conservador que rescate el catéter, si es posible, con el fin de evitar complicaciones y ahorrar recursos sanitarios.

Para que se produzca una bacteriemia relacionada con un catéter, los microorganismos han de acceder al dispositivo para formar una biocapa permanente que, en última instancia, dará lugar a la diseminación hematógena. La colonización inicial ocurre por una de las tres vías siguientes: *1)* por la superficie extraluminal del catéter, a través de la solución de continuidad generada en la piel adyacente al punto de inserción; *2)* por la superficie endoluminal del catéter, al manipular la línea o sus conexiones, o *3)* por vía hematógena, a partir de focos distantes de infección que emiten microorganismos al torrente circulatorio. La gran mayoría de las bacteriemias en los pacientes portadores de dispositivos vasculares permanentes se producen por la colonización de éstos por vía endoluminal, por lo que en tal caso parece razonable abordar su tratamiento de manera conservadora.[3]

El tratamiento de elección de la bacteriemia relacionada con un catéter consiste en la administración de antimicrobianos por vía sistémica, junto con la retirada precoz del catéter y su reemplazamiento en una vena diferente, si sigue siendo necesaria la canalización vascular. Sin embargo, en los enfermos con un catéter venoso central de larga permanencia ha de valorarse siempre la conveniencia de realizar un tratamiento conservador sin retirar el catéter, mediante el uso combinado de tratamiento sistémico y local con los antimicrobianos indicados en cada situación clínica. Esta última modalidad se conoce como *antibiotic (anti-infective) lock therapy* (ALT).[3]

La ALT se propuso durante los años 1980 como una opción para el tratamiento adyuvante de las bacteriemias relacionadas con catéteres en aquellos pacientes, fundamentalmente portadores de catéteres para nutrición parenteral total domiciliaria, con escasas posibilidades de retirada de sus dispositivos. Su base científica es la aceptación de la vía intraluminal como mecanismo de colonización inicial del catéter y, por ello, la posibilidad de que la instilación de antimicrobianos y su permanencia en la luz durante la mayor parte de las horas del día puedan condicionar una curación de la bacteriemia sin necesidad de retirar el catéter.[4-6]

1   Técnica de la *antibiotic lock therapy*

El concepto de ALT se desarrolló hace unos 20 años como una técnica similar al sellado de los catéteres con soluciones heparinizadas para evitar su trombosis endoluminal. Este método consiste en la instilación de una solución antimicrobiana, con una alta concentración del fármaco (en general 100 a 1.000 veces superior a la utilizada por vía sistémica), en el interior de la luz del catéter, de modo que ésta quede rellena por completo durante un determinado tiempo con el objetivo de conseguir su esterilización. Mediante esta técnica se pretende evitar la retirada del catéter venoso permanente causante de la sepsis, para disminuir los riesgos, el tiempo y los costes asociados, ya que a menudo se realiza en la zona quirúrgica.

Las posibles ventajas de la ALT son la disminución del riesgo relacionado con los efectos adversos de los antimicrobianos (en especial si no se utilizan por vía sistémica de manera concomitante), permitir la administración local de concentraciones muy altas de fármacos que no serían posibles por ninguna otra vía, proporcionar una manera fácil de administración de los fármacos en solución y posibilitar el tratamiento en régimen ambulatorio. Además de ofrecer ventajas terapéuticas, parece claro que la ALT es una técnica que puede tener un perfil favorable de coste-beneficio respecto al recambio quirúrgico de un catéter vascular permanente o a la necesidad de tratamiento antibiótico sistémico prolongado.

Algunos inconvenientes de la ALT serían la ausencia de actividad en sitios distantes de la infección, la compatibilidad de los antimicrobianos utilizados en la solución con otros fármacos (como la heparina) y los posibles retrasos en la curación de la infección si el tratamiento conservador fracasa. En esta última circunstancia pueden producirse complicaciones sistémicas graves, por lo que esta modalidad de tratamiento conservador de la sepsis relacionada con un catéter sólo debería plantearse en instituciones con experiencia previa y con posibilidades de mantener una monitorización cercana y continua de la respuesta clínica del paciente.[7-17]

2 Fundamentos patogénicos del tratamiento conservador de la sepsis relacionada con un catéter

El tratamiento clínico de las infecciones relacionadas con catéteres requiere una toma de decisiones en relación con la necesidad de su retirada y de la administración de antimicrobianos. La determinación de proceder a mantener un catéter causante de una infección sistémica depende, al menos, de tres factores fundamentales: el tipo de catéter, el agente causante de la infección y el estado clínico del paciente.

Los fundamentos patogénicos de la utilización de un tratamiento conservador en los pacientes con sepsis relacionada con un catéter son:

- En los catéteres venosos centrales permanentes está bien demostrado que, transcurridas las primeras semanas desde su implantación, los microorganismos progresan por la superficie intraluminal, donde se forma una biopelícula en la cual pueden sobrevivir y proliferar para causar una infección.[18]
- Aunque la bacteriemia relacionada con un catéter venoso central permanente puede ser una complicación grave, se dispone de evidencia científica, procedente de modelos *in vitro* y de experimentación animal, sobre la eficacia de determinados fármacos para erradicar las bacterias existentes en las biopelículas. El desprendimiento de éstas ocasiona las manifestaciones clínicas sistémicas de la infección.
- Los antimicrobianos administrados exclusivamente por vía sistémica no consiguen erradicar los microorganismos presentes en las biopelículas. En los pacientes con bacteriemia que han sido tratados únicamente con tratamiento sistémico, la curación no ha superado el 30 % de los casos y ha sido necesario retirar los catéteres, incluso en casos de infecciones causadas por patógenos de poca virulencia (especies de estafilococos coagulasa negativos).[19]

- La administración local de determinados fármacos, en general a concentraciones que superan al menos de 100 a 1.000 veces el valor de la concentración mínima inhibitoria (CMI) para el agente causante de la bacteriemia, ha demostrado su eficacia en numerosas situaciones clínicas en humanos.[4,6,20]

Por las consideraciones patogénicas antes mencionadas, es evidente que este tipo de tratamiento debe ser considerado para cualquier catéter venoso central permanente cuya utilidad clínica sea de especial relevancia para el paciente (depuración renal, tratamientos oncológicos, o con inmunosupresores o inmunomoduladores, y nutrición parenteral crónica). Es absolutamente fundamental realizar un diagnóstico adecuado y comprobar la estabilidad clínica y hemodinámica de los pacientes, así como la ausencia de complicaciones locales o sistémicas de la infección.[3]

3 Indicaciones del tratamiento conservador

Las recomendaciones de la ALT para el tratamiento de las bacteriemias relacionadas con catéteres han sido publicadas recientemente.[3] A pesar de que el nivel de evidencia para la mayoría de ellas es moderado, en la guía establecida se señala que:

- La ALT estaría indicada para el tratamiento conservador de las bacteriemias asociadas a catéteres venosos centrales permanentes, en caso de no haber signos de infección en el punto de inserción, el túnel subcutáneo o la piel adyacente a los reservorios, siempre que se considere como objetivo la salvación del catéter. Es imprescindible que el paciente presente signos claros de estabilidad clínica y hemodinámica, tanto al inicio como durante todo el tiempo de la administración de esta modalidad terapéutica. Asimismo, es aconsejable que una vez iniciado el tratamiento conservador se compruebe la negativización de los hemocultivos de sangre periférica. Sin embargo, la comprobación de la negatividad de los hemocultivos con sangre obtenida de la luz del catéter tras el inicio de la ALT no es un factor predictor de su eficacia terapéutica.
- La ALT ha de utilizarse siempre asociada a un tratamiento antimicrobiano sistémico adecuado, durante un período que no ha de ser inferior a siete días para ambos sistemas de administración. En los casos en que sólo se documente de manera repetida la positividad de los hemocultivos de sangre obtenida a través de la luz del catéter (para patógenos como las especies coagulasa negativas de estafilococos o bacilos gramnegativos), con negatividad concomitante de los hemocultivos de sangre obtenida por venopunción periférica, la ALT puede administrarse durante 10 a 14 días sin tratamiento sistémico asociado.
- La ALT puede administrarse de manera segura y eficaz para cualquier sepsis relacionada con un catéter venoso central permanente, sea cual sea el microorganismo

implicado. Sin embargo, en los casos producidos por *Staphylococcus aureus* y *Candida* spp. únicamente debe aplicarse en circunstancias excepcionales, dada la alta frecuencia de fracasos terapéuticos.

En resumen, la ALT estaría indicada para el tratamiento de la bacteriemia asociada a un catéter venoso central permanente, en ausencia de complicaciones sistémicas (inestabilidad hemodinámica o hipoperfusión tisular, trombosis séptica o endocarditis infecciosa y metástasis sépticas a distancia) o de signos locales de infección. Sus ventajas más relevantes son la posibilidad de evitar la retirada del dispositivo, la administración de concentraciones muy altas de antimicrobianos en el foco de la infección clínica, la práctica ausencia de toxicidad sistémica, el coste asumible y su facilidad de administración, y por último, que permite su aplicación en régimen ambulatorio.

4　Puntos de incertidumbre

4.1　¿Qué fármacos ofrecen la mayor eficacia y cómo deben administrarse?

Numerosos estudios *in vitro* han evaluado diversos antibióticos, a diferentes concentraciones, y su actividad frente a las bacterias presentes en la luz de los catéteres. Estos estudios también proporcionan información respecto a la estabilidad de los antimicrobianos cuando se usan solos, en combinación con otros antibióticos o heparina, y en diferentes tipos de catéter colonizado por bacterias o levaduras, cuando se utiliza la técnica de la ALT. Además, en algunos se demuestra la eficacia antimicrobiana al comprobar una reducción de la colonización microbiana y el mantenimiento de una actividad bactericida estable en el tiempo. Sin embargo, hay una enorme disparidad en cuanto a las concentraciones utilizadas de los diferentes antimicrobianos y el tiempo de permanencia del fármaco (o de sus combinaciones) en el interior de la luz del catéter, por lo que no se dispone de una demostración precisa que pueda aplicarse de manera directa al tratamiento de los pacientes con sepsis relacionada con un catéter, en quienes se plantee un tratamiento conservador.[4]

La distribución de los antimicrobianos en el interior de las biopelículas puede tener un papel fundamental para conseguir la erradicación microbiológica. En un modelo de vegetaciones endocárdicas se ha comprobado que los aminoglucósidos pueden penetrar de manera homogénea en el interior de la vegetación, mientras que los betalactámicos se mantienen en su periferia y los glucopéptidos se distribuyen con heterogeneidad.[21] Recientemente se ha demostrado que la daptomicina penetra con gran rapidez, en pocos minutos, y de forma homogénea, en las biopelículas formadas por *Staphylococcus epidermidis*.[22] Estas características de los antimicrobianos podrían desempeñar un papel importante en su elección para el tratamiento conservador de la sepsis relacionada con un catéter.

En un modelo *in vitro* se ha observado que diversos antimicrobianos muestran diferencias muy relevantes en su actividad frente a *S. aureus* resistente a la meticilina (SARM) presente en las biopelículas de los catéteres vasculares. La daptomicina tiene una rápida e intensa acción bactericida, con una erradicación de las colonias a las 48 horas de su exposición al fármaco. Con minociclina y tigeciclina se obtuvo un efecto similar, aunque levemente inferior en cuanto a tiempo y rapidez de erradicación microbiológica. La vancomicina y el linezolid tuvieron una eficacia bactericida moderada y no consiguieron la erradicación bacteriana hasta transcurridos 5 días de exposición. La rifampicina no tuvo actividad bactericida en ningún momento de la exposición.[23]

En un modelo experimental en conejos con catéteres colonizados causantes de sepsis por *S. aureus*, tratados mediante ALT, se demostró que la gentamicina, a dosis de 40 mg/l, fue el antibiótico más efectivo frente a *S. aureus* tanto sensible como resistente a la meticilina, y que el ciprofloxacino fue superior a la vancomicina y el linezolid.[24] Se han publicado diversos trabajos en los que se ha demostrado, en un modelo en ratones de sepsis por catéter, que la administración concurrente de daptomicina, por vía sistémica y mediante ALT, erradica la colonización de los catéteres y se mantiene durante una semana,[25] y que administrada de manera sistémica es más eficaz que la vancomicina para el tratamiento de las infecciones relacionadas con biopelículas de *S. epidermidis* resistente a la meticilina.[26]

4.2 *¿Cuánto tiempo ha de mantenerse la ALT y cada cuánto debe cambiarse la solución antimicrobiana?*

En los numerosos estudios clínicos de eficacia de la ALT publicados se observa una gran variabilidad en relación con el tiempo de permanencia de la solución en el interior de la luz del catéter, los intervalos para su renovación y la duración total del tratamiento. En general, la solución tiene que contener la concentración deseada del antimicrobiano, habitualmente mezclada con heparina o con solución salina, en un volumen final que permita rellenar por completo la luz del catéter (de 2 a 5 ml).[4-6]

Se ha demostrado que determinados antibióticos, como la vancomicina, la cefazolina y el ciprofloxacino, pero no la ceftazidima, combinados con heparina retienen un 90 % de actividad microbiológica después de la incubación *in vitro* a 25 ºC o 37 ºC durante tiempos superiores a 10 días por bioensayo.[27] En nuestro laboratorio experimental hemos demostrado que los antibióticos utilizados para la ALT, como la vancomicina, la gentamicina, el linezolid y el ciprofloxacino, en solución con heparina o de forma aislada, son estables durante 10 días.[24] Sin embargo, para uno de los fármacos más utilizados como ALT, la vancomicina, se recomienda que con el fin de mantener una concentración local superior a 1.000 veces la CMI_{90} de los estafilococos durante la totalidad del tiempo de relleno, se administren concentraciones muy altas, de 5 mg/ml, y cambiar la solución al menos cada 48 horas.[3] En función de las concentraciones usadas del antimicrobiano y de la dosis de heparina de la solución, algunos fármacos (como la vancomicina, la gentamicina y el ciprofloxacino) pueden llegar a precipitar. Aunque esta situación en general no influye directamente en la actividad antimicrobiana, podría ser una limitación importante para la preparación y la conservación de la solución.[6]

Aunque la duración del tratamiento conservador varía de manera considerable en las series publicadas (de 3 a 30 días), en la mayoría de los casos se mantiene durante dos semanas. Los pacientes con bacteriemia concomitante normalmente son tratados de manera combinada con antimicrobianos sistémicos, al menos hasta comprobar la negativización de los hemocultivos de sangre periférica cuando sean patógenos de escasa virulencia (especies de estafilococos coagulasa negativos), o durante todo el tiempo para el resto de los microorganismos.[4-6]

4.3 ¿Es eficaz la ALT para todas las sepsis relacionadas con catéteres? ¿Siempre es necesario administrar tratamiento sistémico concomitante?

Desde su introducción como nueva modalidad terapéutica, hace más de 20 años, la ALT se ha utilizado en numerosos pacientes portadores de catéteres venosos centrales permanentes destinados sobre todo a la administración de nutrición parenteral total o de agentes de quimioterapia, o para técnicas de depuración renal. Hay numerosos estudios publicados en los cuales se evalúa de manera abierta y no comparativa la eficacia de esta técnica en diferentes situaciones clínicas, de muy diversa etiología y con multitud de variantes en cuanto a la selección de la solución antimicrobiana, la duración del tratamiento y el uso concomitante de antibióticos sistémicos (véase la tabla 1). Globalmente, la eficacia es superior al 80 % en la mayoría de los trabajos, y en casi todos los casos la ALT se administra con tratamiento sistémico acompañante. La experiencia publicada sobre el tratamiento de las infecciones producidas por *S. aureus* demuestra una eficacia claramente inferior, que en general no supera el 50 %, y por ello, en caso de estar implicado este microorganismo, la decisión de administrar un tratamiento conservador debe reservarse para pacientes muy seleccionados.[3,49,50] En relación a las infecciones por *Candida* spp., los trabajos recientes apuntan a un posible efecto beneficioso con la administración de equinocandinas, pero la experiencia aún es limitada.[57]

5 Tratamiento antimicrobiano en función de la etiología de la bacteriemia relacionada con un catéter

Aunque la ALT responde a una idea clara, a la hora de ponerla en práctica hay que tener en cuenta ciertas particularidades de los diferentes microorganismos frente a

Autores, año	N° episodios	Tipo de catéter	Uso del catéter	Tratamiento sistémico	ALT (fármaco y dosis)	Duración (días)	Curación (%)
Messing et al., 1998[7]	22	Tunelizado	NPT	No siempre	VAN 1000 mg/l o AMK 1500 mg/l	12-16	91
Messing et al., 1990[8]	27	Tunelizado	NPT	No siempre	VAN 1000 mg/l o AMK 1500 mg/l o MIN 200 mg/l	7-20	93
Rao et al., 1992[13]	6	Tunelizado	QT	No siempre	AMK 40000 mg/l	7-14	100
Capdevila et al., 1993[9]	13	Tunelizado	HD	Siempre	VAN 100 mg/l o CIP 100 mg/l	15	100
Johnson et al., 1994[14]	12	Tunelizado	Diversos	Nunca	VAN 2000 mg/l o AMK 2000 mg/l	10-14	83
Williams et al., 1994[28]	13	Tunelizado	NPT	Siempre	ND	ND	31
Benoit et al., 1995[10]	7	Tunelizado	NPT	No siempre	VAN 5000 mg/l o GEN 5000 mg/l	7-13	100
Krzywda et al., 1995[15]	22	Tunelizado	NPT	Nunca	VAN 33000-83000 mg/l o GEN 13300 mg/l	ND	92
McCarthy et al., 1995[29]	11	Tunelizado	QT	No siempre	TEI 133000 mg/l	5-9	100
Capdevila et al., 1998[30]	40	Tunelizado	HD	Siempre	VAN 100 mg/l o CIP 100 mg/l	15	100
Domingo et al., 1999[31]	27	DIT	QT	No siempre	VAN 1000 mg/l o AMK 1000 mg/l	5	63
Piketty et al., 1999[32]	31	DIT	QT	Siempre	AMK 60000 mg/l	1-5	42
Boorgu et al., 2000[33]	14	Tunelizado	HD	Siempre	AMX 5000 mg/l o PEN 50 millones UI/L	14-21	100
Fourcade et al., 2001[34]	12	Tunelizado	HD	Siempre	VAN o TIC-CLAV	30	75
Longuet et al., 2001[35]	20	DIT	QT	Siempre	VAN 5000 mg/l o TEI 5000 mg/l	15	31
Krishnasami et al., 2002[16]	62	Tunelizado	HD	Siempre	VAN 5000 mg/l o GEN 4000 mg/l o CFZ 10000 mg/l	21	64,5
Bailey et al., 2002[36]	10	Tunelizado	HD	No siempre	VAN 100 mg/l o GEN 20 mg/l	12	44
Santarpia et al., 2002[37]	50	Tunelizado/DIT	NPT	Siempre	CLI 300 mg o TEI 100 mg o NET 150 mg o PIP 500 mg	7	83
Reimund et al., 2002[38]	25	Tunelizado/DIT	NPT	Siempre	ND	15	25-50
Guedon et al., 2002[17]	24	Tunelizado	NPT	Siempre	TEI 2500 mg/l	14	37,5
Cuntz et al., 2002[39]	20	Tunelizado	NPT	Siempre	TEI 133000 mg/l	15	92
Vardhan et al., 2002[40]	26	Tunelizado	HD	Siempre	VAN 100 mg/l o GEN 20 mg/l	14	62
Viale et al., 2003[12]	30	Tunelizado/DIT	Diversos	No siempre	VAN 20000 mg/l o AMK 10000 mg/ml	ND	93

Koldehoff *et al.*, 2004[41]	8	DIT	QT	Siempre	TAU 5000 mg/l	1-3	100
Poole *et al.*, 2004[42]	47	Tunelizado	HD	Siempre	VAN 2500 mg/l o CFZ 5000 mg/l	5-21	70
De Sio *et al.*, 2004[43]	10	Tunelizado/DIT	QT	Nunca	VAN 50000 mg/l	6-12	100
Rijnden *et al.*, 2005[44]	21	Tunelizado	Diversos	Siempre	CTZ 500 mg/l o VAN 500 mg/l	7-14	66
Sánchez-Muñoz *et al.*, 2005[45]	14	Tunelizado	QT	Siempre	VAN 5000 mg/l o AMK 5000 mg/l	3	86
Bernardi *et al.*, 2005[46]	11	Tunelizado/DIT	QT	Siempre	VANC o AMK o TEI	5-10	91
Lee *et al.*, 2005[47]	16	Tunelizado	HD	Siempre	VAN 100000 mg/l o IMP 50000 mg/l o CIP 2000 mg/l o CFZ 100000 mg/l	10-14	87,5
Fortún *et al.*, 2006[48]	19	Tunelizado/DIT	Diversos	Siempre	VAN 2000 mg/l o CIP 2000 mg/l o GEN 2000 mg/l	5-14	84
Fernández-Hidalgo *et al.*, 2006[49]	115	Tunelizado/DIT	Diversos	Siempre	VAN 2000 mg/l o CIP 2000 mg/l o AMK 2000 mg/l	12	82
Maya *et al.*, 2007[50]	113	Tunelizado	HD	Siempre	VAN 2500 mg/l o CFZ 5000 mg/l	21	41
Del Pozo *et al.*, 2009[51]	18	DIT	QT	Siempre	VAN 2000 mg/l o TEI 10000 mg/l o GEN 2000 mg/l o LEV 5000 mg/l	10-14	89
Del Pozo *et al.*, 2009[52]	44	DIT	QT	Siempre	VAN 2000 mg/l o TEI 10000 mg/l	10	89
Beigi *et al.*, 2010[53]	28	DIT	HD	Siempre	VAN 5000 mg/l	7	96
Funalleras *et al.*, 2011[54]	46	Tunelizado/DIT	Diversos	Siempre	CIP 2000 mg/l o AMK 2000 mg/l	13	95
Del Pozo *et al.*, 2012[55]	13	DIT	QT	No siempre	DAPTO 5000 mg/l	14	85
Joshi *et al.*, 2012[56]	46	Tunelizado	HD	Siempre	Diversos antibióticos (CFZ, AMK, GEN, CTZ o VAN)	ND	59

ALT: *antibiotic lock therapy*; DIT: dispositivo implantado totalmente; NPT: nutrición parenteral total; QT: quimioterapia; HD: hemodiálisis; VAN: vancomicina; AMK: amikacina; MIN: minociclina; CIP: ciprofloxacino; ND: no determinado; GEN: gentamicina; TEI: teicoplanina; AMX: amoxicilina; PEN: penicilina G sódica; TIC-CLAV: ticarcilina-ácido clavulánico; CFZ: cefazolina; CLI: clindamicina; NET: netilmicina; PIP: piperacilina; TAU: taurolidina; CTZ: ceftazidima; IMP: imipenem; LEV: levofloxacino; DAPTO: daptomicina.

Tabla 1. Sumario de los estudios publicados sobre la efectividad de la ALT para el tratamiento conservador de la bacteriemia asociada a los catéteres vasculares.

los cuales puede utilizarse, tanto en relación con los antimicrobianos a administrar (en la tabla 2 se describen las concentraciones de los más utilizados, así como el uso concomitante de heparina) como con las precauciones especiales que hay que tener en determinadas situaciones (véase la figura 1).

Etiología	Antimicrobiano	Concentración	Heparina	Ref.
Cocos/bacilos grampositivos	Vancomicina	2000 mg/l	20 UI/ml	48,49
	Vancomicina	2000 mg/l	100 UI/ml	51
	Vancomicina	2500 mg/l	2500 UI/ml	42
	Vancomicina	2500 mg/l	5000 UI/ml	50
	Teicoplanina	10000 mg/l	100 UI/ml	51
	Cefazolina	5000 mg/l	2500 UI/ml	42
	Cefazolina	5000 mg/l	5000 UI/ml	50
	Daptomicina[a]	5000 mg/l	100 UI/ml (5000 UI/ml si diálisis)	55
Bacilos gramnegativos	Amikacina	2000 mg/l	Heparina sódica 20 UI/ml	49,54
	Gentamicina	2000 mg/l	Heparina sódica 20 UI/ml	48
	Ceftazidima	5000 mg/l	Heparina 2500 UI/ml	42
	Ciprofloxacino[b]	2000 mg/l	Heparina sódica 20 UI/ml	49,54
	Levofloxacino[c]	5000 mg/l		51
Infecciones mixtras (cocos grampositivos y bacilos gramnegativos)	Vancomicina Ciprofloxacino	1000 mg/l 1000 mg/l	Heparina sódica 20 UI/ml	49
	Vancomicina Ceftazidima	2500 mg/l 2500 mg/l	Heparina 2500 UI/ml	42
Candida spp.	Amfotericina B liposomal	2670 mg/l		57
	Amfotericina B liposomal	5000 mg/l		10
	Amfotericina B liposomal	5000 mg/l		12

[a] Antibiótico reconstituido en solución Ringer lactato con una concentración de calcio de 0,045 mg/ml.
[b] Precipitación macroscópica sin implicación clínica.
[c] Sin heparina porque se observaba precipitación macroscópica del compuesto.

Tabla 2. Antimicrobianos más comúnmente utilizados en la ALT en función de la etiología. Concentraciones y uso concomitante de heparina.

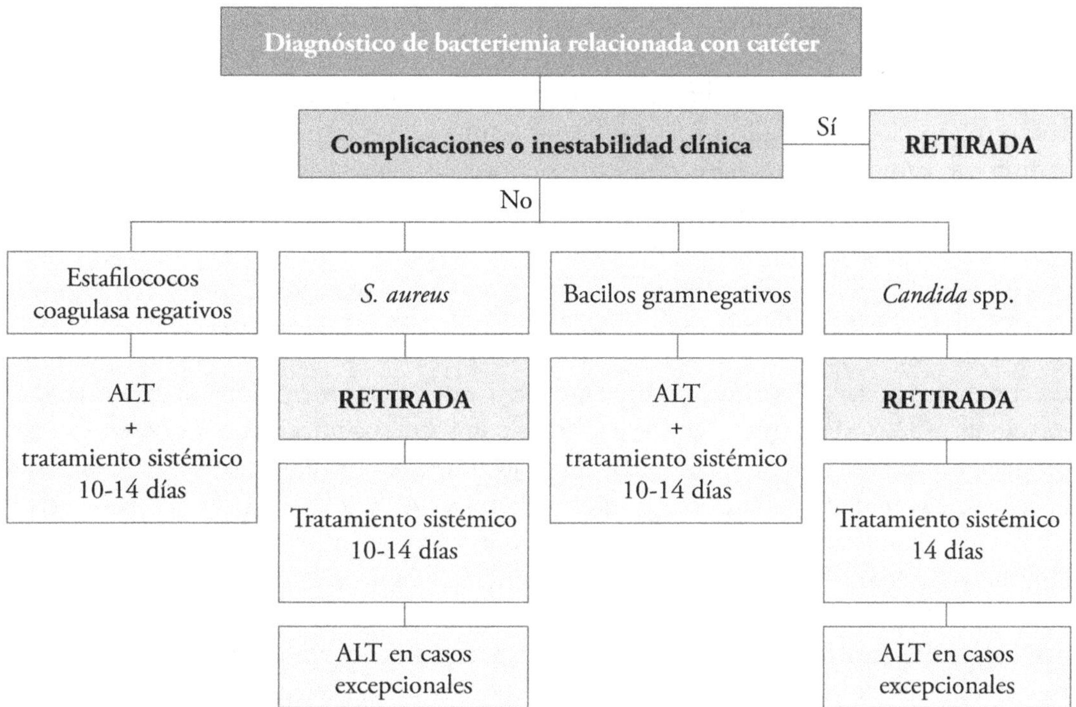

Figura 1. Algoritmo de decisión terapéutica en las bacteriemias relacionadas con los catéteres vasculares.

5.1 Cocos grampositivos

Los cocos grampositivos son los microorganismos que más a menudo están involucrados en las infecciones relacionadas con catéteres vasculares, y los estafilococos coagulasa negativos son más frecuentes que *S. aureus*. El tratamiento de las bacteriemias relacionadas con catéteres por cocos grampositivos no puede ser abordado de manera uniforme, ya que los diferentes microorganismos tienen comportamientos desiguales que obligan a individualizar el tratamiento de estos pacientes.

5.1.1 Estafilococos coagulasa negativos

Los estafilococos coagulasa negativos son los microorganismos más frecuentemente detectados en las bacteriemias relacionadas con catéteres. Además, éstas constituyen un grupo especial de infecciones sobre el cual hay más consenso, y más seguridad, a la hora de tratarlas de manera conservadora, por lo que ocupan la mayor proporción de episodios (de un 43 % a un 74 %) en las series generales de tratamiento conservador.[42]

La efectividad de la ALT en las bacteriemias relacionadas con catéteres causadas por estafilococos coagulasa negativos es alta, entre el 79 % y el 84 %, y los fracasos se deben a recidivas durante el primer mes de seguimiento. Sin embargo, estos estudios tienen una limitación metodológica importante, ya que un nuevo episodio por el mismo microorganismo más allá de 30 días tras la retirada del tratamiento antibiótico se consideró como reinfección, sin realizar un estudio molecular de las cepas involucradas.[48,49] En el estudio de Fernández-Hidalgo *et al.*[49] hubo cinco pacientes con más de un episodio de bacteriemia relacionada con un catéter por estafilococos coagulasa negativos separados por más de un mes. Si se hubieran considerado como recidivas en vez de como reinfecciones, el porcentaje de curación habría bajado del 84 % al 71 %.[49]

Pese al no despreciable porcentaje de pacientes en quienes se documenta o se sospecha un fracaso terapéutico frente a los estafilococos coagulasa negativos, la ALT es una técnica a tener siempre en cuenta, ya que son muy raras las complicaciones a distancia y la mortalidad relacionada. De todas formas, en los pacientes con sucesivas infecciones por estafilococos coagulasa negativos, pese a que puedan estar justificadas por reinfecciones secundarias a las continuas manipulaciones del catéter, debería plantearse la retirada del dispositivo.

En esta circunstancia, el antibiótico que con más frecuencia se utiliza, tanto en la ALT como en el tratamiento sistémico, es la vancomicina, durante 10 a 14 días.[42,48,49] Recientemente se ha publicado la experiencia con el sellado antibiótico con daptomicina en 11 casos de bacteriemia relacionada con catéteres por estafilococos coagulasa negativos, con una efectividad del 82 %.[55] La daptomicina puede ser una alternativa válida para el tratamiento conservador de la bacteriemia relacionada con catéteres por estafilococos coagulasa negativos. Para la ALT, la solución con este antibiótico debe prepararse con suero Ringer lactato, que aporta los iones Ca^{++} necesarios para permitir su actividad antimicrobiana.

5.1.2   Staphylococcus aureus

En el caso de la bacteriemia por *S. aureus* asociada a un catéter venoso central de larga duración, la guía elaborada por la Infectious Diseases Society of America (IDSA) recomienda no realizar tratamiento conservador sino retirar de inmediato la vía venosa infectada, con independencia de la presencia o no de resistencia a la cloxacilina.[3] Esta recomendación se basa en el alto porcentaje de fracasos de esta estrategia en las experiencias publicadas, que oscila entre el 45 % y el 60 %,[42,49,50] incluso con algún caso de mortalidad asociada.[49] En la serie más extensa de tratamiento conservador de la bacteriemia relacionada con catéteres venosos centrales de larga duración debida a *S. aureus* (catéteres para hemodiálisis), la combinación de tratamiento antibiótico sistémico y sellado antibiótico fracasó en 67 de 113 episodios (59 %). En concreto, en 40 episodios el fracaso se debió a fiebre persistente tras 48 horas de tratamiento antibiótico adecuado, y en 27 a recidiva de la bacteriemia durante un seguimiento de 90 días.[50]

Pese a la baja probabilidad de curación de la bacteriemia por *S. aureus* mediante tratamiento conservador con ALT, hay situaciones en las cuales la retirada del catéter no es fácilmente asumible, tales como la pérdida del único acceso venoso posible o la existencia de plaquetopenia o de alteraciones de la coagulación. La guía de la IDSA contempla esta circunstancia.[3] Aun así, en estos casos hay que poner especial atención, ya que la presencia de complicaciones locales (infección del punto de inserción o del trayecto del túnel) o a distancia (endocarditis o osteomielitis, entre otras), así como la inestabilidad hemodinámica, la persistencia de la fiebre o los hemocultivos de control positivos a las 72 horas de haber iniciado el tratamiento antibiótico dirigido, son motivos inexcusables para retirar el catéter de inmediato.

La cefazolina es el antibiótico que con más frecuencia se utiliza para la ALT en las infecciones por *S. aureus* sensible a la meticilina, y la vancomicina en las causadas por SARM,[42,50] aunque también se ha utilizado para el tratamiento conservador en infecciones causadas por cepas sensibles.[48,49] El papel de otros antibióticos con más actividad que la vancomicina frente a las biocapas, como la daptomicina, todavía está por establecer.

La elección del tratamiento sistémico dependerá de la sensibilidad a la meticilina de la cepa de *S. aureus*. En caso de cepas sensibles, el tratamiento de elección es la cloxacilina a dosis de 2 g cada 4 horas por vía intravenosa. Si las cepas son resistentes, hay que tener en cuenta la CMI de la vancomicina para decidir el tratamiento definitivo, ya que existe una evidencia creciente de que el tratamiento estándar con vancomicina (15 mg/kg cada 12 h, i.v.) puede ser subóptimo para aislados con CMI > 1 mg/l.[58] En esta circunstancia habría que considerar alternativas terapéuticas, como la daptomicina, a una dosis no inferior a 6 mg/kg cada 24 horas.

No hay consenso sobre la duración de la ALT y del tratamiento antibiótico sistémico en las infecciones por *S. aureus,* y la misma guía de la IDSA hace diferentes recomendaciones a lo largo del texto, llegando hasta las cuatro semanas.[3] Sin embargo, se ha publicado el logro de éxito terapéutico con un tratamiento de dos o tres semanas, por lo que no hay una razón objetiva para alargarlo más allá de 14 días.[49,50]

La necesidad de realizar un ecocardiograma en todos los pacientes con bacteriemia relacionada con un catéter producida por *S. aureus* es una cuestión todavía controvertida. Un estudio realizado en nuestro centro demostró que la aparición de complicaciones tras 10 a 14 días de tratamiento antibiótico era excepcional cuando se había producido buena respuesta clínica en forma de apirexia y negativización de los hemocultivos en las primeras 72 horas tras la retirada del catéter, en ausencia de valvulopatía (previa conocida o diagnosticada durante el episodio) y habiendo instaurado un tratamiento antibiótico adecuado.[59] Sin embargo, en los pacientes en quienes se plantea mantener el catéter y realizar tratamiento conservador es obligatorio realizar un ecocardiograma, que tendrá que ser siempre transesofágico, ya que la presencia de una endocarditis contraindica de forma absoluta esta modalidad terapéutica. Aunque lo más frecuente es que, si hay afectación endocárdica, ésta sea de cavidades derechas, en nuestra experiencia el 20 % de los pacientes con endocarditis derechas tienen además afectación de las válvulas izquierdas. El ecocardiograma transesofágico permite visualizar con gran detalle el trayecto del catéter en la vena cava superior, aspecto a tener en cuenta porque una infección exoluminal obligaría a retirarlo.

5.1.3   Otros microorganismos grampositivos

Existe poca experiencia con el tratamiento conservador de la bacteriemia relacionada con catéteres causada por otros microorganismos grampositivos distintos de los estafilococos, aunque con resultados positivos. En la serie más extensa, este grupo de patógenos representó un 4,3 % de todos los aislados.[49] En concreto, en este estudio se trataron dos casos producidos por *Enterococcus faecalis*, dos por *Corynebacterium* spp. y uno por *Streptococcus oralis*. El antibiótico utilizado para la ALT en todos ellos fue la vancomicina durante 10 a 14 días, y se logró la curación en el 100 % de los pacientes. Un estudio relativamente reciente, centrado en el sellado antibiótico de catéteres colonizados por microorganismos inusuales, refiere la curación de cinco episodios de bacteriemia causados por *Corynebacterium* spp., cuatro por *Enterococcus faecium* y dos por *Propionibacterium* spp. mediante tratamiento conservador con vancomicina o teicoplanina.[51]

5.2   Bacilos gramnegativos

En los trabajos publicados, los bacilos gramnegativos están implicados en un 10 % a un 23 % de todos los episodios de bacteriemia relacionada con catéteres sometidos a tratamiento conservador.[48,49] En la serie más extensa de tratamiento conservador de la sepsis por bacilos gramnegativos asociada a catéter venoso central de larga duración, los microorganismos aislados en los 46 episodios tratados fueron *Pseudomonas* spp. (11 casos), *Escherichia coli* (6), *Enterobacter cloacae* (5), *Klebsiella pneumoniae* (4), *Acinetobacter baumanii* (3), *Proteus* spp. (3) y otros bacilos gramnegativos (4). En 10 casos las infecciones estaban producidas por dos o más bacilos gramnegativos.[54] En un estudio previo, realizado por el mismo grupo, el bacilo gramnegativo predominante fue *E. coli* (11 casos), seguido de *P. aeruginosa* (5 casos).[49] Sin embargo, la distribución microbiológica de estos dos trabajos no tiene por qué ser comparable con la de otras series, en las que predominan *E. cloacae*[56] o *E. coli*.[51] Estas discrepancias pueden explicarse por la diferente epidemiología de cada centro y por la creencia, extendida durante años, de que las bacteriemias relacionadas con catéteres causadas por *P. aeruginosa* y *A. baumanii* no debían tratarse de manera conservadora, lo cual conlleva un claro sesgo de selección.

En la serie más amplia de tratamiento conservador de las bacteriemias relacionadas con catéteres por bacilos gramnegativos, el porcentaje de curación fue del 95 %.[54] Sólo se documentaron recidivas en dos episodios causados por *Proteus vulgaris* y *K. pneumoniae*, y se logró la curación tras una nueva pauta de tratamiento conservador. Es destacable el alto porcentaje de curación en los episodios causados por *P. aeruginosa*, hecho que puede explicarse por una búsqueda sistemática de complicaciones locales y a distancia en el momento del diagnóstico. Esto lleva a la conclusión de que, si se selecciona adecuadamente a los pacientes, el bacilo gramnegativo causante, *per se*, no tiene que ser una limitación a la hora de indicar un tratamiento conservador.

Las fluoroquinolonas[49,51,54] y los aminoglucósidos[49,54,56] son los antibióticos más utilizados para la ALT, aunque algunos autores se decantan por un betalactámico, como la ceftazidima.[42] El tratamiento antimicrobiano sistémico definitivo vendrá establecido por el patrón de sensibilidad del microorganismo causante.

En la actualidad, la duración recomendada del tratamiento antibiótico de la bacteriemia relacionada con un catéter producida por bacilos gramnegativos es de 10 a 14 días.[3] En el mayor estudio publicado, la mediana de duración del tratamiento conservador fue de 12 días. Sin embargo, en siete episodios por bacilos gramnegativos se realizó tratamiento conservador durante menos de una semana, y no hubo ningún fracaso terapéutico.[49]

5.3   Candida *spp.*

Al igual que se ha explicado para *S. aureus*, ante una infección por *Candida* spp. la recomendación universal es proceder a retirar el catéter e instaurar tratamiento antifúngico sistémico. Sin embargo, de manera excepcional (en pacientes sin opciones para otro acceso venoso) se acepta intentar un tratamiento conservador mediante la combinación de ALT y tratamiento sistémico.[3] Para ello es imprescindible que los pacientes estén clínicamente estables, sin signos de complicaciones locales ni a distancia. En el improbable caso de que nos enfrentemos a esta situación, no está bien establecido cuál es el mejor antifúngico para la ALT. Basándose en la escasa evidencia publicada, el fármaco más frecuentemente utilizado es la amfotericina B liposómica.[57]

En cuanto al tratamiento sistémico, para las cepas sensibles puede utilizarse fluconazol a dosis de 400 mg al día hasta 14 días después del primer hemocultivo de control negativo. En caso de sensibilidad disminuida a los azoles, el tratamiento de elección será una equinocandina: caspofungina (50 mg al día, i.v., tras una dosis de carga de 70 mg), micafungina (100 mg al día, i.v.) o anidulafungina (100 mg al día, i.v., tras una dosis de carga de 200 mg).[3]

5.4   *Infecciones polimicrobianas*

En las series de tratamiento conservador de la bacteriemia relacionada con catéteres con menos criterios de exclusión, las infecciones polimicrobianas representan entre un 7 % y un 16 % de todos los episodios,[49] pese a lo cual este hecho recibe poca atención en la literatura. Ante la presencia de infecciones mixtas por microorganismos grampositivos y gramnegativos, se ha utilizado una mezcla de vancomicina más ceftazidima[42] o de vancomicina más ciprofloxacino.[49] Sin embargo, teniendo en cuenta el patrón de sensibilidad, es posible que el uso de un solo fármaco (una quinolona o un aminoglucósido) sea suficiente en gran parte de los episodios. La respuesta clínica en estos casos es favorable, con tasas de curación muy altas.

Bibliografía

1. Sotir MJ, Lewis C, Bisher EW, Ray SM, Soucie JM, Blumberg HM. Epidemiology of device-associated infections related to a long-term implantable vascular access device. Infect Control Hosp Epidemiol. 1999; 20: 187-91.

2. Maki DG, Kluger DM, Crnich CJ. The risk of bloodstream infection in adults with different intravascular devices: a systematic review of 200 published prospective studies. Mayo Clin Proc. 2006; 81: 1159-71.

3. Mermel LA, Allon M, Bouza E, Craven DE, Flynn P, O'Grady NP, *et al.* Clinical practice guidelines for the diagnosis and management of intravascular catheter-related infection: 2009 update by the Infectious Diseases Society of America. Clin Infect Dis. 2009; 49: 1-45.

4. Bestul MB, Vandenbussche HL. Antibiotic lock technique: review of the literature. Pharmacotherapy. 2005; 25: 211-27.

5. Segarra-Newnham M, Martin-Cooper EM. Antibiotic lock technique: a review of the literature. Ann Pharmacother. 2005; 39: 311-8.

6. Del Pozo JL. Role of antibiotic lock therapy for the treatment of catheter-related bloodstream infections. Int J Artif Organs. 2009; 32: 678-88.

7. Messing B, Peitra-Cohen S, Debure A, Beliah M, Bernier JJ. Antibiotic-lock technique: a new approach to optimal therapy for catheter-related sepsis in home-parenteral nutrition patients. J Parenter Enteral Nutr. 1988; 12: 185-9.

8. Messing B. Catheter-sepsis during home parenteral nutrition: use of the antibiotic-lock technique. Nutrition. 1998; 14: 466-8.

9. Capdevila JA, Segarra A, Planes AM, Ramírez-Arellano M, Pahissa A, Piera L, *et al.* Successful treatment of haemodialysis catheter-related sepsis without catheter removal. Nephrol Dial Transplant. 1993; 8: 231-4.

10. Benoit JL, Carandang G, Sitrin M, Arnow PM. Intraluminal antibiotic treatment of central venous catheter infections in patients receiving parenteral nutrition at home. Clin Infect Dis. 1995; 21: 1286-8.

11. Carratalà J. The antibiotic-lock technique for therapy of 'highly needed' infected catheters. Clin Microbiol Infect. 2002; 8: 282-9.

12. Viale P, Pagani L, Petrosillo N, Signorini L, Colombini P, Macri G, *et al.* Antibiotic lock-technique for the treatment of catheter-related bloodstream infections. J Chemother. 2003; 15: 152-6.

13. Rao JS, O'Meara A, Harvey T, Breatnach F. A new approach to the management of Broviac catheter infection. J Hosp Infect. 1992; 22: 109-16.

14. Johnson DC, Johnson FL, Goldman S. Preliminary results treating persistent central venous catheter infections with the antibiotic lock technique in pediatric patients. Pediatr Infect Dis J. 1994; 13: 930-1.

15. Krzywda EA, Andris DA, Edmiston CE Jr, Quebbeman EJ. Treatment of Hickman catheter sepsis using antibiotic lock technique. Infect Control Hosp Epidemiol. 1995; 16: 596-8.

16. Krishnasami Z, Carlton D, Bimbo L, Taylor ME, Balkovetz DF, Barker J, *et al.* Management of hemodialysis catheter-related bacteremia with an adjunctive antibiotic lock solution. Kidney Int. 2002; 61: 1136-42.

17. Guedon C, Nouvellon M, Lalaude O, Lerebours E. Efficacy of antibiotic-lock technique with teicoplanin in Staphylococcus epidermidis catheter-related sepsis during long-term parenteral nutrition. J Parenter Enteral Nutr. 2002; 26: 109-13.

18. Pascual A. Pathogenesis of catheter-related infections: lessons for new designs. Clin Microbiol Infect. 2002; 8: 256-64.

19. Marr KA, Sexton DJ, Conlon PJ, Corey GR, Schwab SJ, Kirkland KB. Catheter-related bacteremia and outcome of attempted catheter salvage in patients undergoing hemodialysis. Ann Intern Med. 1997; 127: 275-80.

20. O'Horo JC, Silva GL, Safdar N. Anti-infective locks for treatment of central line-associated bloodstream infection: a systematic review and meta-analysis. Am J Nephrol. 2011; 34: 415-22.

21. Cremieux AC, Maziere B, Vallois JM, Ottaviani M, Azancot A, Raffoul H, *et al.* Evaluation of antibiotic diffusion into cardiac vegetations by quantitative autoradiography. J Infect Dis. 1989; 159: 938-44.

22. Stewart PS, Davison WM, Steenbergen JN. Daptomycin rapidly penetrates a Staphylococcus epidermidis biofilm. Antimicrob Agents Chemother. 2009; 53: 3505-7.

23. Raad I, Hanna H, Jiang Y, Dvorak T, Reitzel R, Chaiban G, *et al.* Comparative activities of daptomycin, linezolid, and tigecycline against catheter-related methicillin-resistant Staphylococcus bacteremic isolates embedded in biofilm. Antimicrob Agents Chemother. 2007; 51: 1656-60.

24. Fernández-Hidalgo N, Gavaldà J, Almirante B, Martín MT, Onrubia PL, Gomis X, *et al.* Evaluation of linezolid, vancomycin, gentamicin and ciprofloxacin in a rabbit model of antibiotic-lock technique for Staphylococcus aureus catheter-related infection. J Antimicrob Chemother. 2010; 65: 525-30.

25. Van Praagh AD, Li T, Zhang S, Arya A, Chen L, Zhang XX, *et al.* Daptomycin antibiotic lock therapy in a rat model of staphylococcal central venous catheter biofilm infections. Antimicrob Agents Chemother. 2011; 55: 4081-9.

26. Domínguez-Herrera J, Docobo-Pérez F, López-Rojas R, Pichardo C, Ruiz-Valderas R, Lepe JA, *et al.* Efficacy of daptomycin versus vancomycin in an experimental model of foreign-body and systemic infection caused by biofilm producers and methicillin-resistant Staphylococcus epidermidis. Antimicrob Agents Chemother. 2012; 56: 613-7.

27. Anthony TU, Rubin LG. Stability of antibiotics used for antibiotic-lock treatment of infections of implantable venous devices (ports). Antimicrob Agents Chemother. 1999; 43: 2074-6.

28. Williams N, Carlson GL, Scott NA, Irving MH. Incidence and management of catheter-related sepsis in patients receiving home parenteral nutrition. Br J Surg. 1994; 81: 392-4.

29. McCarthy A, Byrne M, Breathnach F, O'Meara A. "In-situ" teicoplanin for central venous catheter infection. Ir J Med Sci. 1995; 164: 125-7.

30. Capdevila JA, Segarra A, Planes AM, Gasser I, Gavaldà J, Ruiz-Valverde P, *et al.* Long-term follow-up of patients with catheter-related bacteremia treated without catheter removal. Clin Microbiol Infect. 1998; 4: 472-6.

31. Domingo P, Fontanet A, Sánchez F, Allende L, Vázquez G. Morbidity associated with long-term use of totally implantable ports in patients with AIDS. Clin Infect Dis. 1999; 29: 346-51.

32. Piketty C, Hoï AB, Gilquin J, Casetta A, Castiel P, Vaupre S, *et al.* Failure of antibiotic therapy in Staphylococcus epidermidis infection of implantable venous access devices in patients with AIDS, as documented by molecular typing. Clin Microbiol Infect. 1999; 5: 190-4.

33. Boorgu R, Dubrow AJ, Levin NW, My H, Canaud BJ, Lentino JR, *et al.* Adjunctive antibiotic/anticoagulant lock therapy in the treatment of bacteremia associated with the use of a subcutaneously implanted hemodialysis access device. ASAIO J. 2000; 46: 767-70.

34. Fourcade J, Mallaval FO, Raffenot D, Mercier D, Maret J, Morel B. [Value of an antibiotic lock for the prevention of bacteremia recurrence from central catheters in chronic hemodialysis]. Nephrologie. 2001; 22: 457-8.

35. Longuet P, Douard MC, Arlet G, Molina JM, Benoit C, Leport C. Venous access port-related bacteremia in patients with acquired immunodeficiency syndrome or cancer: the reservoir as a diagnostic and therapeutic tool. Clin Infect Dis. 2001; 32: 1776-83.

36. Bailey E, Berry N, Cheesbrough JS. Antimicrobial lock therapy for catheter-related bacteraemia among patients on maintenance haemodialysis. J Antimicrob Chemother. 2002; 50: 615-7.

37. Santarpia L, Pasanisi F, Alfonsi L, Violante G, Tiseo D, De Simone G, *et al.* Prevention and treatment of implanted central venous catheter (CVC)-related sepsis: a report after six years of home parenteral nutrition (HPN). Clin Nutr. 2002; 21: 207-11.

38. Reimund JM, Arondel Y, Finck G, Zimmermann F, Duclos B, Baumann R. Catheter-related infection in patients on home parenteral nutrition: results of a prospective survey. Clin Nutr. 2002; 21: 33-8.

39. Cuntz D, Michaud L, Guimber D, Husson MO, Gottrand F, Turck D. Local antibiotic lock for the treatment of infections related to central catheters in parenteral nutrition in children. J Parenter Enteral Nutr. 2002; 26: 104-8.

40. Vardhan A, Davies J, Daryanani I, Crowe A, McClelland P. Treatment of haemodialysis catheter-related infections. Nephrol Dial Transplant. 2002; 17: 1149-50.

41. Koldehoff M, Zakrzewski JL. Taurolidine is effective in the treatment of central venous catheter-related bloodstream infections in cancer patients. Int J Antimicrob Agents. 2004; 24: 491-5.

42. Poole CV, Carlton D, Bimbo L, Allon M. Treatment of catheter-related bacteraemia with an antibiotic lock protocol: effect of bacterial

pathogen. Nephrol Dial Transplant. 2004; 19: 1237-44.

43. De Sio L, Jenkner A, Milano GM, Ilari I, Fidani P, Castellano A, *et al.* Antibiotic lock with vancomycin and urokinase can successfully treat colonized central venous catheters in pediatric cancer patients. Pediatr Infect Dis J. 2004; 23: 963-5.

44. Rijnders BJ, Van Wijngaerden E, Vandecasteele SJ, Stas M, Peetermans WE. Treatment of long-term intravascular catheter-related bacteraemia with antibiotic lock: randomized, placebo-controlled trial. J Antimicrob Chemother. 2005; 55: 90-4.

45. Sánchez-Muñoz A, Aguado JM, López-Martín A, López-Medrano F, Lumbreras C, Rodríguez FJ, *et al.* Usefulness of antibiotic-lock technique in management of oncology patients with uncomplicated bacteremia related to tunneled catheters. Eur J Clin Microbiol Infect Dis. 2005; 24: 291-3.

46. Bernardi M, Cavaliere M, Cesaro S. [The antibiotic-lock therapy in oncoematology pediatric unit]. Assist Inferm Ric. 2005; 24: 127-31.

47. Lee H, Lee Y, Song Y. Treatment of catheter-related bacteremia with an antibiotic lock protocol in hemodialysis patients. Korean J Nephrol 2005; 24: 903-11.

48. Fortún J, Grill F, Martín-Dávila P, Blázquez J, Tato M, Sánchez-Corral J, *et al.* Treatment of long-term intravascular catheter-related bacteraemia with antibiotic-lock therapy. J Antimicrob Chemother. 2006; 58: 816-21.

49. Fernández-Hidalgo N, Almirante B, Calleja R, Ruiz I, Planes AM, Rodríguez D, *et al.* Antibiotic-lock therapy for long-term intravascular catheter-related bacteraemia: results of an open, non-comparative study. J Antimicrob Chemother. 2006; 57: 1172-80.

50. Maya ID, Carlton D, Estrada E, Allon M. Treatment of dialysis catheter-related Staphylococcus aureus bacteremia with an antibiotic lock: a quality improvement report. Am J Kidney Dis. 2007; 50: 289-95.

51. Del Pozo JL, Alonso M, Serrera A, Hernaez S, Aguinaga A, Leiva J. Effectiveness of the antibiotic lock therapy for the treatment of port-related enterococci, Gram-negative, or Gram-positive bacilli bloodstream infections. Diagn Microbiol Infect Dis. 2009; 63: 208-12.

52. Del Pozo JL, García Cenoz M, Hernáez S, Martínez A, Serrera A, Aguinaga A, *et al.* Effectiveness of teicoplanin versus vancomycin lock therapy in the treatment of port-related coagulase-negative Staphylococci bacteraemia: a prospective case-series analysis. Int J Antimicrob Agents. 2009; 34: 482-5.

53. Beigi AA, Khansoltani S, Masoudpour H, Atapour AA, Eshaghian A, Khademi EF. Influence of intralumenal and antibiotic-lock of vancomycin on the rate of catheter removal in the patients with permanent hemodialysis catheters. Saudi J Kidney Dis Transpl. 2010; 21: 54-8.

54. Funalleras G, Fernández-Hidalgo N, Borrego A, Almirante B, Planes AM, Rodríguez D, *et al.* Effectiveness of antibiotic-lock therapy for long-term catheter-related bacteremia due to Gram-negative bacilli: a prospective observational study. Clin Infect Dis. 2011; 53: e129-32.

55. Del Pozo JL, Rodil R, Aguinaga A, Yuste JR, Bustos C, Montero A, *et al.* Daptomycin lock therapy for grampositive long-term catheter-related bloodstream infections. Int J Clin Pract. 2012; 66: 305-8.

56. Joshi AJ, Hart PD. Antibiotic catheter locks in the treatment of tunneled hemodialysis catheter-related blood stream infection. Semin Dial. 2012; doi: 10.1111/j.1525-139X.2012.01115.x.

57. Walraven CJ, Lee SA. Antifungal lock therapy. Antimicrob Agents Chemother. 2013; 57: 1-8.

58. Gudiol F, Aguado JM, Pascual A, Pujol M, Almirante B, Miró JM, *et al.* Documento de consenso sobre el tratamiento de la bacteriemia y la endocarditis causada por Staphylococcus aureus resistente a la meticilina. Enferm Infecc Microbiol Clin. 2009; 27: 105-15.

59. Pigrau C, Rodríguez D, Planes AM, Almirante B, Larrosa N, Ribera E, *et al.* Management of catheter-related Staphylococcus aureus bacteremia: when may sonographic study be unnecessary? Eur J Clin Microbiol Infect Dis. 2003; 22: 713-9.

Capítulo 11

Prevención de las infecciones relacionadas con catéteres vasculares

M. Pujol Rojo,[1] A. Hornero López[2]

[1] **Servicio de Enfermedades Infecciosas**
   Equipo de Control de Infección Hospitalaria
   Hospital Universitario de Bellvitge
   L'Hospitalet de Llobregat (Barcelona)

[2] **Enfermería Clínica**
   Equipo de Control de Infección Hospitalaria
   Hospital Universitario de Bellvitge
   L'Hospitalet de Llobregat (Barcelona)

Correspondencia:
Dr. Miquel Pujol
mpujol@bellvitgehospital.cat

Introducción

Alrededor del 10 % al 20 % de las infecciones nosocomiales se relacionan con el uso de catéteres vasculares, cuya utilización forma parte integral de la asistencia sanitaria, pues permiten la monitorización hemodinámica y la administración de fluidos y de medicación. La cateterización vascular es el procedimiento invasivo que se realiza con mayor frecuencia en los hospitales, y en la práctica, la mayoría de los pacientes habrán sido portadores de un catéter vascular durante la hospitalización.[1] Existen muy diversos tipos de catéteres vasculares que responden a diferentes necesidades: catéter venoso periférico corto o mediano, catéter arterial, catéter venoso central de inserción periférica, catéter venoso central no tunelizado o tunelizado, catéter venoso central con reservorio permanente, etc.[2] La elección está en relación con el uso y su presumible duración. Seleccionar el tipo de catéter adecuado a las necesidades y características del paciente es muy importante, ya que puede evitar la necesidad de repetir un procedimiento invasivo y reducir el riesgo de infección. Cada tipo de catéter vascular se asocia a un riesgo de infección diferente según sus características. Se ha establecido que la menor incidencia de bacteriemias relacionadas con catéteres vasculares corresponde al catéter venoso periférico, y las más altas al catéter venoso central no tunelizado y al catéter arterial pulmonar.[3]

Las medidas de prevención se basan en el conocimiento actual sobre la patogenia de la infección y de la bacteriemia relacionadas con catéteres vasculares. La bacteriemia se produce cuando el microorganismo coloniza el catéter, accede a la punta, por vía extraluminal o intraluminal, y alcanza el torrente sanguíneo. Hay cuatro vías principales de infección del catéter vascular, dos de ellas de mayor relevancia.[4] La vía extraluminal, a través del punto de inserción, es la más frecuente, en especial para los catéteres de corta duración (menos de dos semanas). Los microrganismos acceden al catéter vascular a través del punto de inserción en la piel, bien durante su colocación o a lo largo de los días en que permanece insertado. El segundo lugar en frecuencia lo ocupa la vía intraluminal, a partir de las conexiones, y es más habitual en los catéteres de larga duración o permanentes que se utilizan, por ejemplo, para la administración domiciliaria de nutrición parenteral. La colonización del catéter se produce a partir de la contaminación microbiana de las conexiones durante su utilización. Los microorganismos progresan por vía intraluminal hasta la punta del catéter vascular, y desde allí acceden al torrente sanguíneo. Finalmente, la colonización hematógena en la punta del catéter a partir de un foco distante de infección, y la contaminación de fluidos, como los de nutrición parenteral, son mecanismos que en la actualidad son relativamente infrecuentes y tienen menor relevancia desde el punto de vista de la prevención.

Las medidas de prevención que se exponen en este capítulo están dirigidas a evitar la contaminación que se produce tanto por la vía extraluminal como por la vía intraluminal. Se comenta el impacto que tiene la aplicación de paquetes de medidas preventivas (denominados en terminología anglosajona *bundles* de prevención) y de listados de verificación. Las medidas que se describen se basan en revisiones efectuadas por diversas sociedades y entidades, como The Joint Comission,[5] los Center for Disease Control and Prevention,[6] el Institute for Healthcare Improvement[7] y la Association for Profesionals in Infection Control and Prevention.[8] Se han categorizado las recomendaciones siguiendo el modelo del Healthcare Infection Control Practices Advisory Committee, según la evidencia científica, las bases teóricas, la aplicabilidad y el impacto económico (véase la tabla 1).[6]

1   Estrategias para la prevención de las infecciones relacionadas con catéteres vasculares

La bacteriemia relacionada con un catéter vascular ha de contemplarse como uno de los principales problemas «evitables o prevenibles» relacionados con los programas de seguridad del paciente. La reciente publicación, por parte de la Agency for Healthcare Reseach and Quality, de las diez principales estrategias de seguridad que se han de implementar de forma inmediata en los hospitales, identifica en segunda posición la aplicación de

---

- Categoría IA: implantación muy recomendable, sólidamente avalada por estudios experimentales, clínicos o epidemiológicos bien diseñados
- Categoría IB: implantación recomendable, avalada por algunos estudios experimentales, clínicos o epidemiológicos, y con un fundamento teórico sólido
- Categoría IC: implantación requerida por regulaciones estatales o federales (no aplicable en España)
- Categoría II: se sugiere su implantación por estar avalada por estudios clínicos o epidemiológicos, o por una justificación teórica
- Evidencia insuficiente: incluye situaciones no resueltas, en que la evidencia es insuficiente o no hay un consenso respecto a su eficacia

---

Tabla 1. Categoría de las recomendaciones según el grado de evidencia científica.

paquetes de medidas preventivas y listados de verificación para evitar estas bacteriemias en los pacientes hospitalizados.[9]

Uno de los primeros proyectos en plantear la bacteriemia relacionada con un catéter vascular como un problema de seguridad, implementar paquetes de medidas de prevención y demostrar una reducción de su frecuencia en las unidades de cuidados intensivos (UCI), partió del equipo de investigación de la Johns Hopkins University School of Medicine en Michigan. Este equipo desarrolló un modelo que favoreció un cambio en la cultura de seguridad del paciente entre el personal sanitario, el *Comprehensive Unit-Based Safety Program,* que incluyó una estricta vigilancia de la bacteriemia relacionada con catéteres y la introducción de un paquete de cinco medidas de prevención, todas ellas muy sencillas de aplicar y basadas en la evidencia científica (véase la tabla 2).[10] La iniciativa incluyó un «listado de verificación» de obligado cumplimiento al practicar una inserción de catéter vascular segura, la capacitación del personal de enfermería para detener el proceso si no se cumplen todos los requisitos del listado de verificación, el utillaje en un solo paquete con todo el material necesario para realizar una inserción segura (el catéter vascular, el antiséptico, las tallas, etc.) y una revisión retrospectiva de cada episodio de bacteriemia relacionada con un catéter vascular para establecer en qué grado podría haberse prevenido. Los resultados demostraron una

---

- Higiene de manos
- Medidas máximas de barrera
- Clorhexidina alcohólica para la asepsia de la piel
- Evitar la inserción en las venas femorales
- Retirada precoz de los catéteres

---

*Tabla 2. Paquete de medidas utilizado para la prevención
de la bacteriemia relacionada con catéteres vasculares.*

extraordinaria y persistente reducción de la bacteriemia relacionada con un catéter vascular en dicha unidad, por lo que esta experiencia se hizo extensiva al resto de las UCI del estado de Michigan y se obtuvieron unos resultados similares.[11] Esta y otras experiencias[12] sugieren que en las UCI es posible conseguir reducciones muy significativas en las tasas de bacteriemia relacionada con un catéter vascular si se cumplen unas sencillas medidas de prevención. No está bien establecido si en las unidades de hospitalización convencional pueden ser aplicables medidas similares. Sin embargo, se están haciendo esfuerzos en este sentido y se han conseguido reducciones, aunque más modestas que las observadas en las UCI.[13]

2 Descripción detallada de las principales medidas de prevención

2.1 *Educación, formación y dotación de personal sanitario*

La formación y la actitud del personal sanitario que inserta los catéteres y realiza las curas de mantenimiento son de extraordinaria importancia en la prevención de la bacteriemia relacionada con un catéter vascular. El personal sanitario ha de tener la formación necesaria, tanto en el procedimiento de inserción y de las curas de mantenimiento como sobre los factores de riesgo que favorecen esta bacteriemia. Además, se precisa una evaluación periódica de dichos conocimientos.[14,15]

Se ha constatado que la inserción y el mantenimiento de un catéter vascular por personal inexperto favorecen el riesgo de colonización del catéter y aumentan el riesgo de bacteriemia. Igualmente, la reducción del personal sanitario o que éste no sea fijo puede incrementar la incidencia de infecciones relacionadas con los catéteres. La introducción en los hospitales de equipos especializados en la inserción y el mantenimiento de los catéteres vasculares puede ser eficaz en relación al coste que ocasione, pues puede reducir la incidencia de bacteriemias, de las complicaciones asociadas y de los costes.[16,17]

Las recomendaciones específicas, y su categorización, en este apartado son:

- Es necesaria la formación del personal sanitario en relación a las indicaciones del catéter vascular, a los procedimientos de inserción y mantenimiento, y a las medidas para la prevención de las infecciones relacionadas (categoría IA).
- Evaluar periódicamente en el personal involucrado en la inserción y el mantenimiento del catéter vascular el conocimiento y la adhesión a las directrices de prevención de las infecciones (categoría IA).
- Designar personal cualificado que demuestre competencia para la inserción y el mantenimiento de catéteres vasculares periféricos y centrales (categoría IA).
- Asegurar la dotación necesaria de personal de enfermería en las UCI. Un alto número de profesionales suplentes y una gran proporción de pacientes por enfermera se asocian con una mayor incidencia de bacteriemia relacionada con un catéter vascular (categoría IB).

2.2 Selección del catéter vascular y de la zona de inserción

El uso de un catéter venoso periférico se relaciona con flebitis, extravasación y, con menor frecuencia, con infección. Las intervenciones multimodales pueden reducir el número de complicaciones relacionadas con su inserción.[18] Es conveniente retirar el catéter venoso periférico insertado en los miembros inferiores (véase la figura 1). Los catéteres de poliuretano se han asociado con un menor riesgo de trombosis que los de otros materiales, como el polivinilo o la silicona.[19] En caso de flebitis, es preciso retirar el catéter de inmediato (véase la figura 2).

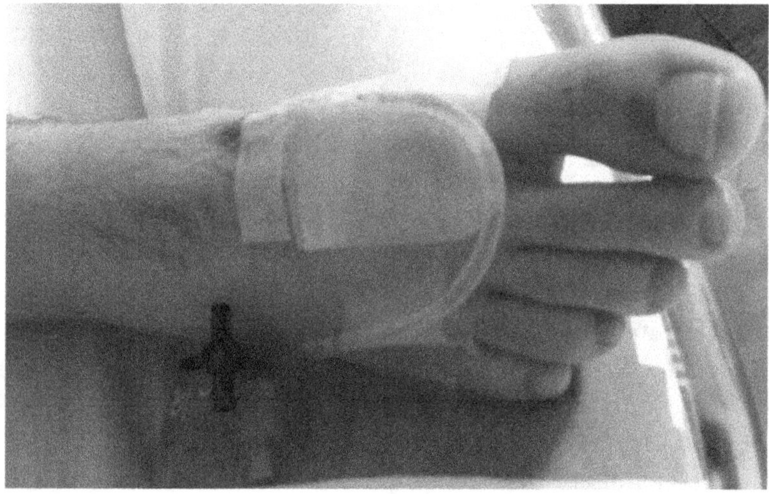

Figura 1. Es conveniente retirar el catéter venoso periférico insertado en el pie.

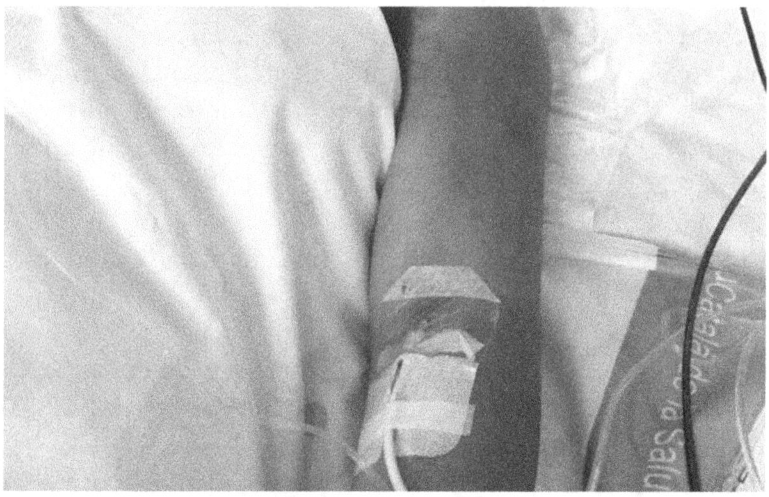

Figura 2. En caso de flebitis, es preciso retirar el catéter de inmediato.

La densidad de la flora microbiana de la piel es el principal factor de riesgo de la bacteriemia relacionada con un catéter vascular. Cuando el catéter se inserta en localizaciones con una gran carga bacteriana, el riesgo aumenta proporcionalmente. El riesgo de trombosis y la carga bacteriana en el territorio de la vena femoral son altos, y por ello, siempre que sea posible ha de evitarse este acceso vascular.

Las recomendaciones específicas, y su categorización, para la utilización de los catéteres venosos periférico cortos y medianos son:

- En los adultos, el catéter ha de insertarse en un miembro superior. Cambiar el catéter vascular insertado en un miembro inferior a un miembro superior lo más rápido posible (categoría II).
- En pacientes pediátricos y en neonatos, los catéteres pueden insertarse en los miembros superiores o inferiores, o en el cuero cabelludo (categoría II).
- Seleccionar el catéter según su función y duración, las posibles complicaciones infecciosas distantes y la experiencia individual del profesional que va a insertarlo (categoría IB).
- Evitar la utilización de palomillas metálicas para la administración de fluidos o medicación que pueda ocasionar necrosis tisular si se produce una extravasación (categoría IA).
- Utilizar un catéter venoso periférico mediano o un catéter venoso central de inserción periférica, en lugar de un catéter venoso periférico corto, cuando la duración del tratamiento intravenoso presumiblemente vaya a exceder los seis días (categoría II).
- Evaluar diariamente las molestias en el punto de inserción, por palpación o por inspección visual, en caso de un apósito transparente. Si no hay signos de infección, los apósitos opacos o de gasa no han de ser cambiados sistemáticamente. Un apósito opaco debe retirarse y el punto de inserción ser inspeccionado visualmente si el paciente refiere molestias en la zona (categoría II).
- Retirar el catéter venoso periférico si el paciente presenta signos de flebitis o infección, o si se detecta un funcionamiento defectuoso del catéter (categoría IB).
- Retirar lo antes posible cualquier catéter venoso periférico que no se utilice (categoría IA).

Las recomendaciones específicas, y su categorización, para la utilización de los catéteres venosos centrales son:

- Valorar los riesgos y los beneficios de la colocación de un catéter venoso central en relación a las complicaciones infecciosas y mecánicas, como neumotórax, laceración, hemotórax y trombosis (categoría IA).
- En los pacientes adultos, evitar el uso de la vena femoral para el acceso venoso central (categoría 1A).

- En los pacientes en hemodiálisis o con enfermedad renal avanzada, evitar el uso de la vena subclavia con el objetivo de no ocasionar una estenosis en ella (categoría IA).
- Para el acceso permanente de diálisis, en pacientes con insuficiencia renal crónica, es recomendable usar una fístula o un injerto vascular en lugar de un catéter venoso central (categoría IA).
- Retirar lo antes posible cualquier catéter venoso central que no se utilice (categoría IA).
- En los pacientes adultos, usar un acceso en la vena subclavia, en lugar de las venas yugular o femoral, para minimizar el riesgo de infección (categoría IB).
- Para colocar un catéter venoso central utilizar la ecografía como guía (si está disponible), con el fin de reducir el número de intentos de inserción y las posibles complicaciones mecánicas (categoría IB).
- Usar un catéter venoso central con el mínimo número de luces y puertos necesarios para el tratamiento del paciente (categoría IB).
- Cuando no puede asegurarse que se haya seguido correctamente una técnica aséptica (en especial para catéteres insertados durante una emergencia médica), es necesario cambiar el catéter tan pronto como sea posible, preferentemente en las 48 horas siguientes (categoría IB).

2.3   Higiene de manos y técnica aséptica

La higiene de manos, con agua y jabón o con soluciones alcohólicas, antes de la inserción y las curas de mantenimiento del catéter vascular, en combinación con una técnica aséptica adecuada, confiere una protección adecuada frente a la infección.[20]

Las recomendaciones específicas, y su categorización, para estas actividades de prevención son:

- Utilizar guantes estériles para la inserción de los catéteres venosos centrales, arteriales o de línea media (categoría IA).
- Realizar una correcta higiene de manos con agua y jabón o con solución alcohólica. La higiene de manos ha de hacerse antes y después de palpar el lugar de inserción del catéter, y antes y después de realizar la inserción, reemplazar, acceder o colocar el apósito del catéter. La palpación de la zona de inserción no debe hacerse después de aplicar el antiséptico, a no ser que se mantenga una técnica aséptica (categoría IB).
- Mantener una técnica aséptica para la inserción y el cuidado de los catéteres vasculares (categoría IB).
- Utilizar guantes limpios o guantes estériles para la inserción del catéter venoso periférico si el lugar de acceso no se toca después de aplicar el antiséptico (categoría IC).

- Utilizar guantes limpios o estériles cuando se cambia el apósito de los catéteres (categoría IC).
- Durante el recambio de un catéter con guía, se recomienda cambiarse los guantes estériles antes de manipular de nuevo el catéter (categoría II).

2.4   *Máximas precauciones de barrera estéril*

La utilización de medidas de barrera máximas (véase la figura 3) durante la inserción de un catéter venoso central reduce la incidencia de bacteriemia relacionada y retrasa su aparición cuando se produce.[21]

Las recomendaciones específicas, y su categorización, para esta actividad preventiva son:

- Utilizar máximas precauciones de barrera estéril, incluyendo gorro, mascarilla, bata estéril, guantes estériles y campo estéril, para la inserción de un catéter venoso central o de un catéter venoso central de inserción periférica, y para el recambio de un catéter con guía (categoría IB).
- Utilizar una funda estéril para proteger los catéteres arteriales pulmonares durante su inserción (categoría IB).

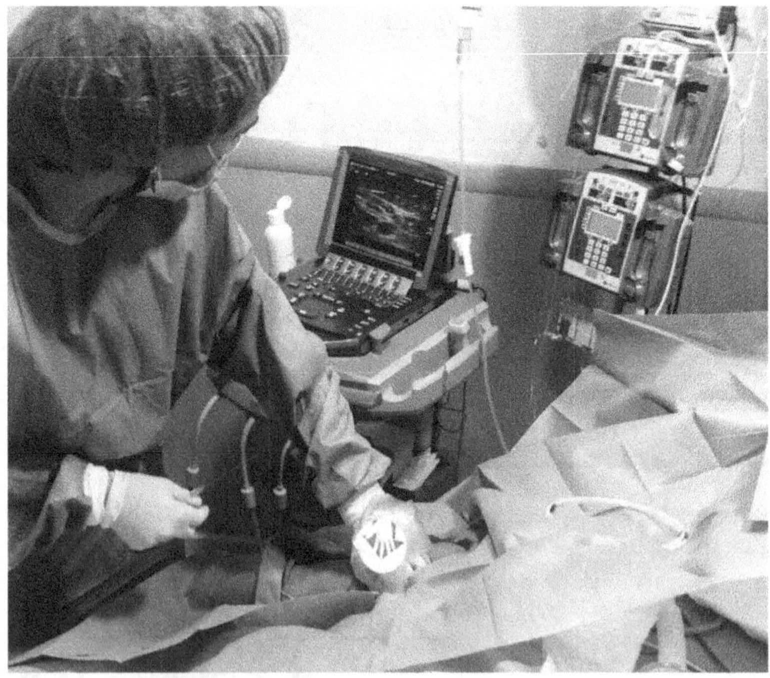

Figura 3. La utilización de medidas de barrera máximas durante la inserción de un catéter venoso central reduce la incidencia de bacteriemia relacionada y retrasa su aparición si se produce.

2.5   Preparación de la piel

La clorhexidina alcohólica es actualmente el estándar para la asepsia de la piel en la inserción de los catéteres vasculares, ya que está demostrada su superioridad respecto a la povidona yodada.[22]

Las recomendaciones específicas, y su categorización, para esta actividad preventiva son:

- Limpiar la piel de la zona de inserción con clorhexidina alcohólica a una concentración superior al 0,5 %, antes de la inserción de un catéter venoso central o de un catéter arterial periférico, así como durante los cambios del apósito. Si la clorhexidina está contraindicada, pueden utilizarse povidona yodada o alcohol al 70 % (categoría IA).
- Limpiar la piel con un antiséptico (clorhexidina alcohólica, alcohol al 70 % o tintura de yodo) antes de la inserción de un catéter venoso periférico (categoría IB).
- Los antisépticos han de dejarse secar, de acuerdo con las recomendaciones del fabricante, antes de insertar el catéter (categoría IB).

2.6   Colocación y recambio de apósitos

Los apósitos semitransparentes de poliuretano son seguros, permiten visualizar el punto de inserción y necesitan menos recambios que los de gasa.[23] Si el punto de inserción está enrojecido (véase la figura 4), es necesario cambiar el catéter lo antes posible. Los apósitos

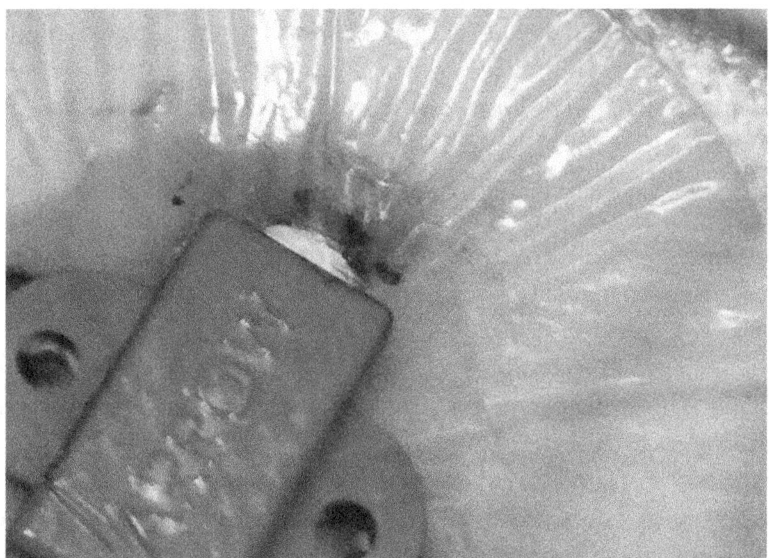

Figura 4. Si el punto de inserción esta enrojecido, es necesario cambiar el catéter lo antes posible.

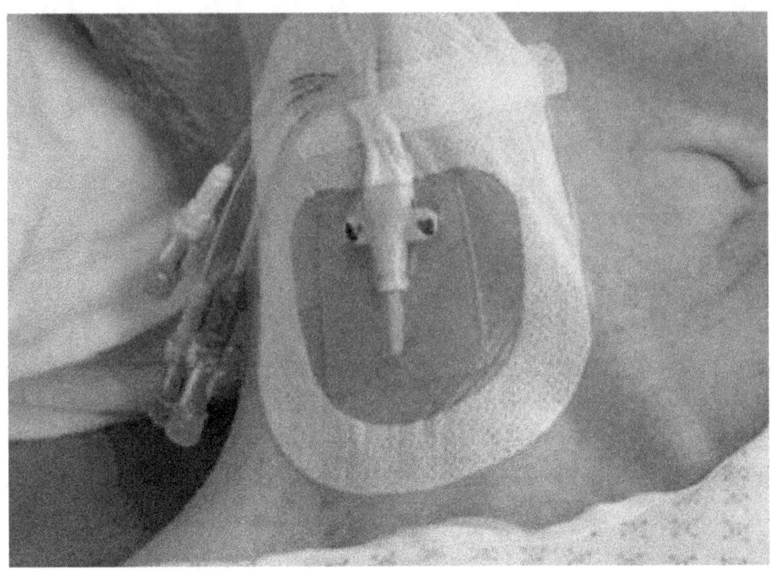

Figura 5. Los apósitos semitransparentes con esponjas de clorhexidina pueden reducir las tasas de bacteriemia cuando ya se han aplicado sin éxito otras medidas de prevención.

semitransparentes con esponjas de clorhexidina pueden reducir las tasas de bacteriemia cuando ya se han aplicado sin éxito otras medidas de prevención (véase la figura 5).[24] Si el punto de inserción no es visible o el apósito está mal colocado, sucio o despegado, es necesario cambiarlo (véase la figura 6).

Las recomendaciones específicas, y su categorización, para esta actividad preventiva son:

- Para cubrir la zona de inserción del catéter utilizar apósitos estériles de gasa o semipermeables transparentes (categoría IA).
- Si el paciente se halla diaforético o si sangra por el punto de inserción, es necesario utilizar un apósito de gasa hasta que el problema esté resuelto (categoría II).
- Cambiar el apósito si está húmedo, despegado o visiblemente sucio (categoría IB).
- No utilizar pomadas ni soluciones tópicas de antibiótico en las zonas de inserción de los catéteres, a excepción de los usados para diálisis, debido al riesgo de infecciones fúngicas secundarias y a la posible aparición de resistencias antimicrobianas (categoría IB).
- No sumergir el catéter en agua. El paciente puede ducharse, pero protegiendo el catéter y las conexiones con una funda impermeable para evitar la posibilidad de contaminación (categoría IB).
- Reemplazar los apósitos de gasa cada dos días (categoría II).
- Reemplazar los apósitos de los catéteres venosos centrales al menos cada siete días, excepto en los pacientes pediátricos, en quienes el riesgo de pérdida del catéter puede superar el beneficio de cambiar el apósito (categoría IB).

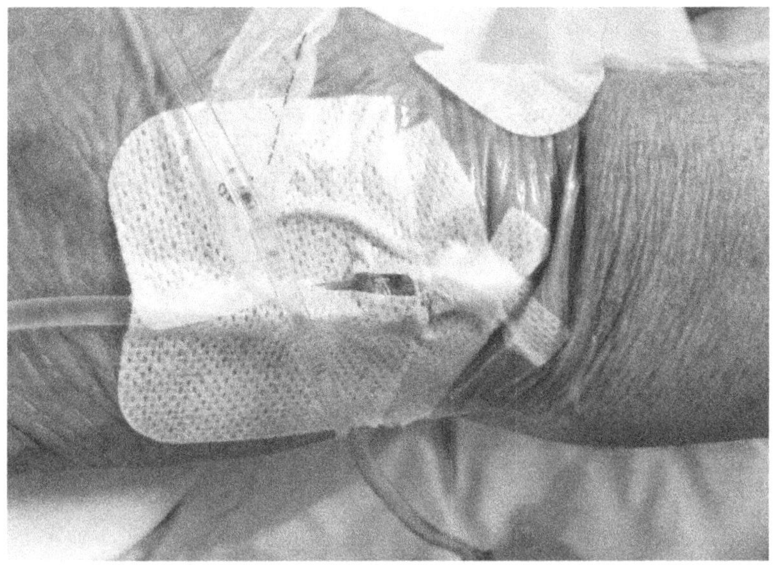

*Figura 6. Si el punto de inserción no es visible o el apósito está mal colocado, sucio o despegado,
hay que cambiarlo inmediatamente.*

- Asegurar que los productos utilizados para el cuidado del catéter sean compatibles con el material de éste (categoría IB).
- Utilizar una funda estéril para el catéter arterial pulmonar (categoría IB).
- En centros con altas tasas de bacteriemias relacionadas con catéteres vasculares y que no se reducen tras la aplicación de las medidas habituales de prevención, es recomendable utilizar esponjas impregnadas de clorhexidina en los catéteres venosos centrales de corta duración colocados en pacientes mayores de dos meses de edad (categoría IB).
- Durante el recambio del apósito, monitorizar visualmente el punto de inserción o inspeccionarlo por palpación a través de un apósito intacto, en función de la situación clínica del paciente. Si el paciente presenta dolor, fiebre sin foco o signos indicativos de sepsis, el apósito debe ser cambiado para permitir la exploración directa del punto de inserción (categoría IB).
- Educar al paciente para que comente con el personal sanitario cualquier molestia relacionada con el punto de inserción del catéter vascular (categoría II).

2.7 Higiene del paciente

En los pacientes ingresados en la UCI, la higiene diaria con toallitas impregnadas de clorhexidina al 2 % puede disminuir la carga bacteriana de la piel y reducir la bacteriemia primaria en comparación con pautas convencionales de higiene diaria con agua y jabón.[25,26]

La recomendación específica, y su categorización, para esta actividad preventiva es:

- Para la higiene diaria de la piel, utilizar jabón de clorhexidina al 2 % con el objetivo de reducir la bacteriemia relacionada con el catéter (categoría II).

2.8 *Dispositivos de sujeción del catéter*

Aunque la evidencia es escasa, pero con una base teórica más consistente, la estabilización del catéter en el punto de inserción disminuye el riesgo de flebitis y de lesiones cutáneas. Los sistemas de sujeción sin sutura pueden disminuir el grado de contaminación cutánea y evitar el sobrecrecimiento bacteriano alrededor del punto de inserción.[27]

La recomendación específica, y su categorización, para esta actividad preventiva es:

- Utilizar un dispositivo de sujeción sin sutura para reducir el riesgo de infección de los catéteres venosos centrales (categoría II).

2.9 *Catéteres impregnados con antisépticos o antimicrobianos*

En centros oncohematológicos, con altas tasas de bacteriemias relacionadas con catéteres venosos centrales y que no se reducen tras la implementación de una estrategia global de prevención, la utilización de catéteres impregnados con una solución de clorhexidina y sulfadiazina argéntica, o de minociclina y rifampicina, cuando se prevea una duración de la cateterización superior a cinco días, puede contribuir a reducir dichas tasas. La estrategia global de prevención ha de incluir al menos los siguientes tres componentes: formación del personal, adhesión estricta a las precauciones de barrera y utilización de clorhexidina alcohólica a concentraciones superiores al 0,5 % para la antisepsia de la piel durante la inserción del catéter venoso central.[28]

La recomendación específica, y su categorización, para esta actividad preventiva es:

- Utilizar catéteres impregnados con solución de clorhexidina y sulfadiazina argéntica, o de minociclina y rifampicina, en los pacientes en quienes se prevea una duración de la cateterización superior a cinco días cuando no se han reducido las tasas después de implementar una estrategia global de prevención (categoría IA).

2.10 *Profilaxis con antibióticos sistémicos*

Aunque alguna revisión ha sugerido un cierto efecto beneficioso de la prevención de las infecciones con los catéteres tunelizados,[29] no se recomienda la administración de antibióticos sistémicos para evitar la presión antibiótica selectiva.

La recomendación específica, y su categorización, para esta actividad preventiva es:

- No administrar profilaxis antibiótica sistémica antes de la inserción ni durante el uso de un catéter vascular, para prevenir su colonización y la bacteriemia relacionada (categoría IB).

2.11 Pomadas de antibióticos o antisépticos

La utilización de pomadas con antibióticos o antisépticos, mupirocina y povidona yodada, en el punto de inserción en pacientes en hemodiálisis, ha demostrado una reducción significativa de las infecciones y de las bacteriemias relacionadas, en especial en los pacientes con colonización nasal por *Staphylococcus aureus*.[30]

La recomendación específica, y su categorización, para esta actividad preventiva es:

- No utilizar pomadas ni cremas de antisépticos o antibióticos en el lugar de inserción del catéter. En los pacientes en hemodiálisis, sólo está indicado al final de cada sesión y siempre que sea compatible con el material del catéter de hemodiálisis y de acuerdo con las recomendaciones del fabricante (categoría IB).

2.12 Sellado del catéter con antimicrobianos

Se han utilizado con éxito diversos antibióticos (vancomicina, gentamicina y ciprofloxacino) y soluciones antisépticas (alcohol y taurolidina) para realizar lavados o sellar la luz del catéter, evitando así la bacteriemia relacionada en los pacientes portadores de un catéter venoso central de larga duración y en aquellos sometidos a hemodiálisis.[31-33]

La recomendación específica, y su categorización, para esta actividad preventiva es:

- En los pacientes con un catéter venoso central de larga duración y con antecedentes de múltiples episodios de bacteriemia relacionada con un catéter venoso central, puede sellarse el catéter con soluciones de antibiótico (categoría II).

2.13 Uso de anticoagulantes

Hay una estrecha relación entre la trombosis venosa y el riesgo de infección relacionada con los catéteres. Diversos estudios han analizado la utilización profiláctica de heparina en la prevención de la bacteriemia relacionada con un catéter vascular. Los resultados discordantes en la prevención de la bacteriemia y el riesgo de aparición de trombocitopenia han desestimado esta opción.[34]

La recomendación específica, y su categorización, para esta actividad preventiva es:

- No utilizar anticoagulantes por vía sistémica para la prevención de la infección relacionada con el catéter (categoría II).

2.14   *Sustitución de los catéteres venosos periféricos*

El reemplazo programado ha sido una estrategia de prevención de las complicaciones producidas por un catéter venoso periférico. Aunque en diversos programas nacionales de prevención de la bacteriemia se contempla un recambio programado a las 72 horas, diversos estudios no han observado diferencias en las tasas de flebitis ni de bacteriemia entre 72 horas o 96 horas desde la inserción, e incluso cuando no se ha programado ningún recambio.[35]

Las recomendaciones específicas, y su categorización, para esta actividad preventiva son:

- No es necesario cambiar los catéteres venosos periféricos con una frecuencia inferior a 72-96 horas desde su inserción para reducir el riesgo de infección y la flebitis en los adultos (categoría IB).
- En los niños, los catéteres venosos periféricos se cambiarán cuando esté clínicamente indicado (categoría IB).

2.15   *Recambio de los catéteres venosos centrales, de los catéteres venosos centrales de inserción periférica y de los catéteres para hemodiálisis*

Diversos estudios realizados con pacientes de UCI no han hallado diferencias en las tasas de infección entre el recambio programado del catéter a los siete días y el recambio según la necesidad.[36]

Las recomendaciones específicas, y su categorización, para esta actividad preventiva son:

- No cambiar sistemáticamente los catéteres venosos centrales, los de inserción periférica, los de hemodiálisis ni los colocados en la arteria pulmonar (categoría IB).
- No utilizar sistemáticamente un fiador o guía para el recambio de los catéteres no tunelizados, y nunca en caso de infección (categoría IB).
- No retirar un catéter venoso central o un catéter venoso central de inserción periférica sólo por la presencia de fiebre. Descartar siempre otras infecciones o una causa no infecciosa de la fiebre (categoría II).

2.16 Catéteres umbilicales

El acceso umbilical se utiliza habitualmente en los neonatos, pues estos vasos son fáciles de canalizar y permiten la extracción de sangre para análisis y para deteerminar la situación hemodinámica. Alrededor de un 3 % a un 5 % de los catéteres pueden ser el foco de origen de una bacteriemia, sin grandes diferencias entre los colocados en la arteria o en la vena umbilical.[37]

Las recomendaciones específicas, y su categorización, para esta actividad preventiva son:

- Retirar y no cambiar los catéteres colocados en la arteria umbilical si hay signos de bacteriemia relacionada o trombosis (categoría II).
- Limpiar la zona umbilical con un antiséptico antes de insertar el catéter. Evitar la tintura de yodo en los recién nacidos, por su posible efecto sobre el tiroides. Pueden utilizarse otros productos que contienen yodo, como la povidona yodada (categoría IB).
- No utilizar pomadas ni cremas antibióticas en los puntos de inserción de los catéteres umbilicales, ya que pueden aumentar el riesgo de infecciones fúngicas y condicionar la aparición de resistencias antimicrobianas (categoría IA).
- Añadir dosis bajas de heparina (de 0,25 a 1 UI/ml) a los fluidos que se infunden a través de los catéteres umbilicales arteriales (categoría IB).
- Retirar los catéteres umbilicales tan pronto como sea posible, y si hay signos de insuficiencia vascular en los miembros inferiores. Es recomendable que los catéteres en la arteria umbilical no permanezcan más de cinco días (categoría II).
- Los catéteres umbilicales venosos deben retirarse tan pronto como sea posible, pero pueden utilizarse hasta 14 días si se manipulan asépticamente (categoría II).

2.17 Catéteres arteriales periféricos y de monitorización de presión

El riesgo de bacteriemia asociada al catéter arterial es menor que el asociado al catéter venoso central.[3] No ha podido demostrarse la utilidad de las medidas de barrera estéril máximas para disminuir la bacteriemia producida por este tipo de catéter. Cuando la inserción es en la arteria femoral se asocia con un riesgo más alto de infección, que con mayor frecuencia está producida por bacilos gramnegativos.[38]

Las recomendaciones específicas, y su categorización, para esta actividad preventiva son:

- En los adultos, para reducir el riesgo de infección es preferible el acceso a través de las arterias radial, braquial o pedia, en lugar de por vía femoral o axilar (categoría IB).
- No utilizar la arteria braquial en los niños. Las arterias radial, pedia y tibial posterior son preferibles a la inserción por vía femoral o axilar (categoría II).

- Utilizar gorro, mascarilla, guantes estériles y una talla pequeña fenestrada durante la inserción de un catéter arterial periférico (categoría IB).
- Utilizar máximas precauciones de barrera durante la inserción de un catéter arterial axilar o femoral (categoría II).
- No cambiar sistemáticamente los catéteres arteriales para prevenir la bacteriemia relacionada (categoría II).
- Volver a colocar el catéter arterial sólo cuando haya una indicación clínica (categoría II).
- Retirar el catéter arterial tan pronto como sea posible (categoría II).
- Utilizar, siempre que sea posible, un transductor desechable (categoría IB)
- Si no es posible el uso de transductores desechables, los transductores reutilizables deben esterilizarse según las instrucciones del fabricante (categoría IA).
- Mantener estériles todos los componentes del sistema de control de presión, incluyendo el dispositivo de calibración y la solución de lavado (categoría IA).
- Minimizar el número de manipulaciones del sistema de monitorización de presiones (categoría II).
- Cuando se utiliza una conexión de membrana en lugar de la llave de tres pasos, es necesario desinfectar la membrana con un antiséptico apropiado antes de acceder al sistema de control de la presión (categoría IA).
- No administrar glucosa ni soluciones de nutrición parenteral a través del circuito de control de la presión (categoría IA).
- Cambiar los transductores desechables a intervalos de 96 horas, al igual que los otros componentes del sistema (categoría IB).
- Minimizar las manipulaciones del dispositivo. Utilizar sistemas de circuito cerrado para mantener la permeabilidad de los catéteres de monitorización de la presión (categoría II).

2.18 *Recambio de los equipos de administración de medicación*

El recambio óptimo de los equipos de administración se ha establecido en algunos estudios y en metaanálisis. Los resultados principales señalan que no es necesario un recambio más frecuente que cada 72-96 horas.[39] Cuando se administran fluidos que facilitan el crecimiento bacteriano, como nutrición o lípidos, es necesario un recambio más frecuente del equipo.

Las recomendaciones específicas, y su categorización, para esta actividad preventiva son:

- Cambiar los equipos de administración de infusión continua, incluidos los equipos secundarios adicionales, con una frecuencia no inferior a 96 horas, y como máximo cada siete días (categoría IA).

- Sustituir los equipos de infusión de propofol cada 6-12 horas y cada vez que se cambie el frasco (categoría IA).
- Sustituir los equipos de infusión de sangre, hemoderivados o emulsiones lipídicas (tanto si se administran solas o en combinación con aminoácidos y glucosa) durante las primeras 24 horas (categoría IB).

2.19   Sistemas de infusión sin aguja

Las llaves de tres pasos, utilizadas para la administración de medicación y fluidos, y para la extracción de muestras de sangre, representan una potencial fuente de contaminación intraluminal del catéter. Sin embargo, la utilización de conectores sin aguja se ha relacionado con un aumento en las tasas de incidencia de las bacteriemias relacionadas con catéteres vasculares por una desinfección inapropiada del conector.[40]

La recomendaciones específicas, y su categorización, para esta actividad preventiva son:

- Minimizar el riesgo de contaminación de los conectores sin aguja y de los puntos de inyección. Desinfectarlos cuidadosamente con un antiséptico adecuado (clorhexidina, povidona yodada o alcohol al 70 %) y acceder al sistema utilizando sólo dispositivos estériles (categoría IA).
- Usar conectores sin aguja para el acceso al sistema de infusión (categoría IC).
- Cambiar los conectores sin aguja con la misma frecuencia que el equipo de infusión. No se ha demostrado ningún beneficio si se cambian los equipos con una frecuencia inferior a 72 horas (categoría II).
- Asegurar que todos los componentes del sistema son compatibles, para minimizar las fugas y roturas (categoría II).
- Cuando se utilizan conectores sin aguja, son preferibles los de tipo *split septum* que otros de válvulas mecánicas, ya que algunas de estas válvulas pueden aumentar el riesgo de infección (categoría II).

2.20   Estrategias para mejorar el rendimiento

Diversos estudios han puesto de manifiesto la eficacia de intervenciones consistentes en la introducción de paquetes de medidas de fácil aplicación.[11]

La recomendación específica, y su categorización, para esta actividad preventiva es:

- Las intervenciones para la prevención de la bacteriemia relacionada con un catéter vascular han de incluir paquetes de medidas *(bundles)* de eficacia probada. Se fomentará la adhesión y el cumplimiento de las medidas por parte del personal sanitario (categoría IB).

Bibliografía

1. Eggimann P. Prevention of intravascular catheter infection. Curr Opin Infect Dis. 2007; 20: 360-9.
2. Edgeworth J. Intravascular catheter infections. J Hosp Infect. 2009; 73: 323-30.
3. Maki DG, Kluger DM, Crnich CJ. The risk of bloodstream infection in adults with different intravascular devices: a systematic review of 200 published prospective studies. Mayo Clin Proc. 2006; 81: 1159-71.
4. Mermel LA. What is the predominant source of intravascular catheter infections? Clin Infect Dis. 2011; 52: 211-2.
5. The Joint Comission. Preventing central-line-associated bloodstream infections. A global challenge, a global perspective. Oak Brook, IL: Joint Comission Resources; 2012.
6. 2011 Guidelines for the prevention of intravascular catheter-related infections. (Consultado el 1 de marzo de 2013.) Disponible en: http://www.cdc.gov/hicpac/BSI/01-BSI-guidelines-2011.html.
7. How to guide: prevent central line-associated bloodstream infections (CLABSI). MA: Institute for Healthcare Improvement; 2012. Disponible en: www.ihi.org.
8. Guideline to elimination of catheter-related bloodstream infections, an APIC guide, 2009. (Consultado el 1 de marzo de 2013.) Disponible en: http://www.apic.org/Resource_/EliminationGuideForm/259c0594-17b0-459d-b395-fb143321414a/File/APIC-CRBSI-Elimination-Guide.pdf.
9. Shekelle PG, Pronovost PJ, Wachter RM, McDonald KM, Schoelles K, Dy SM, et al. The top patient safety strategies that can be encouraged for adoption now. Ann Intern Med. 2013; 158: 365-8.
10. Pronovost PJ, Berenholtz SM, Goeschel C, Thom I, Watson SR, Holzmueller CG, et al. Improving patient safety in intensive care units in Michigan. J Crit Care. 2008; 23: 207-21.
11. Pronovost P, Needham D, Berenholtz S, Sinopoli D, Chu H, Cosgrove S, et al. An intervention to decrease catheter-related bloodstream infections in the ICU. N Engl J Med. 2006; 355: 2725-32.
12. World Health Organization. Bacteremia zero: preventing bloostream infections from central line venous catheter in Spanish ICUs. (Consultado el 1 de marzo de 2013.) Disponible en: http://www.who.int/patientsafety/implementation/bsi/bacteriemia_zero/en/.
13. Freixas N, Bella F, Limón E, Pujol M, Almirante B, Gudiol F. Impact of a multimodal intervention to reduce bloodstream infections related to vascular catheters in non-ICU wards: a multicentre study. Clin Microbiol Infect. 2012; doi: 10.1111/1469-0691.12049.
14. Warren DK, Zack JE, Mayfield JL, Chen A, Prentice D, Fraser VJ, et al. The effect of an education program on the incidence of central venous catheter-associated bloodstream infection in a medical ICU. Chest. 2004; 126: 1612-8.
15. Zingg W, Imhof A, Maggiorini M, Stocker R, Keller E, Ruef C. Impact of a prevention strategy targeting hand hygiene and catheter care on the incidence of catheter-related bloodstream infections. Crit Care Med. 2009; 37: 2167-73.
16. Fridkin SK, Pear SM, Williamson TH, Galgiani JN, Jarvis WR. The role of understaffing in central venous catheter-associated bloodstream infections. Infect Control Hosp Epidemiol. 1996; 17: 150-8.
17. Stone PW, Pogorzelska M, Kunches L, Hirschhorn LR. Hospital staffing and health care-associated infections: a systematic review of the literature. Clin Infect Dis. 2008; 47: 937-44.
18. Mestre G, Berbel C, Tortajada P, Alarcia M, Coca R, Fernández MM, et al. Successful multifaceted intervention aimed to reduce short peripheral venous catheter-related adverse events: a quasiexperimental cohort study. Am J Infect Control. 2012; doi: 10.1016/j.ajic.2012.07.014.
19. Maki DG, Ringer M. Risk factors for infusion-related phlebitis with small peripheral venous catheters. A randomized controlled trial. Ann Intern Med. 1991; 114: 845-54.
20. Pittet D, Hugonnet S, Harbarth S, Mourouga P, Sauvan V, Touveneau S, et al. Effectiveness of a hospital-wide programme to improve compliance with hand hygiene. Infection Control Programme. Lancet. 2000; 356: 1307-12.
21. Raad II, Hohn DC, Gilbreath BJ, Suleiman N, Hill LA, Bruso PA, et al. Prevention of central venous catheter-related infections by using

maximal sterile barrier precautions during insertion. Infect Control Hosp Epidemiol. 1994; 15: 231-8.

22. Mimoz O, Pieroni L, Lawrence C, Edouard A, Costa Y, Samii K, *et al.* Prospective, randomized trial of two antiseptic solutions for prevention of central venous or arterial catheter colonization and infection in intensive care unit patients. Crit Care Med. 1996; 24: 1818-23.

23. Maki DG, Ringer M. Evaluation of dressing regimens for prevention of infection with peripheral intravenous catheters. Gauze, a transparent polyurethane dressing, and an iodophor-transparent dressing. JAMA. 1987; 258: 2396-403.

24. Timsit JF, Mimoz O, Mourvillier B, Souweine B, Garrouste-Orgeas M, Alfandari S, *et al.* Randomized controlled trial of chlorhexidine dressing and highly adhesive dressing for preventing catheter-related infections in critically ill adults. Am J Respir Crit Care Med. 2012; 186: 1272-8.

25. Bleasdale SC, Trick WE, González IM, Lyles RD, Hayden MK, Weinstein RA. Effectiveness of chlorhexidine bathing to reduce catheter-associated bloodstream infections in medical intensive care unit patients. Arch Intern Med. 2007; 167: 2073-9.

26. Climo MW, Yokoe DS, Warren DK, Perl TM, Bolon M, Herwaldt LA, *et al.* Effect of daily chlorhexidine bathing on hospital-acquired infection. N Engl J Med. 2013; 368: 533-42.

27. Yamamoto AJ, Solomon JA, Soulen MC, Tang J, Parkinson K, Lin R, *et al.* Sutureless securement device reduces complications of peripherally inserted central venous catheters. J Vasc Interv Radiol. 2002; 13: 77-81.

28. Raad I, Hanna H. Intravascular catheters impregnated with antimicrobial agents: a milestone in the prevention of bloodstream infections. Support Care Cancer. 1999; 7: 386-90.

29. Van de Wetering MD, van Woensel JB. Prophylactic antibiotics for preventing early central venous catheter Gram positive infections in oncology patients. Cochrane Database Syst Rev. 2007; (1): CD003295.

30. McCann M, Moore ZE. Interventions for preventing infectious complications in haemodialysis patients with central venous catheters. Cochrane Database Syst Rev. 2010; (1): CD006894.

31. Carratalà J, Niubó J, Fernández-Sevilla A, Juvé E, Castellsagué X, Berlanga J, *et al.* Randomized, double-blind trial of an antibiotic-lock technique for prevention of Gram-positive central venous catheter-related infection in neutropenic patients with cancer. Antimicrob Agents Chemother. 1999; 43: 2200-4.

32. Yahav D, Rozen-Zvi B, Gafter-Gvili A, Leibovici L, Gafter U, Paul M. Antimicrobial lock solutions for the prevention of infections associated with intravascular catheters in patients undergoing hemodialysis: systematic review and meta-analysis of randomized, controlled trials. Clin Infect Dis. 2008; 47: 83-93.

33. Safdar N, Maki DG. Use of vancomycin-containing lock or flush solutions for prevention of bloodstream infection associated with central venous access devices: a meta-analysis of prospective, randomized trials. Clin Infect Dis. 2006; 43: 474-84.

34. Levy JH, Hursting MJ. Heparin-induced thrombocytopenia, a prothrombotic disease. Hematol Oncol Clin North Am. 2007; 21: 65-88.

35. Rickard CM, Webster J, Wallis MC, Marsh N, McGrail MR, French V, *et al.* Routine versus clinically indicated replacement of peripheral intravenous catheters: a randomised controlled equivalence trial. Lancet. 2012; 380: 1066-74.

36. Eyer S, Brummitt C, Crossley K, Siegel R, Cerra F. Catheter-related sepsis: prospective, randomized study of three methods of long-term catheter maintenance. Crit Care Med. 1990; 18: 1073-9.

37. Butler-O'Hara M, Buzzard CJ, Reubens L, McDermott MP, DiGrazio W, D'Angio CT. A randomized trial comparing long-term and short-term use of umbilical venous catheters in premature infants with birth weights of less than 1251 grams. Pediatrics. 2006; 118: e25-35.

38. Lorente L, Santacreu R, Martín MM, Jiménez A, Mora ML. Arterial catheter-related infection of 2,949 catheters. Crit Care. 2006; 10: R83.

39. Maki DG, Botticelli JT, LeRoy ML, Thielke TS. Prospective study of replacing administration sets for intravenous therapy at 48- vs 72-hour intervals. 72 hours is safe and cost-effective. JAMA. 1987; 258: 1777-81.

40. Esteve F, Pujol M, Limón E, Saballs M, Argerich MJ, Verdaguer R, *et al.* Bloodstream infection related to catheter connections: a prospective trial of two connection systems. J Hosp Infect. 2007; 67: 30-4.

Capítulo 12

Eficacia de los programas preventivos multimodales para la reducción de las bacteriemias relacionadas con catéteres en los servicios de medicina intensiva

M. Palomar Martínez,[1] F. Álvarez Lerma[2]

[1] **Unidad de Críticos**
Hospital Universitari Arnau de Vilanova
Lleida

[2] **Servicio de Medicina Intensiva**
Hospital Universitari del Mar
Parc de Salut
Barcelona

Correspondencia:
Dra. Mercedes Palomar
mpalomarmartinez@gmail.com

Introducción

En el año 2001, el Institute for Healthcare Improvement (IHI) y la Voluntary Hospital Assocation desarrollaron el concepto de *bundle* (paquete de medidas) para mejorar el proceso de los cuidados críticos en la implementación de una iniciativa llamada *Idealized Design of the Intensive Care Unit*.[1]

Un paquete de medidas consiste en un número reducido de intervenciones basadas en la evidencia científica que, aplicadas de forma simultánea en una población definida de pacientes, proporciona un resultado significativamente mejor que cuando cada una de ellas se aplica de forma individual. Se ha recomendado centrar su aplicación en las áreas de mayor potencial de daño y costes, así como en aquellas en que la evidencia es mayor. Entre los primeros objetivos de estos paquetes de medidas se encuentran las infecciones asociadas a los cuidados sanitarios, en especial las relacionadas con dispositivos médicos, como los catéteres vasculares o los aparatos para ventilación mecánica,[2,3] si bien su aplicación también se ha recomendado y ha sido efectiva para la sepsis.[4]

La prevención de las infecciones nosocomiales incluye una serie de medidas generales comunes para todas ellas y otras específicas para la localización, que se basan en la fisiopatología propia de cada infección, de las que se escogerán las más relevantes para ser incluidas en el paquete de medidas.[5]

Para aplicar los paquetes de medidas y buscar más eficacia en su implementación, se requiere un trabajo que fomente la cultura de la seguridad.[1,6] Ésta se ha definido como «el producto de los valores individuales y de grupo, actitudes, percepciones, competencias y patrones de comportamiento que determinan el compromiso, estilo y dominio de una organización sanitaria y su gestión de la seguridad».[7] Intervenciones como la formación, la implementación de listas de control, las órdenes estandarizadas, la evaluación de competencias y las herramientas de supervisión, han desempeñado un importante papel en este cambio de cultura. Y aún más importante, la reducción de las infecciones asociadas a los cuidados sanitarios se ha convertido en una tarea más multidisciplinaria basada en el trabajo en equipo, incluyendo el apoyo administrativo de los equipos directivos.

Uno de los ejemplos más exitosos de la iniciativa del IHI fue la experiencia del estado de Michigan (EE.UU) con la aplicación de un paquete de medidas para evitar las bacteriemias relacionadas con catéteres venosos centrales, al lograr que 105 unidades de cuidados intensivos (UCI) de todo el estado consiguieran reducir, transcurridos 18 meses, la tasa media de estas bacteriemias desde 7,4 a 1,5 episodios por mil días de utilización de los catéteres, y mantenerla.[8] Este modelo se ha replicado en diferentes escenarios, incluyendo España. La primera experiencia a gran escala de aplicación de un paquete de medidas para la prevención de las bacteriemias relacionadas con catéteres en las UCI de nuestro país ha sido el *Proyecto Bacteriemia Zero*, una iniciativa promovida y liderada por la Sociedad Española de Medicina Intensiva, Crítica y Unidades Coronarias que ha contado con el apoyo de la Agencia de Calidad del Ministerio de Sanidad, Seguridad Social e Igualdad y la Organización Mundial de la Salud. Esta experiencia se ha extendido posteriormente a la prevención de la neumonía asociada a ventilación mecánica en un segundo programa llamado *Neumonía Zero*.

El diseño y la aplicación de un paquete de medidas requieren cumplir una serie de condiciones que teóricamente son imprescindibles para su éxito, y que a continuación se describen.[1]

1   Diseño del paquete de medidas

En primer lugar, se aconseja que el número de intervenciones o elementos que lo constituyan sea de tres a cinco, y que estos elementos estén bien basados en la evidencia científica y aceptados por los clínicos. Por otra parte, cada intervención tiene que ser relativamente independiente del resto. El paquete de medidas ha de aplicarse a una población definida y en circunstancias también definidas.

El desarrollo del paquete tiene que ser llevado a cabo por un equipo multidisciplinario, y los elementos recomendados serán más descriptivos que prescriptivos para permitir una adaptación local y un juicio clínico apropiados. Por último, y en teoría, el cumplimiento de las recomendaciones incluidas en el paquete ha de medirse como «todo o nada» con el objetivo de alcanzar al menos un 95 % de aplicación.[9] Pero en la realidad, cuando se verifica el grado de cumplimiento se comprueba que es difícil alcanzar esos objetivos. Aunque de manera individual cada una de las medidas pueda tener un seguimiento alto, es frecuente que el total de los elementos se cumpla en un porcentaje muy inferior.

2   Implementación del paquete de medidas

Entre los puntos clave para la implementación se encuentran los que recoge la tabla 1, que a continuación se detallan.

2.1   *Elección de los elementos prioritarios a recomendar*

En primer lugar tienen que identificarse los componentes del paquete. Éste es un punto clave, pues las medidas preventivas posibles son numerosas, decenas incluso, y hacer énfasis en todas ellas es casi imposible.[10,12] Los elementos escogidos han de ser aquellos con mayor evidencia científica y cuya aplicación sea más sencilla, incluyendo el coste.

En la prevención de la bacteriemia relacionada con catéteres, las medidas escogidas por el IHI y aplicadas en el programa de Michigan estaban dirigidas a mejorar la práctica clínica en el momento de la inserción del catéter (prevenir la vía exoluminal de colonización del catéter), y a acortar la duración de la cateterización, planteando la retirada del catéter venoso central tan pronto como fuera posible.[8]

En el *Proyecto Bacteriemia Zero* se hicieron ligeras modificaciones en la composición del paquete de medidas para adaptarse a la realidad de nuestro país. En nuestras UCI, la estancia de los pacientes es más larga que en las americanas (hay un menor número de camas de críticos por 100.000 habitantes), la tasa de uso de catéteres venosos centrales es mayor (80 % frente a 50 % del tiempo de estancia en la UCI) y probablemente también su permanencia (según los datos del Estudio Nacional de Vigilancia de la Infección No-

---

- Identificar los elementos prioritarios a recomendar
- Elaborar el paquete de medidas junto a un plan de implementación
- Diseñar cuidadosamente cómo se presenta el paquete de medidas
- Involucrar a los directivos en la elaboración del plan de implementación
- Probar en un estudio piloto tanto el paquete de medidas como el plan de implementación, y redefinirlos antes de llevarlos a cabo
- Registrar el cumplimiento de cada elemento, analizar las barreras que limitan su aplicación e informar de los resultados

Tabla 1. Puntos clave para la implementación de paquetes de medidas.

socomial en UCI [ENVIN-HELICS], el tiempo medio de aparición de una bacteriemia relacionada con un catéter en España es superior a las dos semanas tras el ingreso en la UCI). Por ello, era importante dedicar medidas preventivas dirigidas al mantenimiento de los catéteres (prevenir la vía endoluminal de colonización) y añadir un elemento más al paquete de medidas: el manejo higiénico de los catéteres, incluyendo la higiene de manos antes de la manipulación, la reducción al mínimo de dichas manipulaciones y la desinfección de los puertos sin aguja antes de la administración de los fármacos (véase la tabla 2).

En los pacientes pediátricos, con una mayor limitación para los accesos vasculares, y por tanto con más necesidad de preservarlos, se han seguido estrategias similares a la descrita, con elementos específicos dedicados al mantenimiento del catéter.[13]

2.2 *Elaboración de un plan de implementación*

La base teórica que justificaría el efecto de los paquetes de medidas es que su aplicación estimula el trabajo en equipo y la comunicación en los grupos multidisciplinarios, creando las condiciones necesarias para el desarrollo de un cuidado fiable y seguro en las UCI.

Sin embargo, el diseño de un paquete de medidas, por muy acertado que sea, será poco eficaz si no se acompaña de una estrategia de implementación.[14-16] La simple publicación de las recomendaciones o la introducción pasiva conducen con frecuencia al fracaso, como ilustran algunas experiencias. En una UCI escocesa se introdujo el paquete de medidas para la prevención de la neumonía asociada a ventilación mecánica promocionado por el IHI.[17] A pesar de disponer de una copia de éste en la cabecera de cada enfermo con ventilación, el cumplimiento fue mínimo en las ocasiones en que periódicamente se monitorizó, y las tasas de neumonía asociada a ventilación mecánica no se redujeron respecto al período

Michigan	Proyecto Bacteriemia Zero
Higiene adecuada de manos	Higiene adecuada de manos
Uso de clorhexidina en la preparación de la piel	Uso de clorhexidina en la preparación de la piel
Uso de medidas de barrera durante la inserción de los catéteres	Uso de medidas de barrera durante la inserción de los catéteres
Evitar la localización femoral	Preferencia de la vena subclavia
Retirada de los catéteres innecesarios	Retirada de los catéteres innecesarios
	Manejo higiénico de los catéteres

Tabla 2. Paquetes de medidas para prevenir las bacteriemias relacionadas con catéteres. Comparación de las estrategias de Michigan y España (Proyecto Bacteriemia Zero).

previo a su implantación. Al comprobar el fracaso, se inició una actividad educativa mediante talleres formativos, información de los resultados del cumplimiento, análisis de las barreras y discusión de la adherencia en las rondas diarias. El cumplimiento ascendió del 0 % al 54 %, y las tasas de incidencia de neumonía descendieron desde 19,1 a 7,5 episodios por mil días de uso de la ventilación mecánica. Esta experiencia validaría el éxito del programa de Michigan, que introdujo de manera simultánea la parte técnica (paquete de medidas específico) y un programa de seguridad integral.[18] Entre los componentes de los programas de seguridad se encuentran, además de la formación, intervenciones dirigidas a mejorar la comunicación entre estamentos y reordenar el trabajo, para que se realice en equipo mediante listas de comprobación, monitorización de procedimientos e indicadores. En el *Proyecto Bacteriemia Zero*[19] se adaptó la estrategia de Michigan con la implantación simultánea de los dos brazos: el técnico (denominado STOP-BRC) y el de seguridad (denominado Plan Integral de Seguridad) (véase la figura 1).

Las barreras que pueden surgir al tratar de trasladar el conocimiento a la práctica habitual son numerosas e incluyen aspectos tanto de conocimiento como de actitud, y finalmente de comportamiento,[16] que los programas de seguridad pueden combatir.

Dentro de las barreras relacionadas con el conocimiento, podemos encontrar que el personal no esté familiarizado con la evidencia científica, ya sea por el volumen de información existente, por falta de tiempo para estar informado o por cuestiones de acce-

---

Bacteriemia zero

STOP-BRC

a. Higiene adecuada de manos
b. Uso de clorhexidina en la preparación de la piel
c. Uso de medidas de barrera total durante la inserción de los catéteres
d. Preferencia de la vena subclavia como lugar de inserción
e. Retirada de catéteres innecesarios
f. Manejo higiénico de los catéteres

Plan de seguridad integral: PSI

1. Evaluar la cultura de seguridad (medición basal y periódica)
2. Formación en seguridad del paciente
3. Identificar errores en la práctica habitual (por los profesionales)
4. Establecer alianzas con la dirección de la institución para la mejora de la seguridad
5. Aprender de los errores

Figura 1. Componentes del Proyecto Bacteriemia Zero.

sibilidad. Los programas educativos organizados institucionalmente neutralizarán esta carencia. En el *Proyecto Bacteriemia Zero,* la formación se realizó en línea a través de un *web* específico que incluía tanto las cuestiones relacionadas con el impacto de las bacteriemias relacionadas con catéteres y las principales estrategias de prevención, como nociones generales de seguridad del paciente.

Otras barreras tienen que ver con las actitudes. Los profesionales sanitarios pueden no estar de acuerdo con las guías en general o en particular, creer que la interpretación de la evidencia científica no es correcta o que no es aplicable a sus pacientes, que las medidas recomendadas no son prácticas o que incluso representan un reto para su autonomía. A veces se duda de que las medidas recomendadas tengan el efecto deseado, o de que personalmente se sea capaz de ponerlas en práctica, aunque la barrera más frecuente a este respecto es la falta de motivación que lleva a perpetuar los viejos hábitos y prácticas asistenciales. La aplicación de las herramientas incluidas en los programas de seguridad ayuda a superar estas barreras, al reforzar la comunicación entre los profesionales, identificar errores en las prácticas diarias y promover objetivos de mejora dirigidos a optimizar la atención a los pacientes.

2.3 *Diseño cuidadoso de la presentación del paquete de medidas*

El comportamiento de las personas está influenciado por sus creencias. Por ello, para acelerar la adopción del paquete de medidas es esencial presentarlo con un razonamiento claro y convincente que lo justifique, mostrando las consecuencias que tendría el desarrollo de la infección en contraposición a las ventajas que supondría incorporar cada una de las medidas. En el *Proyecto Bacteriemia Zero,* la estrategia para lograr la aceptación y el cumplimiento del programa se basó en cuatro puntos: implicar al personal sanitario, educar en la evidencia científica, ejecutar el programa y evaluar los resultados (véase la tabla 3). Para

---

- Comprometer:
  - Casos de la unidad, mostrar datos iniciales de bacteriemias relacionadas con catéteres
- Educar al personal en la evidencia
- Ejecutar:
  - Crear un equipo de material para colocar catéteres
  - Crear una lista de comprobación de inserción de catéteres
  - Reforzar a la enfermería para controlar el proceso de colocación (y manejo) de los catéteres
- Evaluar:
  - Informar de los resultados (tasas de bacteriemias relacionadas con catéteres, encuestas de seguridad)
  - Considerar las infecciones como defectos

Tabla 3. Estrategias para implantar el Proyecto Bacteriemia Zero.

motivar al personal se recomendaba presentar las tasas de bacteriemias relacionadas con catéteres de la unidad y compararlas con las tasas nacionales o de otras UCI conocidas. Además, se valoró que mostrar casos de pacientes de la propia unidad y el impacto que en ellos había tenido el desarrollo de la infección era especialmente motivador.

La presentación del proyecto ha de orientarse y adaptarse a las necesidades de los usuarios (personal sanitario), lo cual implica proveer de herramientas que faciliten la adopción, tal y como materiales educativos, carteles informativos recordando el contenido del paquete de medidas u otras herramientas, del tipo de listas de comprobación y modelos de análisis de errores o de objetivos diarios (véanse las figuras 2 y 3). Todos estos elementos se incluían en el *Proyecto Bacteriemia Zero,* con la posibilidad de adaptarlos a las características propias de cada unidad. La formación se ofrecía en un módulo en la página *web* e incluía tanto formación técnica relacionada con la prevención de las infecciones relacionadas con catéteres como formación básica en seguridad del paciente. Además, se recomendaba realizar sesiones informativas y formativas presenciales. Para articular la presentación y el desarrollo del programa, en cada unidad tenía que crearse un núcleo responsable del cual tenían que formar parte al menos un médico y una enfermera, y se aconsejaba implicar también a algún directivo.

Tienen que identificarse las prioridades y los objetivos, así como los recursos para los usuarios, que habrían de acompañar al documento del programa. En Michigan, los encargados de implementar el programa disponían de un mínimo de cuatro horas semanales de dedicación. Por desgracia, en la mayoría de los hospitales españoles no se destinaron recursos extra para desarrollar el programa; tan sólo, la mayor parte de las veces, se concedieron permisos para asistir a las reuniones nacionales o autonómicas que se celebraron.

2.4　*Involucrar a los directivos en la elaboración del plan de implementación*

La participación activa de los directivos es necesaria tanto para motivar al personal sanitario como para ayudar a eliminar las barreras funcionales o de otro tipo que pudiera haber en cada servicio. Pero el compromiso no debería ser sólo de las direcciones asistenciales o de las gerencias, sino también de estructuras superiores como el ministerio de sanidad y las consejerías de salud de las comunidades autónomas. Los directivos pueden tener un papel decisivo en la introducción del paquete de medidas en la práctica hospitalaria, mediante la inclusión en los acuerdos de gestión con los servicios de determinados programas con paquetes de medidas y facilitando los recursos de tiempo y personal para desarrollar todas las actividades incluidas en ellos, como las formativas, de monitorización, etc.

En la experiencia del *Proyecto Bacteriemia Zero* se observó una importante variabilidad en la implicación de los directivos, tanto en los hospitales como en las comunidades autónomas, desde intervenciones muy activas hasta un total desinterés por el proyecto. Entre los indicadores de seguridad incluidos se encontraba la realización de rondas de

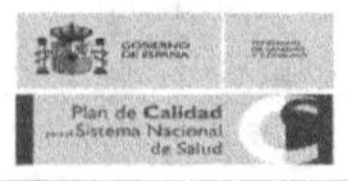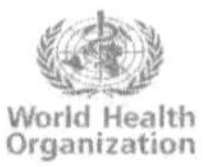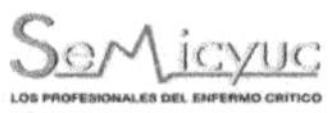

Bacteriemia zero

LISTA DE VERIFICACIÓN DE OBJETIVOS DIARIOS

Paciente:	Nº Habitación	Fecha. ___/___/___
	Turno de mañana *	Turno de tarde
¿Qué se necesita para el alta del paciente en UCI? *		
¿Cuál es el mayor riesgo para el paciente y cómo puede reducirse? *		
Tto dolor/sedación		
Cardio/volemia; objetivo neto para medianoche; bloqueo beta; examen de los ECG		
Neumo/ventilador (cabecero de la cama elevado 30º, profilaxis úlcera péptica y trombosis venosa profunda, desconexión, control de la glucemia); no encamado		
Infección: sospecha o confirmada (hemocultivos, antibióticos adecuados y a tiempo, esteroides,) Cultivos, Niveles fármacos		
GI/nutrición/régimen intestinal		
¿Puede suspenderse alguna medicación? ¿Pasarse a v.o.? ¿Ajustarse según la función renal? *		
Pruebas/procedimientos hoy ¿Qué pruebas de laboratorio previstas se necesitan? ¿Qué pruebas se necesitan? ¿RX de tórax?		
Catéteres * ¿Pueden retirase catéteres/tubos? ¿Se puede sustituir el catéter femoral/yugular por otro de menor riesgo (subclavia, mediana-basílica)? ¿Puede disminuirse el número de luces? ¿Puede suprimirse alguna de las soluciones lipídicas (NPT/ Propofol)? ¿Se ha manejado higiénicamente el catéter (limpieza con alcohol o clorhexidina de los puntos de inyección; cambio apósito, etc..)?.		
¿El paciente está recibiendo **profilaxis** contra la trombosis venosa profunda/úlcera péptica?		
Interconsultas		
¿Está informado el servicio responsable?		
¿Se ha informado a la familia? ¿Se han abordado cuestiones sociales?		
¿Hay eventos o desviaciones que notificar? ¿Cuestiones para el Sistema de información sobre seguridad de UCI?		

La presente lista de objetivos diarios puede ser adaptada al contexto de cada Hospital. Se consideran básicos los ítems marcados con *

Instrumento PSI

Figura 2. Modelo de lista de objetivos diarios.

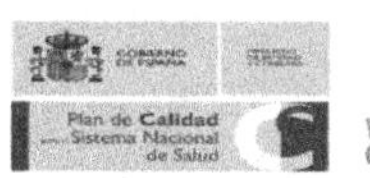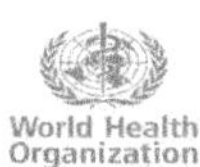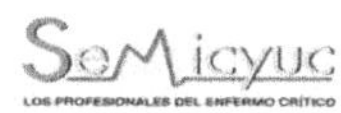

Bacteriemia zero

LISTA DE VERIFICACIÓN EN LA INSERCIÓN DE VÍAS CENTRALES

Paciente		Nº Habitación	
Fecha ____/____/____	**Turno:** ☐ Mañana ☐ Tarde ☐ Noche	**Nivel de urgencia** ☐ Urgente ☐ Electiva	
Lugar inserción ☐ Subclavia ☐ Yugular ☐ Femoral ☐ Mediana-Basílica		**Recambio con guía** ☐ Sí ☐ No	

Se requiere un mínimo de 5 procedimientos supervisados, **tanto torácicos como femorales** (10 en total). Si un médico coloca con éxito 5 vías en un único lugar, sólo se le considerará independiente para realizar el procedimiento en ese lugar.

Función de asistente: Enfermera asistente en la colocación de la vía es el encargado de rellenar la lista de comprobación.

En caso de desviación en cualquiera de los pasos fundamentales, se notificará inmediatamente al médico que lo está realizando (operador) y se detendrá el procedimiento hasta que se haya corregido. Si es necesaria alguna corrección, márquese la casilla "Sí con aviso" y anótese en el campo "Observaciones" la corrección realizada, si procede

Pasos fundamentales	Sí	Sí con aviso	Observaciones:
Antes del procedimiento			
Consentimiento informado y/o información al paciente			
Confirmó la realización de higiene de manos adecuada			
Operador(es): gorro, mascarilla, bata/guantes estéril(es), protección ocular			
Asistente: gorro, mascarilla, bata/guantes estéril(es), protección ocular			
Ayudantes /observadores: gorro, mascarilla			
Desinfectó el lugar de inserción con clorhexidina			
Utilizó técnica aséptica para cubrir al paciente de pies a cabeza			
Durante el procedimiento			
Mantuvo el campo estéril			
Necesitó un segundo operador cualificado después de 3 punciones sin éxito (excepto en caso de emergencia)			
Después del procedimiento:			
Limpió con antiséptico (clorhexidina) los restos de sangre en el lugar y colocó apósito estéril			

Enfermera que supervisa________________________________

Bacteriemia zero, 1ª edición, 2009. Basado en el proyecto "Keystone ICU" desarrollado por la Universidad Johns Hopkins (Pronovost el al., N Eng J Med, 2006; 2725:32). Adaptado al español con permiso de la Universidad Johns Hopkins por el Ministerio de Sanidad y Consumo de España y el Departamento de Seguridad del Paciente de la Organización Mundial de la Salud. Publicado por el Ministerio de Sanidad y Consumo de España. "Keystone ICU" es propiedad de la Facultad de Medicina de la Universidad Johns Hopkins. En la adaptación de los instrumentos de "Bacteriemia zero" ha colaborado la SEMICYUC mediante un contrato con el Ministerio de Sanidad y Consumo.

Instrumento STOP BRC

Figura 3. Esquema para aprender de los errores.

seguridad; de largo, este indicador fue el de menor cumplimiento y, con el tiempo, de los que más abandonos ha experimentado.

La ausencia de implicación de los órganos directivos se reflejaba en la encuesta inicial de valoración del clima de seguridad que realizaron los participantes en el proyecto. Sin embargo, esta valoración mejoró en la segunda edición de la encuesta al finalizar el programa, reflejando la incorporación en diversos hospitales y comunidades autónomas. En general, la participación y la mejoría de los indicadores, tanto de seguridad como en especial las tasas de bacteriemias relacionadas con catéteres, fueron superiores en aquellos hospitales y territorios con mayor compromiso de los directivos.

2.5 *Probar el proyecto en un estudio piloto y redefinir tanto el paquete elegido como el plan de implementación antes de llevarlo a cabo*

Este punto es relevante por varias razones. En primer lugar, lo que en teoría funciona puede ser un fracaso en la práctica. Por otra parte, las condiciones locales pueden ser muy variables y lo que ha sido un éxito en un hospital, o en un país, es posible que no funcione en otros. Todas las posibles barreras que se han descrito pueden tener más o menos presencia local, por lo que antes de lanzar un programa tiene que probarse para corregir los elementos necesarios, sea en su contenido o en la forma de introducirlo.

En España, antes de desarrollar el *Proyecto Bacteriemia Zero* en el ámbito nacional se realizó un estudio piloto durante el último trimestre de 2007, en 17 UCI de tres comunidades autónomas, que mostró la viabilidad del proyecto (reducción de la tasa de bacteriemias relacionadas con catéteres en un 50 %) y algunas de las dificultades para su implantación. El protocolo se modificó para que su extensión a la mayoría de las UCI españolas presentara las menores dificultades posibles,[20] se elaboró una guía de implantación y se desarrollaron todas las herramientas necesarias, incluyendo una presentación en formato electrónico (con el programa *PowerPoint* de Microsoft Office®) para su introducción en los servicios.

Además, se habilitó una plataforma de comunicación *(EZcollab)* que permitió disponer de una biblioteca de documentos y manuales, y que facilitó el intercambio de experiencias y de respuestas a problemas que encontraban los participantes en la aplicación del programa. Esta plataforma fue especialmente útil en los primeros meses, y permitió resolver cuestiones como dónde conseguir la solución de clorhexidina y cómo obtener modelos alternativos de objetivos diarios, y aclarar dudas de registro o definiciones, entre otras.

2.6 *Registrar el cumplimiento de cada elemento, analizando las barreras para su aplicación, e informar de los resultados*

La creciente promoción de los paquetes de medidas mantiene la incógnita de cuál es realmente su grado de adopción y eficacia, tanto global como de cada uno de los elementos que los componen. En la experiencia de Michigan no se notificaron datos del cumplimiento del paquete de medidas de prevención de las bacteriemias relacionadas con catéteres centrales. Más recientemente, un estudio de la National Healthcare Safety Network de Estados Unidos, realizado en 250 UCI que reunían un mínimo de 500 días de utilización del dispositivo, investigó el grado de cumplimiento global y de cada elemento del paquete de medidas. Tan sólo el 38 % de las UCI comunicaron un cumplimiento alto. En estas UCI con mejor adhesión, el cumplimiento de cada elemento osciló entre un mínimo del 44 % (la optimización del lugar de inserción de los catéteres) y un máximo del 73 % (el uso de la solución de clorhexidina). Un dato destacable es que sólo las UCI con una política escrita del paquete de medidas, una monitorización del cumplimiento y que éste alcanzara el 95 %, obtenían una reducción de las tasas.[21]

En el *Proyecto Bacteriemia Zero* se realizó una monitorización del paquete de medidas y de los seis indicadores de seguridad integral. La cuantificación se realizó mediante cumplimentación mensual *on line,* tanto de la bacteriemia (tasas por paciente, por días de estancia y por días de cateterización) como de la seguridad (porcentaje de UCI que disponían de solución de clorhexidina, de carros de inserción, de listas de comprobación de la inserción del catéter, de objetivos diarios, de sesiones de aprender de los errores y de rondas de seguridad).

3   Impacto del *Proyecto Bacteriemia Zero*

El *Proyecto Bacteriemia Zero* se inició en enero de 2009. De forma progresiva, todas las comunidades autónomas se adhirieron al proyecto y finalmente participaron en el programa 192 UCI.

El objetivo principal era reducir la media estatal de la densidad de incidencia de las bacteriemias relacionadas con catéteres a menos de cuatro episodios por mil días de uso de catéter (una reducción del 40 % respecto a la tasa media registrada en dichas unidades en los cinco años previos). Este objetivo se alcanzó ampliamente, pues la mediana de incidencia estimada descendió en las UCI participantes de una inicial en 2008 de 3,07 episodios por mil días de cateterización a 1,12 tras 16 a 18 meses de participar en el programa, es decir, aproximadamente un 50 % de reducción. Las tasas eran más altas en las UCI de hospitales grandes y universitarios, en comparación con los medianos o pequeños y los no docentes, pero la reducción de las tasas fue significativa en todos los tipos de institución.

Otro punto importante era la sostenibilidad de la mejoría, circunstancia que el proyecto original había comunicado.[22] El *Proyecto Bacteriemia Zero* ha mostrado también que, tras acabar el programa activo de 18 meses (en junio de 2010) y con una incorporación de nuevas UCI (en un número importante de mayor complejidad, entendido como pertenecientes a hospitales de más 500 camas), las tasas de bacteriemias relacionadas con catéteres se han mantenido e incluso han mejorado. La figura 4 muestra las tasas de bacteriemias relacionadas con catéteres (expresadas como media) del registro ENVIN-HELICS desde el año 2000, y puede apreciarse la reducción mantenida de la incidencia nacional en los meses de abril a junio de esos años, en los que se incluyen datos correspondientes a UCI que no han participado en el *Proyecto Bacteriemia Zero*.

Cuando se analizan los datos del registro del *Proyecto Bacteriemia Zero* procedentes de las UCI que aportan información de sus tasas de manera continuada (219 UCI en 2011) se comprueba que, desde la cifra inicial (media) de 4,89 episodios por mil días de uso de catéter en 2008, se pasó a 2,78 en el período de intervención 2009-2010, a 2,61 en 2011 y a 2,23 de enero a octubre de 2012 (periodos de seguimiento tras finalizar la intervención). A través de la página *web*, en la cual se encuentra la base de datos, cada UCI disponía de todos sus datos en tiempo real, y para las tasas de bacteriemias relacionadas con catéteres centrales también de los de su comunidad autónoma y los nacionales, lo que permitía la consiguiente inmediata comparación.

La participación de las UCI en el proyecto fue desigual. Aquellas que se adhirieron desde el primer momento y colaboraron durante más de 12 meses seguidos han obtenido mejores tasas o una mayor reducción proporcional que las que participaron menos tiempo o sólo informaron de sus tasas en los períodos de registro del ENVIN-HELICS (tres meses en 2009 y tres meses en 2010). Estos datos confirman que es el mantenimiento de una estrategia lo que permite cambiar culturas y hábitos.

Además de la reducción de las tasas, en el *Proyecto Bacteriemia Zero* había unos objetivos secundarios: *1)* promover y reforzar la cultura de seguridad en las UCI del Sistema Nacional de Salud, *2)* crear una red de aquellas UCI, a través de las comunidades autónomas, que aplicaran prácticas seguras de efectividad demostrada, y *3)* documentar todos los episodios de bacteriemia, incluidas las de orígenes diferentes a los catéteres, así como sus causas y las características de los pacientes que las desarrollan.

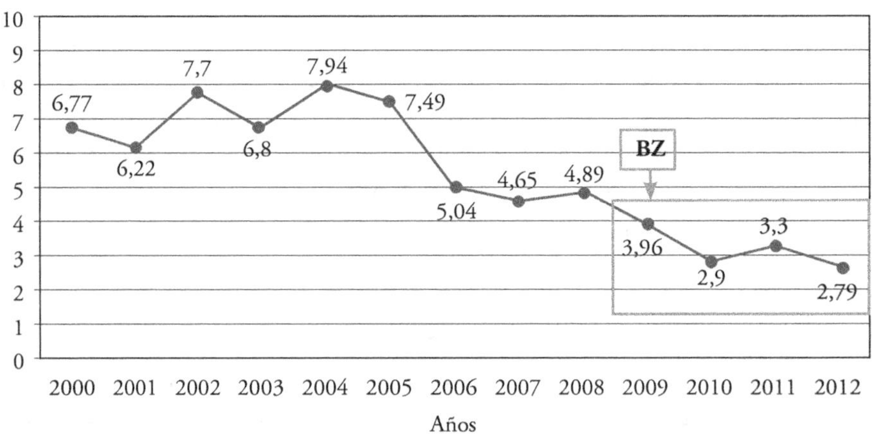

Figura 4. Evolución de la tasa de bacteriemias relacionadas con catéteres adquiridas en UCI en el registro ENVIN-HELICS (tasas expresadas en número de episodios por mil días de cateterización).

Las herramientas para aplicar el paquete de medidas para la prevención de la bacteriemia relacionada con la inserción (STOP-BRC) incluyeron: lista de comprobación durante la inserción de los catéteres; módulo de formación, en el cual se incluían las normas básicas de inserción y mantenimiento de los catéteres; lista de comprobación de objetivos diarios; carro exclusivo con el material necesario para la colocación de los accesos venosos; carteles informativos con los seis procedimientos propuestos para disminuir las bacteriemias; equipos para la seguridad del paciente en cada hospital (médico y enfermera) que garantizaran la aplicación de las intervenciones; y reconocimiento de autoridad para las enfermeras que siguen la lista de comprobación durante la inserción de los catéteres.

Las recomendaciones del *Proyecto Bacteriemia Zero* han supuesto cambios importantes en la asistencia diaria de las UCI españolas, con un incremento de las prácticas más seguras. El 92 % de las UCI participantes comunicaron, además de las tasas de bacteriemias relacionadas con catéteres, la monitorización del paquete de medidas y de los seis indicadores de seguridad integral al menos en una ocasión. El 41,7 % de las UCI cumplieron los seis indicadores, el 24,7 % cinco y sólo el 4 % uno o dos indicadores.

Se dispuso de los datos de 35.400 listas de comprobación de la inserción de catéteres. La recomendación de optimizar el lugar de inserción fue muy seguida, ya que el acceso fue por vía subclavia en el 40 % de los casos y por vía femoral únicamente en el 17 %.

Las medidas de esterilidad máximas durante la inserción, incluyendo el uso de guantes, bata, gorro y paños cubriendo totalmente al paciente, han sido uno de los aspectos, junto al uso de la solución de clorhexidina como antiséptico, que más se han modificado respecto a la práctica previa en España, y ha requerido cambios no sólo educativos sino también en el material disponible en los hospitales, que ha incorporado sábanas estériles para mantener un campo adecuado. Hasta ahora, el desinfectante más usado en la inserción y el mantenimiento de los catéteres había sido la povidona yodada; sin embargo, la evidencia científica, tanto en estudios individuales como en metaanálisis, apoya fuertemente su sustitución por soluciones de clorhexidina. La transparencia del producto ha hecho que algunos sanitarios la rechazaran, por lo que la opción de usar una solución tintada es una alternativa de creciente implantación. El uso de clorhexidina, las medidas de barrera máxima y la higiene de manos correcta antes de la técnica tuvieron un cumplimiento, en los 35.400 casos monitorizados en el *Proyecto Bacteriemia Zero,* por encima del 94 %.

Está claro que el cumplimiento técnico ha sido muy superior al de seguridad. Aunque se han creado equipos de seguridad en las UCI y se ha introducido el plan de seguridad integral, tiene que trabajarse más en este aspecto. Por ejemplo, las rondas de seguridad con directivos han sido el indicador de menos cumplimiento (inferior al 50 %), mientras que algo mejores resultaron el seguimiento de objetivos diarios y las sesiones de aprender de los errores.

La motivación del equipo líder en las unidades y en las comunidades autónomas ha sido el principal motor para conseguir los objetivos. Expresar los resultados en términos de ganancias (vidas salvadas, reducción de estancias y euros ahorrados) ha sido especialmente motivador

El *Proyecto Bacteriemia Zero* tuvo un impacto positivo en otras tasas de infección asociadas a dispositivos, en concreto la densidad de incidencia de la neumonía asociada a ventilación mecánica disminuyó en el primer año sin más explicación que el beneficio del programa de seguridad integral. El estancamiento posterior de la tasa de estas neumonías mostró la necesidad de un paquete de medidas específico de prevención, que mantuviera la estructura del *Proyecto Bacteriemia Zero*, y fue el motor para iniciar el programa *Neumonía Zero*.

Los sistemas de vigilancia son necesarios para cuantificar de manera eficaz las infecciones asociadas a los cuidados sanitarios y las razones por las que se desarrollan, así como la eficacia de las intervenciones para combatirlas. Considerar la infección nosocomial como un error evitable es el primer paso hacia la erradicación. Diferentes experiencias de aplicación de paquetes de medidas, dentro de programas de actuación estructurados, han conseguido reducir de manera significativa las tasas en ámbitos muy variados.[23-30]

Un resumen final sería que los paquetes de medidas por sí mismos, sin una planificación y un esfuerzo adicional de implantación, no mejoran el cuidado. La mejoría es el resultado de las estrategias del equipo para «rediseñar» el trabajo, comunicarse mejor y trabajar más eficazmente.

Bibliografía

1. Resar R, Griffin FA, Hapden C, Nolan TW. Using care bundles to improve healthcare quality. IHI Innovation series. White paper. Cambridge, MA: Institute for Healthcare Improvement; 2012.

2. How-to guide: prevent ventilator-associated pneumonia. Cambridge, MA: Institute for Healthcare Improvement; 2012. Disponible en: http: //www.ihi.org/knowledge/Pages/Tools/HowtoGuidePreventVAP.aspx

3. How-to guide: prevent central line-associated bloodstream infections. Cambridge, MA: Institute for Healthcare Improvement; 2012. Disponible en: http: //www.ihi.org/knowledge/Pages/Tools/HowtoGuidePreventCentralLineAssociatedBloodstreamInfection.aspx

4. Institute for Healthcare Improvement. Sepsis resuscitation bundle. Disponible en: http://www.ihi.org/knowledge/Pages/Changes/ImplementtheSepsisResuscitationBundle.aspx

5. Palomar M, Rodríguez P, Nieto M, Sancho S. Prevención de la infección nosocomial en el paciente crítico. Med Intensiva. 2010; 34: 523-33.

6. Carey M, Buchan H, Sanson-Fisher R. The cycle of change: implementing best-evidence clinical practice. Int J Qual Health Care. 2009; 21: 37-43.

7. Healht - EU. Patient safety. (Consultado el 20-3-2013.) Disponible en: http://ec.europa.eu/health-eu/care_for_me/patient_safety/index_en.htm

8. Pronovost P, Needham D, Berenholtz S, Sinopoli D, Chu H, Cosgrove S, *et al.* An intervention to decrease catheter-related bloodstream infections in the ICU. N Engl J Med. 2006; 355: 2725-32.

9. Nolan T, Berwick DM. All-or-none measurement raises the bar on performance. JAMA. 2006; 295: 1168-70.

10. O'Grady NP, Alexander M, Dellinger EP, Gerberding JL, Heard SO, Maki DG, *et al.* Guidelines for the prevention of intravascular catheter-related infections. Centers for Disease

Control and Prevention. MMWR Recomm Rep. 2002; 51: 1-29.

11. León C, Ariza J. Guías para el tratamiento de las infecciones relacionadas con catéteres intravasculares de corta permanencia en adultos: conferencia de consenso SEIMC-SEMICYUC. Enferm Infecc Microbiol Clin. 2004; 22: 92-101.

12. Mermel LA, Allon M, Bouza E, Craven DE, Flynn P, O'Grady NP, *et al.* Clinical practice guidelines for the diagnosis and management of intravascular catheter-related infection: 2009 update by the Infectious Diseases of America. Clin Infect Dis. 2009; 49: 1-45.

13. Miller MR, Griswold M, Harris II JR, Yenokyan G, Huskins WC, Moss M, *et al.* Decreasing PICU catheter-associated bloodstream infections: NACHRI's quality transformation efforts. Pediatrics. 2010; 125: 206-13.

14. Kaier K, Wilson C, Hulscher M, Wollersheim H, Huis A, Borg M, *et al.* Implementing strategic bundles for infection prevention and management. Infection. 2012; 40: 225-8.

15. Rubinson L, Wu AW, Haponik EE, Diette GB. Why is it that internists do not follow guidelines for preventing intravascular catheter infections? Infect Control Hosp Epidemiol. 2005; 26: 525-33.

16. Cabana MD, Rand CS, Powe NR, Wu AW, Wilson MH, Abboud PA, *et al.* Why don't physicians follow clinical practice guidelines? A framework for improvement. JAMA. 1999; 282: 1458-65.

17. Hawe CS, Ellis KS, Cairns CJ, Longmate A. Reduction of ventilator-associated pneumonia: active versus passive guideline implementation. Intensive Care Med. 2009; 35: 1180-6.

18. Roming M, Goeschel C, Pronovost P, Berenholz SM. Integrating CUSP and TRIP to improve patient safety. Hospital Pract. 2010; 38: 114-21.

19. Proyecto Bacteriemia Zero. Disponible en: http://hws.vhebron.net/bacteriemia-zero/bzero.asp

20. Palomar Martínez M, Álvarez Lerma F, Riera Badía MA, León Gil C, López Pueyo MJ, Díaz Tobajas C, *et al.* Prevención de la bacteriemia relacionada con catéteres en UCI mediante una intervención multifactorial. Informe del estudio piloto. Med Intensiva. 2010; 34: 581-9.

21. Furuya EY, Dick A, Perencevich EN, Pogorzelska M. Pogorzelska M, Goldmann D, *et al.* Central line bundle implementation in US intensive care units and impact on bloodstream infections. PLoS One. 2011; 6: e15452.

22. Pronovost P, Goeschel CA, Colantuoni E, Watson S, Lubomski LH, Berenholtz S, *et al.* Sustaining reductions in catheter related bloodstream infections in Michigan intensive care units: observational study. BMJ. 2010; 340: c309.

23. Rosenthal CD, Maki DG, Rodrigues C, Álvarez-Moreno C, Leblebicioglu H, Sobreyra-Oropeza M, *et al.* Impact of International Nosocomial Infection Control Consortium (INICC) strategy on central line-associated bloodstream infection rates in the intensive care units of 15 developing countries. Infect Control Hosp Epidemiol. 2010; 31: 1264-72.

24. Jarvis WR. The Lowbury Lecture. The United States approach to strategies in the battle against healthcare-associated infections, 2006: transitioning from benchmarking to zero tolerance and clinician accountability. J Hosp Infect. 2007; 65: 3-9.

25. Agency for Healthcare Research and Quality. AHRQ patient safety project reduces bloodstream infections by 40 percent. September 10, 2012. Disponible en: http: //www.ahrq.gov/news/press/pr2012/pspclabsipr.htm

26. Peredo R, Sabatier C, Villagrá A, González J, Hernández C, Pérez F, *et al.* Reduction in catheter-related bloodstream infections in critically ill patients through a multiple system intervention. Eur J Clin Microbiol Infect Dis. 2010; 29: 1173-7.

27. Marra AR, Cal RG, Durão MS, Correa L, Guastelli LR, Moura DF Jr, *et al.* Impact of a program to prevent central line-associated bloodstream infection in the zero tolerance era. Am J Infect Control. 2010; 38: 434-9.

28. DePalo VA, McNicoll L, Cornell M, Rocha JM, Adams L, Pronovost PJ. The Rhode Island ICU collaborative: a model for reducing central line-associated bloodstream infection and ventilator-associated pneumonia statewide. Qual Saf Health Care. 2010; 19: 555-61.

29. Guerin K, Wagner J, Rains K, Bessesen M. Reduction in central line-associated bloodstream infections by implementation of a postinsertion care bundle. Am J Infect Control. 2010; 38: 430-3.

30. Shuman EK, Washer LL, Arndt JL, Zalewski CA, Hyzy RC, Napolitano LM, *et al.* Analysis of central line-associated bloodstream infections in the intensive care unit after implementation of central line bundles. Infect Control Hosp Epidemiol. 2010; 31: 551-3.